W9-AZX-515

Handbook of Symptom-Oriented Neurology

Second Edition

Handbook of Symptom-Oriented Neurology

Second Edition

WILLIAM H. OLSON, M.D.
Professor and Chairman of Neurology
Associate Professor of Anatomy
University of Louisville School of Medicine
Louisville, Kentucky

ROGER A. BRUMBACK, M.D.
Professor of Pathology, Neurology, Pediatrics, and
Psychiatry and Behavioral Sciences
Director of Neuropathology
University of Oklahoma College of Medicine
Neuropathologist, Laboratory Service
Veterans Affairs Medical Center
Oklahoma City, Oklahoma

GENEROSO GASCON, M.D.
Professor of Pediatrics
King Faisal Specialist Hospital and Research Centre
Riyadh, Kingdom of Saudi Arabia

VASUDEVA IYER, M.D.
Professor of Neurology
Chief, Division of Clinical Neurophysiology
University of Louisville School of Medicine
Louisville, Kentucky

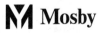 **Mosby**

St. Louis Baltimore Boston Chicago London Philadelphia Sydney Toronto

Mosby

Dedicated to Publishing Excellence

Publisher: George Stamathis
Editor: Susie Baxter
Developmental Editor: Ellen Baker Geisel
Project Manager: Nancy C. Baker
Production Editor: Jill Waite
Proofroom Manager: Barbara M. Kelly
Designer: Nancy C. Baker
Manufacturing Supervisor: Karen Lewis

Copyright © 1994, 1989 by Mosby–Year Book, Inc.

All rights reserved. No part of this publication may be reproduced, stored
in a retrieval system, or transmitted, in any form or by any means, elec-
tronic, mechanical, photocopying, recording, or otherwise, without prior
written permission from the publisher.

Permission to photocopy or reproduce solely for internal or personal use is
permitted for libraries or other users registered with the Copyright Clearance Center, provided that the base fee of $4.00 per chapter plus $.10 per
page is paid directly to the Copyright Clearance Center, 27 Congress Street,
Salem, MA 01970. This consent does not extend to other kinds of copying,
such as copying for general distribution, for advertising or promotional purposes, for creating new collected works, or for resale.

Printed in the United States of America
Composition by Clarinda Printing/binding by Malloy

Mosby–Year Book, Inc., 11830 Westline Industrial Drive, St. Louis, Mis-
souri 63146

Library of Congress Cataloging in Publication Data
Olson, William H., 1936-
    Handbook of symptom–oriented neurology / William H. Olson,
Roger A. Brumback.—2nd ed.
        p.   cm.
    Rev. ed of: Handbook of symptom-oriented neurology / William H.
Olson . . . [et al.]. c1989.
    Includes bibliographical references and index.
    ISBN 0-8016-7779-3
    1. Nervous system—Diseases.   2. Symptomatology.   3. Family
medicine.   I. Brumback, Roger A.   II. Title.
    [DNLM: 1. Nervous System Diseases—diagnosis—outlines.
2. Nervous System Diseases—therapy—outlines.   3. Primary Health
Care—outlines.   WL 18 052h 1993]
RC346.H235 1993
616.8—dc20
DNLM/DLC
for Library of Congress   93-33852
                                                                      CIP

    1   2   3   4   5   6   7   8   9   0   98   97   96   95   94

PREFACE TO THE SECOND EDITION

This is the third version of a book first published in 1980. The purpose now is the same as it was then: to assist the primary care physician in managing common, treatable, and emergency neurologic problems. No attempt has been made in this text to write an exhaustive treatise of neurologic disease, present neurologic pathophysiology, or detail the diagnosis of rare, untreatable neurologic conditions. We believe that this book will enable primary care physicians to note a neurologic symptom and, in most cases, arrive at a neurologic diagnosis and institute an appropriate therapeutic regimen.

The content and philosophy of this manual were based on a paper by Dr. T. J. Murray (Concepts in undergraduate teaching. *Clin Neurol Neurosurg* 79:237–284, 1976) which addressed the issue of common neurologic complaints presenting to family physicians in Canada. Although at least 10% of all patients seen by primary care physicians in family practice have neurologic complaints, many physicians feel uneasy with neurologic problems because medical school curricula devote far less than 10% of the time to these types of problems.

Since 1980 major advances have been made in the clinical neurosciences. Superb images of the brain generated by either computed tomography (CT) or magnetic resonance imaging (MRI) are available in most communities throughout the United States. Lumbar puncture is no longer necessary to determine if a stroke is hemorrhagic, and in most cases the diagnosis of multiple sclerosis is simple with an MRI. Plasmapheresis is routinely used to treat myasthenia gravis and other autoimmune diseases, and in the near future at least a half dozen more anticonvulsants will be available for the treatment of seizures. The treatment of Parkinson's disease has been improved with the introduction of monoamine oxidase-B (MAO-B) inhibitors and dopamine agonists.

Also since the first edition, two diseases—Alzheimer's disease and acquired immune deficiency syndrome (AIDS)—have moved to the forefront of the health concerns of the general public. With our increasingly aged population, more and more cases of the progressive dementing disorder, Alzheimer's disease, are being recognized. With greater public awareness of this devastating and currently untreatable condition, it is imperative that physicians not only recognize the clinical symptoms and provide patient counseling, but also identify treatable conditions with similar symptoms. On the other hand, AIDS currently provides a much more difficult problem, because the causative viral agent is highly neurotropic and can produce a wide variety of symptoms related to the infection. In many respects this infection deserves the appellation once applied to syphilis—"the great imitator."

Special recognition needs to be given to Mr. Gary Baune, who continues to be our superb medical illustrator. We also wish to recognize specific persons who have reviewed chapters relative to their area of expertise: Dr. Jannice Aaron on neuroradiology, Dr. Walter Olson on movement disorders, Dr. David Changaris on those areas of neurosurgical importance, and Dr. Martin Raff on infectious disease. Mary H. Brumback provided invaluable assistance in proofreading.

William H. Olson, M.D.
Roger A. Brumback, M.D.
Generoso Gascon, M.D.
Vasudeva Iyer, M.D.

CONTENTS

Scattered through the text are triangular markers, ▶,
which highlight the key diagnostic features for each specific
disease.

NEUROLOGIC EXAMINATION

1

Contrary to popular opinion, there is no "standard" neurologic examination. When we are requested to teach the neurologic examination, our response is, The neurologic examination of whom? The ambulatory adult? The infant? The comatose patient? A neurologic examination should be *problem oriented,* and in reality there are different examinations for different clinical situations. Therefore we have included many of our suggestions for the neurologic examination under specific chapter headings. In most circumstances, common sense should prevail. For example, testing the sense of smell is of little help in the diagnosis of a primary muscle disease, and testing the anal wink is of little value in diagnosing the average headache. In essence, the neurologic examination is a process of gathering objective data relating to the hypotheses formed during the process of history taking.

This chapter is intended to provide hints on the more commonly used (and abused) portions of the neurologic examination. It is not a complete guide to the entire procedure. A more complete guide to the "standard" problem-oriented neurologic examination is found in Appendix B.

I. SCREENING OF NEUROLOGIC ABNORMALITIES.

A. **Station and gait.** Table 1–1 outlines and Figure 1–1 illustrates the procedure for station and gait testing, which usually can be performed in less than 1 minute. Virtually every aspect of the central and peripheral nervous system is tested. A patient with a normal station and gait is unlikely to have any serious structural neurologic abnormality. Twenty feet of straight walking space is desirable, and the patient should be barefooted and clothed only in underwear or a gown.

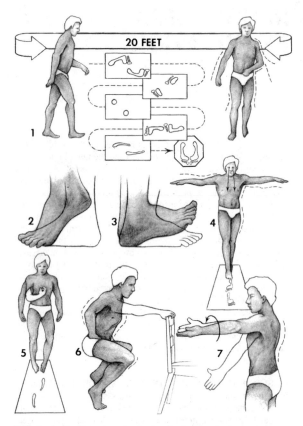

FIG 1–1. Testing of station and gait. Pay particular attention to arm swing, arm posture, body posture, instability while turning around, tendency to look at floor. See text for additional information.

TABLE 1–1.
Procedure for Station and Gait Testing

Instructions	Things to Note
Walk the distance normally	Asymmetric arm swing, abnormal arm and hand postures, and instability of the trunk
Rapidly turn around and walk on tiptoe	Extra steps while turning around and inability to rise completely on the tips of the toes
Rapidly turn and walk on heels	Foot drop
Turn and walk with heels touching toes (tandem walk)	Instability characteristic of midline cerebellar lesions
Turn and "walk on outsides of feet like a bowlegged cowboy does" (walking on lateral aspects of feet)	This maneuver specifically brings out hemiplegic posturing of an arm from subtle or old upper motor neuron damage
Do a deep knee bend (preferably with hands on hips; if there is an obvious balance problem, patient may hold onto an object, such as a chair)	Loss of balance indicates cerebellar difficulties; inability to rise indicates proximal weakness
Stand with feet together, eyes closed, arms outstretched with palms facing ceiling and fingers spread apart	Increased swaying with eyes closed indicates either posterior column disease or a peripheral neuropathy; with subtle hemiparesis affected arm will pronate, while in more obvious hemiparesis the arm will pronate and then drift downward and outward

1. Abnormalities of station and gait.
   a. *Abnormal mentation:* Patient follows directions poorly, slowly; needs examiner to demonstrate instructions; tendency to continue doing same task (perseveration).
   b. *Hemiplegia:* Decreased arm swing on affected side, circumduction of leg, pronation of arms when held outstretched with palms up, flexion of arm when walking on sides of feet.
   c. *Cerebellar ataxia:* Unsteadiness when turning around, in tandem walking, and in deep knee bending.

    d. *Sensory ataxia:* Increased swaying when eyes are closed (positive Romberg test).

    e. *Muscle disease:* Difficulty with deep knee bend, waddling gait.

    f. *Basal ganglia disorders:* Abnormal postures and movement (e.g., Parkinson's disease, Huntington's disease).

    g. *Lumbar disk disease:* Inability to walk on heels or toes on one side; spinal list.

    h. *Peripheral neuropathy:* Bilateral footdrop; cannot walk on heels.

2. By observing station and gait, a skillful examiner can obtain in 1 minute a glimpse of mental status (how well the patient comprehends and follows instructions), upper motor neuron function (posturing of arms and gait), lower motor neuron function (muscle atrophy and weakness), muscle disease (proximal weakness), basal ganglia function (abnormal posture and movement), cerebellar function (balance and tandem walk), and the sensory system (poor balance with eyes closed [Romberg test]). A patient who can perform all the maneuvers normally will rarely have a significant neurologic abnormality. Abnormalities noted can be more specifically tested in the remainder of the neurologic examination. For example, if station and gait testing suggests a cerebellar abnormality, more specific cerebellar tests should be performed.

B. Deep tendon reflexes (muscle stretch reflexes). The most difficult part of the neurologic examination to perform correctly (and that medical students think is easiest!) is evaluation of deep tendon reflexes (Figs 1–2 to 1–5). If possible, have the patient undressed and sitting with legs dangling freely over the edge of the table. The reflex elicited will depend on: (1) whether the tendon is struck, (2) how hard the tendon is struck, and (3) how quickly the tendon is struck. To avoid striking an improper area, the tendon should first be palpated. The lightest tap that will still elicit the response should be given. A hammer with a relatively soft rubber end and a flexible handle will best allow the rapid, light tap. The examiner will most often find asymmetry of reflexes rather than gross hyperactivity or absence of reflexes. Reflexes may be normal, hyperactive or hypoactive, clonic or absent, or symmetric or asymmetric, and

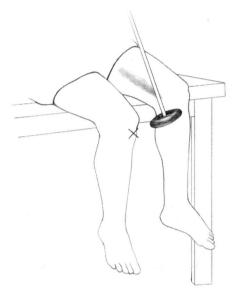

FIG 1–2. Patellar reflex. Note that feet do not touch the floor. The type of hammer illustrated was developed in England and is especially effective. Look not only for reflex contraction of the quadriceps but also contralateral contraction of the adductor muscle and the number of swings the leg makes. *Remember:* dysfunction of either the afferent or efferent nerves may diminish the reflex.

should be recorded as such. Recording pluses, minuses, and such, unless carefully defined, does little to convey accurate information on the chart.

C. **The Babinski reflex.** The Babinski reflex (Fig 1–6), or plantar response, may be present depending on: (1) type of stimulation used, (2) rapidity with which the stimulus is delivered, and (3) position of the patient. A sharp object (safety pin or sharpened end of some hammers) will produce little more than

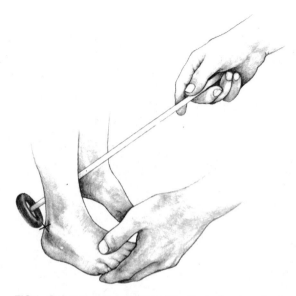

FIG 1–3. Achilles reflex. While striking the tendon, have the patient apply *light* pressure with the sole of the foot to the palm of the examiner.

a withdrawal response, whereas too light a touch will produce no response. We find a key to be the most readily available, appropriate stimulus. The key is used to stimulate the *lateral* aspect of the plantar surface of the foot, beginning at the heel and moving up to the ball of the foot but staying lateral to the great toe. Examples of some responses to plantar stimulation are shown in Table 1–2. Because the abnormal response is such an important sign of nervous system disease, the best approach to recording the results, if in doubt, is to record exactly the observed movements. It is totally inadequate to say simply "Babinski absent." Of course he is! He died more than 60 years ago.

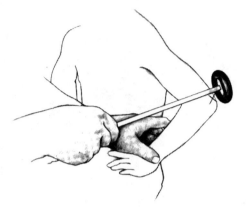

FIG 1–4. Triceps reflex. This reflex is most easily elicited when the patient rests the arms on the hips.

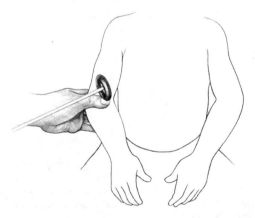

FIG 1–5. Biceps reflex. It is important that the arms be symmetrically flexed and relaxed, as illustrated.

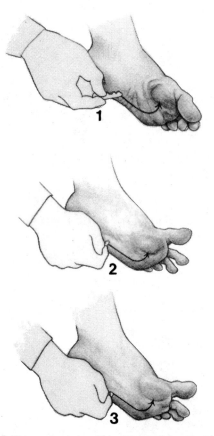

FIG 1–6. Plantar stimulation. Note that only two of the five possibilities constitute a positive Babinski response. See text for additional information.

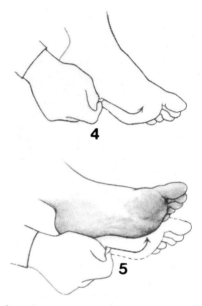

FIG 1–6 (cont.).

D. **Examination of optic fundus.** Ophthalmoscopic examination of the optic fundus is the only opportunity the physician has to look directly at the brain, and it is imperative to do so in *every* patient with neurologic symptoms. This should be done even in difficult cases, such as a crying, hyperactive 4-year-old child. Mentally make a list of those parts of the fundus that must be seen to confirm the hypotheses formed during the history. For example, in the patient with suspected multiple sclerosis, look particularly for temporal pallor of the optic disk. Adjust the size of the beam to match the size of the pupil (too large a beam causes light to reflect off the iris). Using too bright

TABLE 1–2.
Responses to Plantar Stimulation

Name	Observation	Interpretation
Normal response (flexor plantar response)	First movement of great toe is flexion	Normal
Classic Babinski reflex (classic extensor plantar response)	Extension of great toe with extension and fanning of other toes	Most often seen in upper motor neuron lesions (below the foramen magnum)
Babinski reflex (extensor plantar response)	First movement of great toe is extension (there may be subsequent flexion of great toes); other toes either show no movement or flexion	Seen in all types of upper motor neuron lesions (especially above the foramen magnum)
Mute plantar response	Nothing happens	Severe sensory loss or paralysis of foot
Withdrawal	Patient pulls foot away	Often seen in toxic-metabolic peripheral neuropathies
Asymmetric response	Mute plantar response on one side and flexor plantar response on other side	Indication of need to look for other signs of neurologic disease

a beam may cause excessive pupillary constriction. In general, use the brightest light possible that still allows visualization of the retina. Darkening the room is usually not helpful, since it prevents the patient from fixating on a target. Pupillary dilating agents are generally not necessary.

E. Pharyngeal reflex. The pharyngeal reflex (Fig 1–7) should be tested on each side by stimulating the pharyngeal pillars with a cotton applicator swab. After observing the motor response (elevation of the palate), ask the patient if the sensation was the same on both sides of the pharynx. (Simply jamming a tongue depressor down the patient's throat not only gives very little neurologic information but is downright rude.) Response

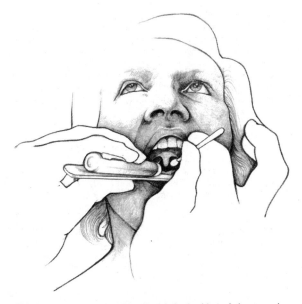

FIG 1–7. Pharyngeal reflex. Touch both sides of the posterior pharynx and watch for elevation of the palate. Ask the patient if the sensation on both sides is the same. In some patients it may be necessary, as illustrated, to press down on the tongue by holding the tongue blade and flashlight in one hand.

is significant only if it is asymmetric; normal responses run the gamut from hyperactive to hypoactive.

F. Sensory examination. The sensory examination under most clinical conditions does not produce objective, "hard" data because it involves subjective judgment by both the patient and the examiner. Beginning medical students are often fascinated by the sensory examination and spend an inordinate amount of time performing it. If pinprick, vibration, light touch, and position sensation are present in the feet, and if the patient can recognize numbers written on the palms of the hands with eyes closed, a major sensory deficit is unlikely. On the other hand, if given a pin and a marking pencil, an intelligent, cooperative patient can often accurately define a circumscribed sensory deficit. Likewise, when testing a sensory level, have the patient run his or her own finger up the body until sensation changes. When a peripheral neuropathy is suspected, ask the patient to compare a single pinprick proximally (e.g., on the chest) with a single pinprick distally (e.g., on the foot). Use a disposable pin, and allow the shaft to slide through the finger to deliver a relatively quantitative response (Fig 1–8). Simply comparing sharp and dull sensation on the foot is inadequate. The examiner should attempt to quantitate any difference between the proximal and distal stimulation sites. For example, ask, "If this [chest] pinprick is worth $100, how much is this [foot] pinprick worth?," and consider a response less than $75 as significant. A useful, objective sign of sensory loss is *summation;* that is, repeated quick pinpricks of the same intensity will suddenly become very painful and the patient will withdraw the extremity and grimace (normally, repeated pricking does not become more painful). This phenomenon is most frequently present in toxic-metabolic peripheral neuropathies such as associated with diabetes mellitus.

G. Non-routine examination. Only when the examination basics (mental status, cranial nerves, reflexes, motor system, sensory system) have been thoroughly mastered are the "curiosities" (e.g., Hoffmann reflex) and "toys" (e.g., optokinetic drums)

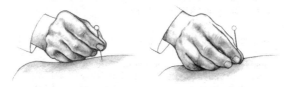

FIG 1–8. Testing sensation of pain. Grasp pin shaft and allow the pin to slide through the fingers until it makes contact with the skin. Compare the response in a normal area (e.g., chest) with that in a suspected area of involvement (e.g., foot).

used. In specialized situations these may be useful, but need not be routinely used by the student or the time-pressed physician.

BIBLIOGRAPHY

Barrows H: Neurologic examination (videotape), Chicago, Division of Marketing Services, American Medical Association.

Caselli RJ: Rediscovering tactile agnosia. *Mayo Clin Proc* 1991; 66:129–213.

DeMyer W: *Technique of the Neurologic Examination, A Programmed Text,* ed 4. New York, McGraw-Hill, 1993.

Goldberg S: Principles of neurologic localization. *Am Fam Physician* 1981; 23:131–141.

Haerer AF: *DeJong's The Neurologic Examination,* ed 5. Philadelphia, JB Lippincott, 1992.

Mayo Clinic Foundation: *Clinical Examinations in Neurology,* ed 6. Philadelphia, WB Saunders, 1991.

Perkin D: *Atlas of Clinical Neurology.* Philadelphia, JB Lippincott Co, 1986.

Rodnitizky RL: *Van Allen's Pictorial Manual of Neurologic Tests.* St Louis, Mosby–Year Book, 1988.

NEURODIAGNOSTIC **2** PROCEDURES

A well-elicited history and an adequate neurologic examination should enable the physician to form a provisional diagnosis. Such a diagnosis will include the probable site of the lesion and the probable type or cause of the neurologic disorder. There will be a number of differential diagnoses, particularly with regard to the type of lesion and these can often be settled only by suitable investigative procedures. It is essential for the physician to have a clear idea regarding the indications as well as the specificity and sensitivity of the various procedures. The goal is to put the patient through minimal discomfort (choosing the least invasive investigations) and obtain the most specific information that will point to the correct diagnosis. The neurodiagnostic procedures may not only be diagnostic but sometimes serve as prognostic indicators as well. In this chapter, brief descriptions of the common neurologic procedures are given, along with their indications and side effects. Table 2–1 lists various neurodiagnostic procedures and their indications.

I. LUMBAR PUNCTURE.
A. Lumbar puncture (LP) is perhaps the commonest neurodiagnostic procedure that a physician must personally perform.
  1. Indications.
    a. Suspected central nervous system (CNS) infection (meningitis or encephalitis): Cerebrospinal fluid (CSF) study should be done *without delay* when meningitis or encephalitis is suspected.

    Caveat: If there are focal findings, such as a hemiplegia, or if there is papilledema, a computed tomography (CT) scan or magnetic resonance imaging

TABLE 2-1.
Diagnostic Tests in Neurologic Disorders

Test	Anatomic/Physiologic Basis	Most Useful In
Electroencephalogram (EEG)	Spontaneous electrical activity of cerebral cortical neurons	Seizure disorders Metabolic encephalopathy Tumors Infectious encephalopathy Dementia Brain death determination
Visual evoked potentials (VEP)	Arrival of electrical signals at the visual cortex through the visual pathways, when the retina is stimulated	Multiple sclerosis Disorders of optic nerve Lesions of optic tract, radiations, or occipital cortex
Brainstem auditory evoked potentials (BAEP)	Passage of electrical signals through auditory nerve, auditory nuclei, lateral lemniscus, and inferior colliculus to auditory cortex	Acoustic neurilemmoma (neuroma) Brainstem tumor Brainstem infarct Multiple sclerosis
Somatosensory evoked potentials (SSEP)	Passage of electrical signals through peripheral nerves to central somatosensory pathways (including dorsal columns, medial lemnisci, thalamus, thalamocortical pathways) and arrival at sensory cortex	Multiple sclerosis Spinal cord tumors Myelopathy
Nerve conduction studies	Conduction of electrical signals through myelinated nerve fibers (motor or sensory)	Peripheral neuropathy Nerve trauma Nerve compression (e.g., carpal tunnel syndrome)

Procedure	Description	Disorders
Needle electromyography (EMG)	Electrical activity of muscle during rest and voluntary contraction	Denervating disease (e.g., amyotrophic lateral sclerosis) Muscular dystrophy Polymyositis
Repetitive nerve stimulation test (Jolly Test)	Neuromuscular transmission	Myasthenia gravis Lambert-Eaton (myasthenic) syndrome
Muscle biopsy	Morphology and histochemistry of muscle fibers	Muscular dystrophy Polymyositis Metabolic disorders
Nerve biopsy	Quantitative morphology of axons and myelin	Peripheral neuropathy
Cerebrospinal fluid (CSF) study	CSF pressure, biochemistry, cell count, serology, microbiology	Meningitis Encephalitis Subarachnoid hemorrhage Multiple sclerosis CNS syphilis
Myelogram	Radiopaque contrast in subarachnoid CSF space outlines spinal canal and its contents (may be combined with CT scan)	Cervical or lumbar disc herniations Spinal cord tumors
Magnetic resonance imaging (MRI)	Varying proton content of different tissues produces differential responses to high-intensity magnetic fields, providing the basis for computerized imaging.	Multiple sclerosis Tumors (especially in posterior fossa) Spinal cord lesions Infarcts
Computed tomographic (CT) scan	Various tissues and compartments within nervous system have different x-ray absorption coefficients, providing basis for computerized imaging	Malformations Hemorrhage Infarct Tumor Hydrocephalus Dementia Head trauma

(MRI) is strongly recommended prior to the LP in order to identify mass lesions.

b. When subarachnoid hemorrhage is suspected: Most cases of subarachnoid hemorrhage can be diagnosed by CT scan alone. LP is indicated more specifically in those patients in whom the CT scan is negative and a hemorrhage is still suspected on clinical grounds.

c. An LP may be done in those patients in whom alterations in CSF biochemistry can be of diagnostic value: e.g., Guillain-Barré syndrome (albuminocytologic dissociation), multiple sclerosis (oligoclonal bands and myelin basic protein, elevated gamma globulin).

d. To determine CNS involvement in cases of leukemia and lymphoma (cytology).

e. When CNS syphilis is suspected.

f. To introduce contrast media or drugs into the CSF.

g. Measurement of CSF pressure for the diagnosis and management of pseudotumor cerebri.

B. Contraindications.

1. Local infection at the site of puncture (if CSF sample must be obtained in such a patient, a cisternal puncture or lateral cervical puncture can be done).

2. When a cerebral mass lesion is suspected as evidenced by signs of increased intracranial pressure such as papilledema: A sudden decrease in intraspinal CSF pressure can potentially lead to herniation of either the tonsils of the cerebellum through the foramen magnum or portions of the temporal lobe through the tentorium cerebelli; such a complication if not promptly detected and treated will be fatal. This underscores the importance of examining the ocular fundi and doing a CT scan before doing an LP. There are two situations in which LP may still have to be done despite the presence of papilledema: (a) when there is a high index of suspicion of meningitis, and (b) when pseudotumor cerebri is strongly suspected. In either case, a neurologic or neurosurgical consultation needs to be made before LP is done.

Note: When future diagnostic studies, such as myelography, are contemplated, postpone the LP since a sample of CSF can be obtained at the time the radiologic procedure is performed.

C. Technique.
1. Explain the procedure thoroughly to the patient and be sure to ask for a history of allergy to local anesthetics or iodine.
2. Site of puncture: The LP is carried out usually at the L3–4 or L4–5 (same level as the highest point of the iliac crest) interspinous space.
3. Position of patient: Have the patient lie on a hard surface on his or her side with the knees pulled up toward the chest and the head flexed ("fetal position") (see Figs 2–1 through 2–5). Make sure that the spine is straight and not curved (bent) sideways. Alternatively, the patient may be made to sit up; this makes it easier to locate the correct space for puncture. For patients who are agitated or delirious, restraint may be necessary; if sufficient personnel are not available, the patient may be trussed (see Fig 2–4).
4. Prepare the skin surface for puncture by applying povidone-iodine (Betadine), or other equally effective

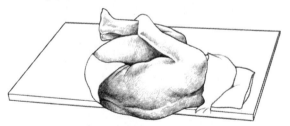

FIG 2–1. Positioning for a lumbar puncture. Note that the patient is placed on a firm surface so that the spinal column is relatively straight. Once the subarachnoid space is entered, the legs should be gently extended in order to relax the patient and relieve pressure on the abdomen.

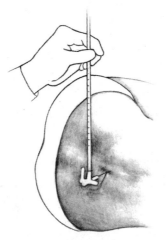

FIG 2-2. Once the subarachnoid space is entered, place the stopcock in an upright position and record the pressure. If a moderately high pressure is recorded (e.g., 250 mm of H_2O), this is most often secondary to patient anxiety. Wait a few minutes and the pressure will frequently return to normal (<200 mm of H_2O).

anti-infective topical solution, with vigorous rubbing. Sterile technique, including gloves and drapes, is very important. Commercially available sterile disposable LP trays and disposable (rather than reusable) spinal needles are preferred. Always use a spinal needle with a stylet.

5. Using local anesthetic, make a skin wheal and then infiltrate more deeply, particularly around the bone. Insert the needle with the bevel parallel to the long axis of the body so that it separates rather than cuts through the fibers of the ligamentum flavum (see Fig 2-5). When the needle enters the subarachnoid space (a pop will be felt as it passes through the posterior spinal ligament and dura), withdraw the stylet, allowing only one drop of CSF to

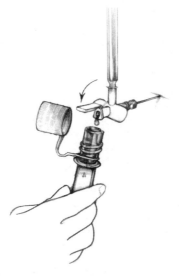

FIG 2–3. After the pressure measurement is taken, turn the stopcock as illustrated and obtain an appropriate amount of fluid.

escape, verifying that the needle is indeed in the subarachnoid space. Reinsert the stylet immediately and tell the patient to relax; have an assistant extend the patient's head and legs. Attach the manometer and record the opening pressure. Normal CSF pressure is less than 200 mm H$_2$O.

6. The needle must be strictly parallel to the bed and the tip is to be pointed toward the patient's umbilicus. If the needle encounters bone, withdraw the needle up to the subcutaneous tissue and then reintroduce it at a different angle. If the needle does not enter the subarachnoid space on the second attempt, it is better to try the procedure in the sitting position which enables one to gauge the midline better. Do not make repeated, unsuccessful attempts

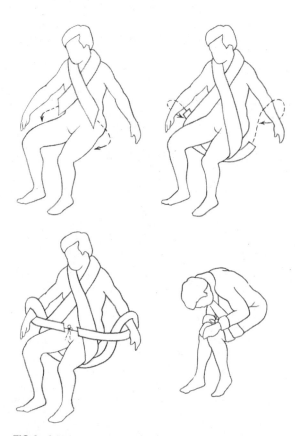

FIG 2–4. Trussing with a sheet: an uncooperative patient may be restrained with a sheet as illustrated.

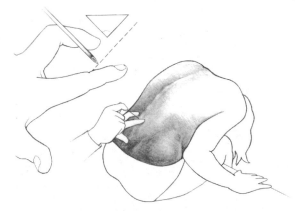

FIG 2–5. In performing a difficult lumbar puncture, it may be necessary for the patient to be in a sitting position, which often makes the landmarks clearer. Increased hydrostatic pressure in the lumbar area tenses the dura, making needle penetration easier. Note that the needle must be inserted with the bevel parallel to the long axis of the spine. Once the needle has entered the subarachnoid space (and with the stylet in place), the patient should be assisted to the lying position; appropriate pressure measurements may then be taken.

to perform an LP, but instead call for more experienced help or perform the procedure under fluoroscopy.

7. After measuring the opening pressure, CSF is removed for laboratory study. Know how much CSF is required before attempting the LP, in order that enough fluid can be obtained for all studies. About 5.5 mL of CSF is required for biochemical studies: determination of glucose (0.5 mL), protein (1 mL), and protein-electrophoresis (4 mL). Microbiologic studies require about 8 mL of CSF for: routine culture (1 mL), acid-fast and fungal cultures (2–3 mL), syphilis serology (1 mL), cryptococcal antigen and antibody (2 mL), Gram's stain (0.5 mL), and

India ink preparation (0.5 mL). Cell count requires 0.5 mL. It is always a good idea to have an extra 2 mL of CSF labeled and frozen, in case the quantity originally sent to the laboratory turns out to be insufficient for the tests ordered, or if confirmation is desired. In general, the first collected tube should go for routine culture and the second tube for protein and other biochemical studies.

Caveat: At the completion of the fluid collection and needle removal there is a hole through the dura into the subcutaneous paravertebral tissue. The continuously produced CSF (at the rate of about 20 mL/hr) may leak through this hole until normal repair processes obliterate the hole. With normal technique the leakage occurs for only a short period, but nonetheless may amount to 30 mL or more. Continuing leakage can result in greater fluid loss and may cause post-LP headache. The fluid removed for the study constitutes only a small proportion of the extra fluid that can be lost with leakage. Therefore one should always be certain to collect adequate amounts for laboratory study and not be concerned about "taking too much." The leakage may be minimized by keeping the bevel of the needle parallel to the long axis of the spine to avoid a dural and posterior ligament tear.

8. If the CSF appears bloody, spin it down *immediately* and compare that tube in the sunlight with an identical tube containing water, looking down from the tops of the tubes (Fig 2–6). If the LP was traumatic, the CSF should appear clear; if the patient has had a subarachnoid hemorrhage, the CSF should appear xanthochromic (yellow). Elevated CSF protein (over 100 mg/dL) or peripheral bilirubin may also result in xanthochromic fluid.
9. Cell count.
   a. A cell count should be done *immediately* (preferably by the physician) since white blood cells (WBCs) lyse quickly at room temperature (at room temperature, there is a 50% loss of cells in the first half-hour after collection).

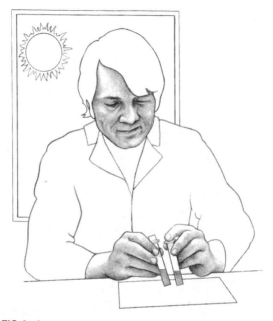

FIG 2–6. Xanthochromia may best be appreciated by comparing CSF with water in sunlight against a white sheet of paper, as illustrated.

    b. Red blood cells (RBCs) in the fluid can be lysed (leaving only the WBCs to be visualized in counting) by drawing acetic acid into a capillary hematocrit tube (or white cell pipette) and then blowing it out; the capillary tube is then introduced into the CSF solution and the CSF drawn up into the capillary tube.

    c. It will be easier to see the cells if they are stained; crystal violet may be used (mix 0.1 g of crystal violet, 1 mL of glacial acetic acid, 50 mL of distilled water, and two drops of phenol). The solution is drawn up into the capillary hematocrit tube (or white cell pipette) and then blown out. The capillary tube is then introduced into the CSF solution. The CSF is drawn up into the capillary tube and after mixing well the CSF is placed in the counting chamber. Under these conditions RBCs appear green and WBCs appear purple.

d. Normal CSF contains less than five lymphocytes and no polymorphonuclear leukocytes per microliter (cubic millimeter). In addition to looking for WBCs and doing a differential count, cytology may be done for the presence of malignant cells. When meningitis or encephalitis is suspected, Gram stain and acid-fast stain (on centrifuged sediment) need to be done.

10. Chemistries.

a. Protein is less than 40 mg/dL in the lumbar subarachnoid fluid and much lower (10–20 mg/dL) in the ventricles. Markedly increased protein (750–1,000 mg/dL) may be seen in spinal block (Froin's syndrome), while mild to moderate elevation may be seen in Guillain-Barré syndrome, meningitis, diabetes, polyneuropathy, and certain types of brain tumors. In multiple sclerosis (MS) the elevation is seldom above 80 to 100 mg/dL. An elevated CSF gamma globulin percentage (normal is less than 13%) by CSF protein electrophoresis indicates the possibility of MS, tuberculosis, myeloma, or other inflammatory or immunologic disorders. An IgG index is a sensitive test of excessive IgG synthesis in the CNS; it is calculated by the formula:

$$\frac{\text{CSF IgG/serum IgG}}{\text{CSF albumin/serum albumin}} = [\text{normal} < 0.7]$$

Demonstration of oligoclonal (IgG) bands and myelin basic protein (>1.0 ng/mL) in the CSF is highly useful in the diagnosis of MS.

b. If meningitis is suspected in a diabetic patient or a patient receiving intravenous (IV) glucose, it may be advantageous to compare the blood sugar and the CSF sugar. The blood should be drawn at least 1 hour prior to the LP for such comparison. The CSF glucose level normally is about two thirds of that in blood.

11. Microbiology. When CNS infection is suspected prompt identification of the etiologic agent is crucial for initiation of appropriate therapy. The following CSF studies should be done:

   a. Gram stain is positive in 90% of patients with bacterial meningitis, although *Haemophilus influenzae* or *Listeria monocytogenes* may be difficult to identify.

   b. Culture is positive in 70% to 90% of untreated bacterial meningitis but the percentage drops if oral antibiotics have been given prior to LP.

   c. Rapid detection of bacterial antigens by latex particle agglutination or countercurrent immunoelectrophoresis is useful in this context. The limulus lysate assay is useful when meningitis due to gram-negative bacteria is suspected.

   d. When tuberculous meningitis is suspected, special stains (such as Ziehl-Neelsen method) should be ordered. Repeated culture or animal inoculation studies may also be necessary.

   e. When viral meningitis is suspected, culture as well as detection of antibodies in CSF is useful.

   f. In suspected fungal meningitis, detection of antigen (e.g., cryptococcal antigen) and culture (with large volumes of CSF) are necessary.

   g. The CSF VDRL (Venereal Disease Research Laboratory) test should be done when neurosyphilis is a possibility.

D. Complications of lumbar puncture.

1. Post-LP headache occurs in about 10% to 20% of patients. The diagnostic feature is marked exacerbation of pain on sitting up and dramatic relief on lying down. Onset is within 1 to 3 days after LP and lasts for days to weeks. Bed rest and liberal fluid intake are useful but in persistent post-LP headache autologous epidural blood patch may be necessary.

2. Iatrogenic meningitis: this complication should not occur if adequate sterile precautions are taken.
3. Herniation: a CT scan easily identifies mass lesions which increase the probability of herniation.

Caveat: Millions of LPs were done safely before the invention of the CT scanner; lack of a CT scan should never delay an LP when acute bacterial meningitis is suspected.

II. Neuroradiologic Procedures.
A. **Computed tomographic scan.** Since its inception, this procedure has totally revolutionized the practice of neurology. CT scans show important anatomy, even though CT scans do not demonstrate most blood vessels adequately enough to exclude vascular disorders. This radiologic examination uses narrow beams of x-rays to penetrate the head in multiple directions with quantification of the absorption of the x-rays by various structures and tissues. Using computer analysis, an entire cross section of the brain can be depicted with clear differentiation of the densities of all areas. Such tomographic "slices" can be visualized as a picture on a cathode ray tube (television screen) where a gray scale shading of each picture point is proportional to its density. Intravenous injection of iodinated contrast material ("IVP dye") may be used to enhance the density of vascular or pathologic structures. Pathologic conditions such as an infarct will cause breakdown of the blood-brain barrier allowing the contrast material to seep into normal brain tissue drawing attention to abnormalities that might otherwise not be apparent on the CT scan. Injection of a water-soluble iodinated contrast material into the subarachnoid space permits improved visualization of the spinal cord and subarachnoid space on a CT scan.

1. Indications: A CT scan is indicated in patients presenting with focal neurologic deficits, altered mental status, head trauma, new-onset seizures, increased intracranial pressure, and suspected mass lesions or subarachnoid hemorrhage. A CT scan done after injection of contrast will improve diagnostic yield in the case of intracranial tumor, abscess, chronic subdural hematoma, infarct, and vascular malformation. While a CT scan is highly sensitive and

somewhat specific in documenting many types of intra-cranial pathologic conditions, its limitations include an inability to show very small lesions and those lesions that are isodense with brain tissue. Thus small plaques of MS may not be visible on CT scans, whereas they are easily visualized by MRI. Similarly an infarct in the first 24 to 48 hours may not be seen on CT scan. Subdural hematomas that are bilateral and isodense may be totally missed by CT scan.

Caveat: A normal CT scan does not rule out an intracranial disorder. Also, a CT scan may show lesions that may not be relevant to the patient's current illness (e.g., agenesis of corpus callosum, old infarcts in a patient presenting with unrelated new symptoms). Remember that symptoms and signs must be correlated with lesions found on the CT scan.

B. **Magnetic resonance imaging.** Magnetic resonance imaging affords visualization of the anatomy of the brain and spinal cord with clarity and detail that is unmatched by any other test. Sagittal, coronal, and horizontal (axial) views can be obtained. The patient is placed in a powerful magnetic field which tends to make the protons of the tissues align themselves in the orientation of the magnetic field. A specific radiofrequency signal (RF pulse) is introduced into the magnetic field which makes the protons resonate; subsequently they return to their original positions when the radiofrequency pulse is discontinued. By computer analysis of the radiofrequency energy emitted by the protons, an image of the tissue is created. Tissue-specific differences in the energy emission allow delineation of the different components such as white matter, gray matter, and CSF. MRI is superior to the CT scan in every way except for imaging acute hemorrhage or when bony detail is desired. It is especially valuable in diagnosing MS, posterior fossa lesions, temporal lobe lesions, and spinal cord lesions. Like CT scans, IV contrast materials (paramagnetic agents such as gadolinium) add valuable information to the detection of disease processes. Further developments, such as MRI angiography and tissue spectroscopy, make the procedure even more valuable.

C. **Myelography.** Myelography is indicated when external pressure on the spinal dura and its contents or when a mass within the spinal subarachnoid space is suspected. Radiopaque material is injected into the subarachnoid space through a spinal (lumbar or lateral cervical) puncture or cisternal puncture. Contrast media is heavier than spinal fluid, and by tilting the patient it can be made to travel up and down the subarachnoid space. It will outline anything deforming the thecal sac. Water-soluble nonionic contrast media are used, and with the newer contrast agents complications are few. However, the major complication is the occurrence of seizures and encephalopathy, if a significant amount of the material escapes into the cranial subarachnoid space. It is advisable to discontinue drugs like phenothiazines and antidepressants before water-soluble myelography to reduce the chance of seizures, since those agents also lower the seizure threshold. Myelography is commonly used to demonstrate a herniated intervertebral disc, extrinsic tumors compressing the spinal cord, or intramedullary lesions. More information can be obtained if CT scanning is combined with myelography. However, since the advent of MRI, the number of myelograms performed has markedly decreased.

D. **Cerebral angiography (arteriography).** The most important indication for cerebral angiography is suspicion of an abnormality of the blood vessels of the brain which cannot be seen on CT scan or MRI. The most common indications are suspected aneurysm or arteriovenous malformation, evaluation of extracranial and intracranial portions of cerebral blood vessels in patients with a transient ischemic attack (TIA) prior to surgical treatment, arteritis involving intracranial vessels, and to assess vascularity and vessel configuration in tumors such as meningioma. During angiography the catheter is inserted into the femoral artery and threaded up the aorta. At the aortic arch the carotid and vertebral arteries and their branches are individually catheterized. A series of radiographs is taken during injection of a radiopaque contrast material. Fine detail of cerebral vessels can be seen as well as the configuration of the larger arteries in the chest and neck. Arteriography is the best method for demonstrating aneurysms, arteriovenous malformations (AVMs), tumor vascularity, occlusive vascular diseases, and abnormal vascular shunts (such as the subclavian steal phenomenon). In addition to anatomic detail much physiology can be assessed including collateral circulation and the primary feeding vessels to AVMs and tumors. Interventional angiography can obliterate AVMs and aneurysms by injecting particles into the lesions through special catheters, at times making surgery unnecessary.

E. **Spinal radiographs.** Spinal radiographs (x-ray films) are often taken for any complaint referable to the spine or the spinal cord. Films of the spine are only as useful as the technical competence of the x-ray technician in obtaining correctly positioned views and the ability of the radiologist to interpret the films. Especially important in cervical spine films are views of all seven vertebrae. In cervical and lumbar spine films, good oblique views are important. Remember when ordering the films that the segmental spinal cord levels are higher than the vertebral spine levels (in adults, the cord ends at approximately L2). Pathologic conditions producing changes seen on spinal films include congenital lesions (e.g., fusion, anomalies, syringomyelia), tuberculosis, fractures, spondylolisthesis, tumors, metabolic bone disease, and degenerative disc disease.

F. **Skull radiographs.** Skull radiographs are most useful in assessing abnormalities in cranial bones, pituitary fossa, abnormal calcifications, and shifts of normal calcified structures. They are occasionally useful in picking up abnormalities in facial bones, vertebrae, and pericranial structures. They usually are not necessary when a patient has had a CT scan or MRI of the head. Pathologic conditions that produce abnormalities that can be seen on skull films include changes in bone structure (single or multiple areas of destruction as in metastases and multiple myeloma), fractures, intracranial calcifications (normal: e.g., pineal, choroid plexus; or abnormal: e.g., tuberous sclerosis, Sturge-Weber syndrome, certain tumors), increased intracranial pressure, craniostenosis, cerebellopontine angle tumor, enlarged sella from pituitary masses, sinus changes, and congenital or acquired disorders of the skull base. If the odontoid process is not seen on spinal films, it should be included in the skull series. There is controversy about the need for routine skull films for minor head injuries, since the yield of therapeutically useful information is very low.

G. **Isotope cisternography.** Isotope cisternography, formerly called radioiodinated serum albumin (RISA) scan, consists of the injection of a radioactive nuclide into the lumbar subarachnoid space. The substance usually employed is technetium 99m. It may be useful in the investigation of normal-pressure hydrocephalus (NPH), CSF leakage, and the patency of ventricular shunts.

III. NEUROPHYSIOLOGIC TESTS.

A. **Electroencephalography.** Electroencephalography records the spontaneous electrical activity of the brain. Electrodes are placed on the scalp in a specific pattern, and the electrical voltage fluctuations between any pair of these electrodes are amplified and recorded permanently on moving paper. Indications include: (1) finding the origin and type of electrical discharge associated with clinical seizures and more often in detecting epileptiform abnormalities in between seizures (interictal tracing); (2) localizing and assessing changes resulting from trauma, neoplasm, infection, or vascular disease; (3) assisting in the diagnosis of coma and dementia; and (4) assisting in the diagnosis of cerebral death. It is particularly useful in the diagnosis of herpes simplex encephalitis and Creutzfeldt-Jakob disease in which diagnostic patterns may be seen. This technique is only as good as the skills of the technician recording the tracing and those of the physician (electroencephalographer) interpreting the tracing. In addition, during the short time of the recording, an intermittent abnormality (e.g., epileptiform abnormality) may or may not occur.

Caveat: A normal EEG does not necessarily rule out a true seizure. In order to increase the chances of recording epileptiform abnormalities in the interictal EEG, it is recommended that the patient be sleep-deprived on the previous night and that both waking and sleep tracings be obtained. Other measures include use of special electrodes such as nasopharyngeal and sphenoidal electrodes, long-term ambulatory cassette EEG monitoring, or in-hospital video EEG with or without telemetry.

B. **Electromyography.** Electromyography refers to the recording of the electrical activity of muscle fibers through a needle electrode inserted into the muscle belly. Abnormal spontaneous electrical activity in the form of fasciculations, fibrillations, or positive sharp waves may be recorded. Fasciculations are seen most often in chronic anterior horn cell disorders like amyotrophic lateral sclerosis (ALS). Fibrillations and positive sharp waves are detected 3 to 6 weeks after the motor nerve is injured. Reinnervation of denervated muscle fibers may be documented by detecting polyphasic motor units during volitional contraction. Changes in the morphology of motor units are helpful in the detection of myopathies and neurogenic disorders. Certain EMG abnormalities, such as myotonia (myotonia congenita, myotonic dystrophy), are diagnostic. By delineating the distribution of denervation changes among different muscles, the site of the lesion (nerve, plexus, nerve root, anterior horn cell) can be accurately localized. For instance, in doubtful cases, objective evidence for a nerve root compression can be obtained by documenting denervation changes limited to those muscles supplied by that particular nerve root. Recovery from a nerve injury can also be predicted or confirmed on the basis of serial EMG studies.

C. **Nerve conduction study.** A nerve conduction study consists of stimulation of a nerve (motor or sensory) at different points and calculating the velocity of conduction of the propagated impulse. The measured velocity is that of the fastest conducting nerve fibers (large myelinated axons) and will be normal if the myelin sheath is intact. Demyelination leads to a decrease in conduction velocity. However, there may be no slowing if the conduction measurement is not through the area of myelin destruction. For example, a conduction study distal to the site of pressure injury to the nerve may initially be normal. In Guillain-Barré syndrome, in which the nerve roots are involved early in the course of the disease, distal conduction may be normal, while proximal conduction (measured as F-wave latency, H-reflex latency, or both) tends to be abnormal. Nerve conduction studies are useful in the diagnosis of:

   1. Entrapment neuropathies: i.e., median nerve at the wrist (carpal tunnel syndrome), tibial nerve at the ankle (tarsal tunnel syndrome), ulnar nerve at the elbow, etc.

2. Confirming the presence of peripheral neuropathies and distinguishing predominantly demyelinating from predominantly axonal polyneuropathies (see Chapter 15, section II.A).

3. Localization of site of injury and follow-up of recovery in nerve trauma.

> *Remember:* Normal nerve velocity does not rule out the existence of polyneuropathy; it only excludes a demyelinating neuropathy involving the larger, thickly myelinated nerve fibers. Small-fiber neuropathies (involving only thinly myelinated or unmyelinated nerve fibers) or axonal neuropathies may not cause significant slowing of nerve conduction.

D. Evoked potentials. Evoked potentials are a recording of the electrical activity in the CNS produced by stimulation of peripheral sensory receptors. Signals are recorded by placing electrodes over the scalp (as in an EEG) or over the spine and are analyzed by a computer that averages and amplifies the signal. Auditory stimuli are delivered by clicks through earphones and visual stimuli by stroboscopic flash, or more reliably by a changing checkerboard pattern on a television screen (pattern shift visual evoked potential). For somatosensory evoked potentials, electric stimuli are delivered to peripheral nerves, such as the median, peroneal, or tibial nerves.

E. Neurosonography.

1. Diagnostic ultrasound was originally used to detect shift of midline structures or hydrocephalus (A-mode echoencephalography). With the advent of the CT scan, this imaging modality was abandoned. Recently, high-resolution, portable, real-time ultrasound scanners have become available and have proved useful in detecting intracranial hemorrhage in premature infants (ultrasound is passed through the fontanels).

2. Duplex scan: B-mode ultrasound with pulsed Doppler ultrasound has been used frequently to investigate the extracranial carotid arteries. This noninvasive technique gives a graphic image of the arterial wall and analyzes the velocity pattern of the blood flow, providing information about stenosis and plaques.

F. Muscle and nerve biopsy. Muscle and nerve biopsy specimens are very fragile, and special care must be taken in obtaining and processing the tissue. Muscle biopsies should only be done where the specimen can be quick-frozen and histochemistry performed. Nerve biopsy should only be done where facilities are available for electron microscopy and teased fiber preparation of the specimen.

Note: Muscle and nerve biopsies should be done under local anesthetic, since general anesthesia in susceptible patients may precipitate malignant hyperthermia (see Chapter 15, section II.D.5).

1. Muscle biopsy. Muscle biopsy may be of value in:
    a. Evaluation of congenital weakness, proximal or distal weakness, or muscle wasting without sensory loss.
    b. Diagnosis of lipid and glycogen storage diseases, sarcoidosis, vasculitis, and polymyositis.
    c. Searching for microscopic changes seen in myotonic disorders, endocrine myopathies, and congenital myopathies.
2. Nerve biopsy. Nerve biopsy may be of value in:
    a. Differentiating between axonal and demyelinating neuropathies.
    b. Showing infiltration of peripheral nerves as in myeloma, carcinoma, sarcoidosis, amyloidosis, vasculitis, and leprosy.
    c. Characterizing congenital hypertrophic neuropathies.

BIBLIOGRAPHY

Aminoff MJ: *Electrodiagnosis in Clinical Neurology,* ed 3. New York, Churchill Livingstone, 1992.

Bronen RA, Sze G: Magnetic resonance imaging contrast agents: Theory and application to the central nervous system. *J Neurosurg* 1990; 73: 820–839.

Davis KR, Kistler JP, Buonanno SF: Clinical neuroimaging approaches to cerebrovascular diseases. *Neurol Clin* 1984; 2:655–665.

Duffy FH, Iyer VG, Surwillo WW: *Clinical EEG and Topographic Brain Mapping.* New York, Springer-Verlag, 1989.

Fishman RA: *Cerebrospinal Fluid in Diseases of the Nervous System,* ed 2. Philadelphia, WB Saunders, 1992.

Gilman S: Advances in neurology. *N Engl J Med* 1992; 326:671–675, 1608–1615.

Grant EG, White EM: Pediatric neurosonography. *J Child Neurol* 1986; 1:319–337.

Iyer VG: Understanding nerve conductions and electromyographic studies. *Hand Clinics* 1993; 9:273–287.

Jablecki CK: Electromyography in infants and children. *J Child Neurol* 1986; 1:297–318.

Kirkwood RJ: *Essentials of Neuroimaging.* New York, Churchill Livingstone, 1990.

Kovanen J, Sulkava R: Duration of postural headache after lumbar puncture. *Headache* 1986; 26:224–226.

Kughn MJ: *Atlas of Neuroradiology.* New York, Gower Medical Publishers, 1992.

Mazziotta JC, Gilman S: *Clinical Brain Imaging.* Philadelphia, FA Davis, 1992.

Miller GM: Magnetic resonance imaging of the spine. *Mayo Clin Proc* 1989; 64:986–1004.

Sato S, Rose DF: The electroencephalogram in the evaluation of the patient with epilepsy. *Neurol Clin* 1986; 4:509–529.

Strokes HD, O'Hara CM, Buchanan RD, et al: An improved method for examination of cerebrospinal fluid cells. *Neurology* 1975; 25:901–906.

Zisfein J, Tuchman AJ: Risks of lumbar puncture in the presence of intracranial mass lesions. *Mt Sinai J Med* 1988; 55:283–287.

HEADACHE 3

Headache is one of the commonest conditions for which patients seek medical treatment and is the fifth commonest reason for outpatient visits. Remember that headache is *a symptom, not a disease,* and successful therapy depends on correct diagnosis. The physician who simply prescribes an analgesic or tranquilizer does the patient no service and runs the risk of causing an iatrogenic drug dependency problem. *NEVER* treat chronic or recurrent headaches with narcotics. A minimum of 30 minutes should be scheduled and spent with each patient complaining of headache. The primary aim is to differentiate serious or life-threatening conditions that present with headache (e.g., brain tumor, subarachnoid hemorrhage, meningitis) from relatively benign conditions (e.g., migraine, tension headache), and develop appropriate strategies for treatment.

I. **HISTORY AND EXAMINATION OF THE PATIENT WITH HEADACHE.**
A. **History.** The determination of the cause of headache is most often made from the history. During the course of the interview, the following information should be obtained (avoid leading questions):
   1. Location of pain.
      a. Frontal, temporal, occipital, or vertex.
      b. Unilateral, bilateral, or shifting.
   2. Type of pain.
      a. Constant or throbbing.
      b. Mixed (constant and throbbing; which is first?).
   3. Duration and timing of pain.
      a. Worse in morning or evening.
      b. Worse with a Valsalva maneuver (bowel movement, coughing, sneezing).
      c. Consistent associations (premenstrual, weekends,

emotional stress, alcohol intake, seasonal, specific foods).

4. Severity of pain: Pain severe enough to wake the patient from sleep may be seen with increased intracranial pressure, cluster headache, and intracranial hemorrhage. On the other hand, the patient may find it difficult to go to sleep with any form of severe headache.

5. Associated symptoms preceding, accompanying, or following the headache (visual changes, dizziness or other sensations may precede classic migraine).

6. Family history (migraine, epilepsy, psychiatric illness).

7. Past medical history (hypertension, infection, allergy, head trauma, recent lumbar puncture).

8. Medication history (vasodilators, oral contraceptives, alcohol, or street drugs).

Caveat: Sudden onset of a severe headache without past history should be considered ominous and warrants immediate exclusion of potentially life-threatening conditions such as subarachnoid hemorrhage or meningitis.

B. **Physical examination.** On examination, particular attention should be given to the following signs:

1. Blood pressure, pulse rate, temperature.

2. Sharpness of optic discs, intact venous pulsations, presence of retinal hemorrhages.

3. Tenderness of temporal arteries.

4. Presence of spasm and tenderness in cervical muscles.

5. Altered sensation in the scalp.

6. Tenderness to percussion of spinous processes in the upper cervical area.

7. Cranial bruits.

8. Tenderness to percussion over sinuses.

9. "Trigger" areas for pain (as in trigeminal neuralgia).

10. Asymmetry of reflexes or other focal neurologic signs.

II. HEADACHE OF INCREASED INTRACRANIAL PRESSURE.

A. **Diagnostic considerations.**

▶ 1. *The most important diagnostic clue* is a bilateral, nonthrobbing headache that is worse in the morning.

2. Initially mild and intermittent, increasing in severity to steady, nonthrobbing pain.
3. May awaken the patient at night.
4. Worse with Valsalva maneuver.
5. When severe, associated with vomiting.
6. Presence of early papilledema (see Chapter 13, section I.B.1.g).
7. Often associated with focal neurologic signs (asymmetric reflexes, palsy of extraocular muscles, pupillary asymmetry).

B. **Treatment.** Immediate hospitalization and additional diagnostic studies such as a computed tomography (CT) scan or magnetic resonance imaging (MRI) are necessary. Treat the underlying cause.

III. **MIGRAINE HEADACHE.**

A. **Definition.** Migraine is a periodic or cyclic disorder in which recurrent headaches occur, often associated with photophobia and autonomic disturbances such as nausea and vomiting. It is considered to be a disorder involving both intracranial vascular regulation and neuronal electrical disturbances.

B. **Classic migraine (migraine with aura).**

1. Diagnostic considerations.
   ▶a. *The most important diagnostic clue* is an aura followed by the sudden onset of a unilateral throbbing headache.
   b. Aura may consist of transient visual (scotoma, monocular blindness, or hemianopsia), sensory, or motor (paresthesia, weakness) phenomena, or simply an indescribable feeling; prodromal symptoms (sometimes preceding headache by several days) include changes in mood or appetite, or both.
   c. Typically throbbing, but occasionally may evolve to a dull, aching, nonthrobbing discomfort.
   d. Although unilateral, often shifts sides with different attacks; commonly temporal, orbital, frontal or, rarely, occipital.
   e. Occurs at any time of the day.
   f. Usually associated with nausea, and often with vomiting, photophobia, and phonophobia.

g. Is usually relieved by sleep or vomiting.

h. Onset is often in the teens; frequency and severity may diminish after the age of 50 years.

i. Commonly premenstrual in females; usually less frequent during pregnancy.

j. May be precipitated by certain foods or chemicals (especially monosodium glutamate, chocolate, cheddar cheese, red wine, or sodium nitrite as in hot dogs) or with fasting.

k. Onset or exacerbation often follows administration of oral contraceptives or reserpine-containing drugs.

l. Family history of headaches is common.

m. Past history of motion sickness or cyclic vomiting as a child.

n. Neurologic examination normal; if abnormal, the patient should have further studies such as an electroencephalogram (EEG) and CT scan or MRI to exclude a structural lesion.

Caveat: If the headache is always on the same side, if seizures and headache occur together, if the neurologic examination is abnormal, or if a cranial bruit is heard, consider the possibility of an arteriovenous malformation (AVM). Refer for further study including cerebral angiography.

2. Treatment.

a. General measures.

1) Migraine victims often are intelligent, obsessive-compulsive; a thorough explanation of the pathophysiology of the headache is an important part of therapy.

2) Discontinue oral contraceptives and look for other triggering factors such as alcohol, specific foods, etc., taking appropriate measures to reduce exposure.

b. Specific management. Patients with migraine fall into two categories: (1) those who have frequent attacks (one or more per week), or attacks of such severity as to interfere with their life style or work, and (2) those who have infrequent or sporadic attacks. Category 1 patients need regular prophylactic or interval therapy to prevent recurrence of the attacks, while category 2 patients need only abortive treatment at the onset of headache.

1) Abortive treatment: Treatment should be given at the earliest warning of an impending attack, in order to be effective. The following are the usually recommended measures:

a) In children and in those in whom the attacks are seldom severe, prompt administration of analgesics such as aspirin or acetaminophen should be tried as the initial measure. In some patients, sleep alone may abort the attack. If nausea or vomiting is a prominent feature, combine analgesics with metoclopramide hydrochloride (Reglan) 10 mg orally or intramuscularly (IM) or promethazine hydrochloride (Phenergan) suppositories.

b) Ergotamine is the mainstay in the abortive treatment of migraine. Ergot is an α-adrenergic blocking agent with direct stimulating effect on vascular smooth muscle. It may also produce depression of central vasomotor centers and have antiserotonin effects. To be effective, ergot should be administered at the very beginning of an attack. It is available in oral, sublingual, suppository, and injectable forms (Table 3–1).

Caveat: Ergot can induce nausea and vomiting and may lead to ergotism (loss of peripheral pulses with weakness, muscle pain, paresthesia of extremities, precordial distress, and pain) if consumed in large quantities. Use with great care or avoid in organic heart disease, peripheral vascular disease, hypertension, pregnancy, hepatic disease, and septic states.

TABLE 3–1.
Commonly Used Ergot Preparations

Form	Brand Name	Constituents	Dosage
Oral	Cafergot Wigraine	Ergotamine tartrate 1 mg and caffeine 100 mg	2 tablets at onset followed by 1 tablet every half-hour to maximum of 6 tablets per attack
Suppository	Cafergot Wigraine	Ergotamine tartrate 2 mg and caffeine 100 mg	1 at onset followed by 1 every half-hour up to maximum of 3 suppositories per attack
Sublingual	Ergostat	Ergotamine tartrate 2 mg	1 tablet at first warning of impending attack followed by 1 tablet every half-hour if needed to maximum 3 tablets per attack or 5 tablets/wk
Parenteral	DHE-45	Dihydroergotamine mesylate 1 mg/mL	1.0 mL IM at first warning of attack followed by 1.0 mL every hour to maximum of 3.0 mL per attack or 6.0 mL/wk; for more rapid effect initial dose may be given IV

    c) If simple measures (as outlined above) fail to
       stop an attack and the pain persists continu-
       ously for a prolonged period:
       i) Administer dihydroergotamine mesylate
         (DHE-45) 1 mg IM at the onset of head-
         ache; if necessary repeat after 1 hour. The
         maximum dose is 3 mg per attack. Dihy-
         droergotamine mesylate can also be given
         in 0.5–1.0 mg IV doses. Coadministra-

tion of metoclopramide (Reglan) 10 mg helps to reduce nausea and vomiting.

ii) Sumatriptan succinate (Imitrex), a specific serotonin ($5-HT_1$) receptor agonist is highly effective in controlling not only the headache, but also other symptoms that accompany migraine headaches such as nausea and photophobia. It is currently available as a 6 mg self-dose injection unit (for subcutaneous injection by patient). The drug is well-tolerated, but should be avoided in patients with hypertension or ischemic heart disease. It is preferable to administer sumatriptan as the initial drug for severe migraine and not after ergot preparations have been administered.

Note: Sumatriptan is extremely expensive and should be reserved for those patients with severe acute migrane headaches.

iii) Narcotic treatment should only be a last and desperate measure owing to its potential for addiction. If pain is severe enough to require narcotics, meperidine hydrochloride (Demerol) 50 to 100 mg IM may be given.

iv) An occasional patient who is resistant to these measures and goes into "status migrainosus" may respond to high-dose, short-term corticosteroid therapy.

Caveat: Keep in mind that a patient known to have migraine can develop other conditions which cause severe headache and hence if there is any question about the diagnosis, further studies, e.g., a CT scan or MRI, may be necessary.

2) Interval and prophylactic treatment. For patients with one or more attacks per week or those in whom the attacks are of such severity as to interfere with life style and work, prophylactic treatment should be instituted.

   a) Propranolol hydrochloride (Inderal), a nonselective β-adrenergic blocking agent, may be started at a dose of 40 mg orally (PO) bid or 80 mg of the long-acting preparation (Inderal LA). The dose may be increased to 160 to 200 mg gradually or until the headaches are abolished. Maintain therapeutic doses for 6 months and then gradually reduce over a 2-month period. If headaches recur, restart the drug. The aim is to achieve a sustained remission from headache. Common side effects include fatigue, general weakness, insomnia, and mental depression. Contraindications include bradycardia, postural hypotension, bronchial asthma, and congestive heart failure. Use with great caution in diabetic patients since propranolol may mask the warning symptoms of hypoglycemia. Patients prone to depression should not be given propranolol since it may worsen this condition. Other β-adrenergic blockers reported to be useful in migraine are atenolol (component of Tenormin), metoprolol tartrate (Lopressor), and timolol maleate (Blocadren).

   b) Patients who have both depression and migraine benefit from amitriptyline hydrochloride (Elavil, Endep) at an initial dose of 25 mg at bedtime; gradually increase to maximum effectiveness (usually 100 mg at bedtime). Use with caution in patients prone to cardiac arrhythmias. Other tricyclic antidepressants are probably equally effective.

   c) In patients with disabling headaches, methysergide maleate (Sansert), 4 to 8 mg total daily dose with meals is effective. Efficacy should be established in 3 weeks. It should be taken for 8-week intervals with 4 weeks off to avoid retroperitoneal fibrosis or other serious side effects. Cyproheptadine hydrochloride (Periactin) is another antiserotonin agent which has been found to be effective in some patients. Side effects include weight gain and somnolence.

3) Recent studies have shown that calcium channel blocking agents may also be used as prophylactic treatment. The drug most commonly used is verapamil hydrochloride.

4) Other prophylactic drugs include carbamazepine (Tegretol), divalproex sodium (Depakote), and phenytoin (Dilantin), which have been reported to be effective in migraine prophylaxis. Initial dose of carbamazepine is at 200 mg PO tid and initial dose of Depakote is 250 mg PO tid. If necessary, these drugs may be titrated to therapeutic anticonvulsant levels. Baclofen (Lioresal) in divided doses of 20 to 60 mg/day may also be effective.

5) Patient and physician information about migraine can be obtained from the National Headache Foundation, 5252 North Western Ave. Chicago, IL 60625, telephone (312) 878-7715.

C. **Common migraine (migraine without aura).** Common migraine is similar to classic migraine, but the essential difference is the lack of visual and other neurologic symptoms. As the name indicates, this is the commonest form of migraine headache; features of migraine may coexist with those of muscle contraction headache, thus giving rise to a combination of throbbing and constant headaches.

　1. Treatment: Treatment is the same as for classic migraine.

D. **Complicated migraine.**

▶ 1. Headache associated with significant neurologic complications (such as hemiplegia), presumably secondary to ischemia from intracranial vascular constriction. The neurologic complications may outlast the headache phase, and the headache phase may be relatively minor. Very rarely there may be permanent neurologic sequelae. Before making a diagnosis of complicated migraine it may be necessary to rule out an underlying arteriovenous malformation (especially if the deficit always occurs in the same location). The common types of complicated migraine are:

a. *Hemiplegic migraine:* The hemiplegia often shifts from side to side during different attacks.

b. *Ophthalmoplegic migraine:* Oculomotor paralysis occurs on the same side as the headache; recurrent painful oculomotor palsy in a child strongly suggests complicated migraine.

c. *Basilar artery migraine* occurs mostly in children and adolescents; vertigo, tinnitus, diplopia, and ataxia accompany occipital throbbing headache.

d. *Acute confusional migraine* occurs in adolescents, manifested as recurrent episodes of confusion and disorientation along with headache.

e. *Retinal migraine:* monocular visual disturbances lasting for days, not necessarily associated with a headache.

2. Treatment: Prophylactic (interval) treatment, as in classic migraine, is strongly recommended even when the attacks are infrequent.

E. Cluster headache (Horton's headache, histamine cephalgia, migrainous neuralgia).

1. Diagnostic considerations.

▶ a. *The most important diagnostic clue* is the sudden onset of severe unilateral retro-orbital lancinating pain that tends to occur repeatedly.

b. Frequently associated with tearing or unilateral nasal discharge on the side of the headache; other features include partial ptosis and smaller pupil (Horner's syndrome) on the side of the headache.

c. May last from 30 minutes to several hours.

d. Often awakens patient at night.

    e. Tends to occur in a series followed by remission for months or even years (hence the name *cluster* headache).

    f. Often precipitated by a small amount of alcohol.

    g. Usually familial, more frequent in males.

2. Treatment: Patients with cluster headache need two forms of therapy: (1) abortive treatment for an attack and (2) prophylactic treatment to stop future attacks.

    a. Abortive treatment: Ergotamine preparations are often effective if the attacks occur at a predictable time (see section III.B.2 for treatment). Oxygen inhalation (100% oxygen through mask) for 10 to 15 minutes has been found to be effective in most patients.

    b. Prophylactic treatment.

        1) Propranolol may be tried first [see section III.B.2.b.(2).(a) for dosage]. If this fails, methysergide is effective in many patients.

        2) For patients that are resistant to these prophylactic agents, corticosteroid therapy may be useful; prednisone 60 mg daily for 3 days with the dose reduced progressively to the minimum that is effective in stopping the attacks from recurring; continue for the duration of the bout.

        3) This type of headache may occur in chronic form on an almost daily basis; lithium carbonate treatment has been reported to be an effective therapy (300 mg two to three times a day to provide a blood level of $0.7-1.2$ mEq/L).

        Note: Lithium carbonate has a number of side effects and caution is necessary.

        4) In one variety of cluster headache, chronic paroxysmal hemicrania (CPH), in which the clusters are strictly unilateral (do not shift from side to side), indomethacin (Indocin) has been found to be highly effective (dose may vary from $25-100$ mg/day).

IV. TENSION HEADACHE (MUSCLE CONTRACTION HEADACHE).

A. Diagnostic considerations.

▶ 1. *The most important diagnostic clue* is a bilateral, non-throbbing constant headache that begins in the occipital area and spreads to the frontal area. Scalp tenderness is common. Tension headache is the most common type of headache.

2. Although the initial pain is viselike, it may eventually assume a vascular quality.

3. Not affected by a Valsalva maneuver.

4. Worse in the evening.

5. May last for days.

6. Occurs in situations of tension, such as family problems and job stress. Common in patients with history of whiplash, cervical arthritis, and occupations where the head is held for long periods in one position (as in secretaries using word processors).

7. Neurologic examination is normal except for spasm and tenderness of cervical muscles, tenderness to percussion of spinous processes in high cervical area, and decreased sensation to pinprick over scalp. Hyperalgesia of the scalp is occasionally found.

   Note: Whatever the cause, pain is produced by irritation of C2, which becomes the greater occipital nerve innervating the scalp. This is by far the most common type of headache.

B. Treatment.

1. Alter precipitating situations, e.g., a word-processor screen that is adjustable up and down or from right to left.

2. Heat and massage to cervical area combined with high dose of aspirin.

3. Cervical traction (see Fig 3–1 of modified over-the-door traction apparatus).

4. Steroid injections in occipital area near exit of greater occipital nerve.

5. For chronic pain syndrome, a combination of fluoxetine

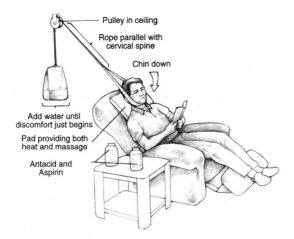

FIG 3–1. Modification of standard "over-the-door" traction for greater occipital nerve entrapment (tension headache) and cervical radiculopathy. Patients are compliant and comfortable.

(Prozac) 20 mg qam and nortriptyline (Pamelor) 25 mg qpm for 6 months is especially effective.

V. SINUS HEADACHE (NASAL HEADACHE).
A. Diagnostic considerations.
▶ 1. *The most important diagnostic clue* is a frontal, non-throbbing headache with tenderness to percussion over the sinus.
  2. Sinus headaches are rare without predisposing nasal abnormality (structural defect, allergy, polyps).
  3. May be unilateral or bilateral; location depends on sinus involved.
  4. Often seasonal, particularly in persons with allergy.
  5. Associated with nasal congestion and discharge, fever, malaise, painful teeth.
  6. Percussion over sinuses exacerbates pain.

7. Sinus radiographs show opacification. CT scan or MRI shows the changes much better.

B. Treatment.

1. Systemic decongestant: pseudoephedrine hydrochloride (Sudafed) 60 mg tid or phenylpropanolamine hydrochloride (component of ENTEX-LA 1 tablet bid).
2. Topical nasal decongestant: 0.25% phenylephrine hydrochloride (Neo-Synephrine Hydrochloride).

    Caveat: Decongestants should be used sparingly as tachyphylaxis and rebound may develop.

3. Antihistamines: The allergic patient usually knows which works best. Terfenadine (Seldane) 60 mg bid or astemizole (Hismanal) 10 mg qd is associated with less drowsiness than other agents.
4. Nonnarcotic analgesics such as aspirin, acetaminophen, or ibuprofen.
5. Systemic antibiotics: cefaclor (Ceclor) 250 mg tid or amoxicillin 250 mg qid (or with clavulanate as Augmentin 250 mg tid) if patient has systemic manifestations such as fever.
6. Intranasal cromolyn sodium (Nasalcrom) bid or qid or intranasal beclomethasone dipropionate (Vancenase) bid or qid, or both in combination, can be used for long-term prophylaxis.
7. Surgical drainage when chronic and severe.

VI. POSTTRAUMATIC HEADACHE.

A. Diagnostic considerations.

1. Posttraumatic headaches occur after significant head trauma (loss of consciousness) and have both organic and psychological components.
2. May be indistinguishable from chronic, recurring tension headaches.
3. Duration is usually from 6 to 12 months but may persist for years.
4. May be associated with dizzy spells.
5. May be part of postconcussion syndrome, which is characterized by fear, anxiety, fatigue, irritability, and inability to concentrate.

Caveat: Symptoms of a subdural hematoma can be insidious and hence a CT scan or MRI should be done.

B. Treatment.
1. Nonnarcotic analgesics such as aspirin, acetaminophen, or ibuprofen.
2. Diazepam 5 mg tid may be used to reduce anxiety and restlessness, but dependence may develop and diazepam should never be used for longer than 6 months.
3. Propranolol or amitriptyline [see section III.B.2.b.(2).(a) and (b)] may sometimes be useful for the more severe and prolonged posttraumatic headache.

Caveat: The physician should be alert to emotional factors or to litigation problems in the patient with prolonged or treatment-unresponsive posttraumatic headache.

VII. POST LUMBAR PUNCTURE (LP) HEADACHE.
A. Diagnostic considerations.
▶ 1. *The most important diagnostic clue* is headache following LP that is precipitated by sitting or standing and relieved promptly by lying down.
2. Often frontal or occipital, may be generalized, and may be associated with nuchal pain.
3. Occurs within 1 to 2 days of LP and is thought to be due to leakage of cerebrospinal fluid (CSF) through the dural hole.
4. Duration varies from 1 to several days.
5. Predisposing factors may include poor LP technique, larger size of needle, and multiple punctures.

B. Treatment.
1. Strict bed rest with feet elevated; let patient try to sit up every 12 hours to determine if headache reappears.
2. Adequate hydration (about 4 L/day).
3. Analgesics are usually ineffective.
4. With persistent headache, an epidural blood patch (usually done by the anesthesiologist) using the patient's venous blood may be highly effective.

VIII. SUBARACHNOID HEMORRHAGE HEADACHE.
A.   **Diagnostic considerations.**
> ▶ 1. *The most important diagnostic clue* is the abrupt onset of a severe occipital or generalized headache in a patient with no previous history of headaches.
>   2. Usually not localized, but definite localization may suggest the site of an underlying leaking aneurysm.
>   3. Associated with *stiff neck,* dizziness, nausea and vomiting, irritability, restlessness, convulsions, drowsiness.
>   4. Altered consciousness is common.
>   5. Signs of localizing neurologic dysfunction may be *absent.*
>   6. Papilledema (see Chapter 13, section I.B.1.g) may develop after hemorrhage depending on the location of the hemorrhage and degree of impedance to venous return around the optic nerve. *Subhyaloid hemorrhages* are pathognomonic.

B.   **Treatment.** CT scan and angiography should be performed as soon as possible, since aneurysms tend to rebleed, leading to fatal outcome. Neurosurgical consultation should be obtained immediately to decide whether the aneurysm can be clipped.

IX. TEMPORAL ARTERITIS.
A.   **Diagnostic considerations.**
> ▶ 1. Onset of severe, continuous unilateral head pain in an elderly person is temporal arteritis until proved otherwise.
>   2. The presence of an elevated erythrocyte sedimentation rate (ESR greater than 40 mm/hr).
>   3. Tender swollen nonpulsatile temporal arteries are often, but not always, present.
>   4. The typical patient is over age 55 years and female.
>   5. Polymyalgia rheumatica (generalized muscle aches and pains) is frequently associated with temporal arteritis.

B.   **Treatment.**
>   1. This is a neurologic emergency because arteritis may involve the ophthalmic or other intracranial arteries, leading to blindness and other focal deficits. Start steroid therapy with prednisone 60 to 80 mg *immediately.*

Continue high-dose steroid therapy until the ESR returns to normal. Then gradually reduce the dose to 20 to 30 mg/day and continue for 6 months to 1 year. Monitor the patient for complications of steroid therapy such as gastrointestinal bleeding, intercurrent infection, osteoporosis, aseptic necrosis of femoral head. Alternate-day therapy may reduce steroid-induced complications.

2. Diagnostic temporal artery biopsy should be scheduled within 2 to 3 days of presentation. A sufficient length of artery should be taken since the arteritis tends to be focal and may be missed. Therapy should not be delayed since instituting treatment with corticosteroids will not alter the histologic findings for a number of days.

X. CENTRAL NERVOUS SYSTEM (CNS) INFECTION HEADACHE (ABSCESS, ENCEPHALITIS, MENINGITIS).

A. Diagnostic considerations.

▶ 1. Any headache associated with fever and altered mentation is CNS infection until proved otherwise.

2. Subacute or acute onset of constant, increasingly severe pain.

3. Usually generalized but may be worse in occipital area.

4. Increases with physical activity.

5. Associated with stiff and painful neck, nausea and vomiting, irritability, restlessness.

6. Altered consciousness may be present.

7. Photophobia, strabismus, ptosis, or pupillary inequality may be present.

8. LP is mandatory for diagnosis and culture of the organism.

Caveat: If an abscess is suspected obtain a CT scan or MRI before performing the LP (see Chapter 14, section VIII.A.

B. Treatment. Treatment depends on culturing the organism and determining antibiotic sensitivity; broad-spectrum par-

enteral antibiotics should be used to treat the patient until the culture result returns. Consider isolation of patient until infectious agent is known (see Chapter 14).

XI. OCULAR HEADACHE.

A. **Causes.** Ocular causes of headache include glaucoma, diplopia with accompanying orbicularis contraction, uncorrected refractive errors such as astigmatism, ocular or retroocular inflammations, or orbital tumors.

▶ 1. Ocular headache starts as a feeling of heaviness in the eyes, gradually becoming more severe.
2. Absent on awakening, appears in afternoon, and gradually worsens.
3. Pain may be dull, bursting, sharp, or throbbing, and is often due to persistent muscle contraction.
4. Bifrontal or periorbital in location.
5. May be associated with prolonged reading or other use of eyes.
6. May be associated with altered visual acuity or reduced ocular motility.

B. **Treatment.** Measurement of intraocular pressure is necessary. Corrective lenses may be helpful. Obtain CT scans of the orbit if retroocular lesion is suspected.

XII. TRIGEMINAL NEURALGIA (TIC DOULOUREUX).

A. **Diagnostic considerations.**

▶ 1. Recurrent paroxysmal pain in the distribution of one or more branches of the trigeminal nerve is most probably trigeminal neuralgia.
2. Pain may radiate to jaw or teeth and present as a dental problem.
3. Precipitated by minimal sensory stimuli to the affected side of the face (especially a localized area or trigger point, which may appear as a dirty or unshaven patch).
4. Occurs after age 40 years; suspect multiple sclerosis when onset is earlier.
5. No sensory loss in trigeminal distribution; if there is sensory loss or decreased corneal reflex look for tumors or vascular abnormalities involving the trigeminal nerve.
6. Occasionally associated with multiple sclerosis.

B. Treatment.
1. Carbamazepine 400 to 1,200 mg/day is the drug of choice; the initial dose, 200 mg bid with meals, is increased gradually to the minimal effective dosage.
2. Phenytoin 300 to 700 mg/day, adjusted to produce a blood level of 10 to 20 μg/mL, may be effective in a few patients.
3. Baclofen in doses of 20 to 80 mg/day may be effective in some patients.
4. Surgical treatment may be considered in resistant cases. Trigeminal gangliolysis by percutaneous radiofrequency technique (80% chance of pain relief for 1 year), injection of glycerol around the gasserian (semilunar) ganglion, and suboccipital craniotomy with decompression of trigeminal nerve are some of the techniques used.

XIII. TEMPOROMANDIBULAR NEURALGIA (TMJ SYNDROME).

A. Diagnostic considerations.
▶1. Recurrent, usually unilateral, severe, constant, aching facial pain around the temporomandibular joint sometimes radiating to the jaws associated with tenderness over the temporomandibular joint.
2. Pain is exacerbated by movement of the lower jaw (chewing, yawning).
3. Patient may report an associated clicking or grating sound.
4. May be associated with bruxism during sleep; depression or insomnia may also be present.
5. Occurs commonly in young women or in elderly patients with severe overbite resulting from the loss of back teeth, or after fracture.
6. Palpation of the temporalis muscle or direct pressure on the temporomandibular joint may result in pain.
7. Special radiologic techniques often reveal asymmetric temporomandibular joints with degenerative changes in the cartilage.

B. Treatment. Treatment is often unsatisfactory. Correction of dental malocclusion may or may not relieve the pain. Conservative therapy includes heat applied to the affected area, a diet of soft foods, limitation of mouth opening, dental prostheses, mild analgesics, muscle relaxants, or antidepressants. Surgical replacement of the temporomandibular joint may be necessary.

XIV. TOXIC HEADACHE.
A. Diagnostic Considerations.
1. Toxic headache has the characteristics of vascular headache.
2. Drugs causing headache include phenacetin, amyl nitrite, reserpine, lithium, dextroamphetamine, ephedrine, disulfiram, digitalis, imipramine.
3. May result following excessive intake of alcohol or coffee.
4. May appear on discontinuation of corticosteroids, barbiturates, ergot, narcotics.
5. Occupational hazards include mechanics and farmers exposed to exhaust fumes (carbon monoxide), refrigerator repairmen exposed to refrigerants, coal miners exposed to mine gases, and persons exposed to insecticides.

B. Treatment.
1. Headache will subside following removal from toxic exposure.
2. Caffeine withdrawal headaches terminate with administration of caffeine.

BIBLIOGRAPHY

Cady RK, Shealy LN: Recent advances in migraine management. *J Fam Pract* 1993; 36:85–91.

Callahan M, Raskin N: A controlled study of DHE in the treatment of acute migraine headaches. *Headache* 1986; 26:168–171.

Dalessio DJ: Classification and treatment of headache during pregnancy. *Clin Neuropharmacol* 1986; 9:121–131.

Diamond S, Dalessio DJ: *The Practicing Physician's Approach to Headache*. Baltimore, Williams & Wilkins, 1992.

Ferrar MO: Treatment of migraine attacks with sumatriptan. *N Engl J Med* 1991; 325:316–321, 322–326.

Gallagher RM: *Drug Therapy for Headache.* New York, Dekker, 1991.

Gascon, G: Chronic and recurrent headaches in childhood and adolescence. *Pediatr Clin North Am* 1984; 31:1027–1051.

Kovanen J, Sulkava R: Duration of postural headache after lumbar puncture. *Headache* 1986; 26:224–226.

Lance JW: Advances in biology and pharmacology of headache. *Neurology* 1993; 43(Suppl. 3):11–47.

Lyons ML, Meyer FB: Cerebrospinal fluid physiology and the management of increased intracranial pressure. *Mayo Clin Proc* 1990; 65: 684–707.

MacDonald JT: Childhood migraine. *Postgrad Med* 1986; 80:301–306.

Mathew NT: Indomethacin sensitive headache syndrome. *Headache* 1981; 21:147–150.

Raskin N: Serotonin receptors and headache. *N Engl J Med* 1991; 325:353–354.

Rovit LR, Murali R, Jannetta PJ: *Trigeminal Neuralgia.* Baltimore, Williams & Wilkins, 1990.

Sjaastad O: *Cluster Headache Syndrome.* Philadelphia, WB Saunders, 1992.

Subcutaneous Sumatriptan International Study Group: Treatment of migraine attacks with sumatriptan. *N Engl J Med* 1991; 325:316–321

Vinken PJ, Bruyn JW, Klawans HL, et al: Headache. In *Handbook of Clinical Neurology,* vol 48. Amsterdam, Elsevier, 1985.

DIZZINESS, VERTIGO, AND LIGHTHEADEDNESS: PROBLEMS OF SPATIAL DISORIENTATION

4

The dictionary definition of *dizziness* is: "a whirling sensation in the head, mental confusion, giddiness." Patients likewise use the word to describe the sensation they feel when they stand upright too quickly, when they look over the edge of a cliff, when they are unsteady on their feet, when they are seasick, or when they generally feel unwell. To some patients dizziness is the sensation one feels after rapidly spinning around or after receiving a severe blow to the head. The differences in these sensations are subtle, and most patients are not eloquent enough to differentiate between them. Patients often use the word "lightheadedness" to describe dizziness. The term *vertigo* should be limited to the sensation of movement, either of oneself or of the environment; a clear-cut history of this type of sensation (vertigo) more often than not indicates that the pathologic process is in the peripheral vestibular system.

I. THE PATIENT WITH DIZZINESS.
A. History. A major responsibility of the primary care physician is to identify the commonest causes of dizziness such as postural hypotension, hyperventilation, multiple sensory deficits, and postinfectious vertigo and thus avoid costly and

time-consuming evaluations by a specialist. The following historical information should be obtained from the patient:

1. Attempt to define the complaint of "dizziness"; a practical approach is to have the patient choose the sensation which is closest to the complaint from the aforementioned examples.

2. The duration and description of the *first* attack is usually most helpful. The frequency of subsequent attacks should also be determined.

3. Associated symptoms include progressive hearing loss, diplopia, paresthesias of the hands and feet, and tinnitus.

4. Positional factors: dizziness on arising from a sitting to a standing position, dizziness with sudden movement of the head, or dizziness associated with hyperextension or rotation of the neck.

5. Precipitating factors: dizziness associated with stressful situations, excessive or low salt intake, or directly related to meals may be diagnostic.

6. Past medical history: Severe head trauma, antecedent viral infections, diabetes, atherosclerotic phenomena, or psychiatric difficulties are especially helpful diagnostic signs.

7. All present and past medications should be reported; particular attention should be paid to antibiotics (especially streptomycin), anticonvulsants, antihypertensives, and high-dose salicylates.

B. **Classic complaints.** Often the cause of dizziness is strongly suggested by the history, and some complaints can be considered nearly diagnostic. Under these circumstances a physical and neurologic examination should be targeted to a specific hypothesis. For example:

1. "I'm dizzy when I get up in the morning." (Patients tend to become dehydrated overnight, making postural hypotension most prominent in the morning.)

2. "I'm dizzy whenever I'm alone at night." (Hyperventilation is strongly associated with anxiety-producing situations.)

3. "Every time I'm dizzy I see double." (Intermittent diplopia is usually caused by ischemia of the midbrain and this suggests basilar artery insufficiency.)

4. "I can't use the phone in my right ear anymore, the right side of my face is numb, and I'm unsteady on my feet." (Unilateral hearing loss without a history of trauma or ear infection is an acoustic neuroma until proved otherwise.)

5. "I suddenly became dizzy, nauseous, and unsteady on my feet, and my left face and right arm felt funny." (Symptoms on one half of the face and opposite side of the body strongly suggest brainstem disease; in this case infarction in the distribution of the posterior inferior cerebellar artery.)

6. "I've had diabetes for many years, I can't read the newspaper because of my cataracts, and my grandchildren tease me about being drunk all the time." (Elderly patients with multiple sensory deficits commonly complain of dizziness.)

7. "I've had fullness in my ear for a week and then suddenly I became so dizzy I had to lie in bed and hold on for fear of falling out." (Ménière's disease presents with a prodrome and dramatic vertigo.)

C. Physical examination.

1. A cardiovascular evaluation should be done (blood pressure in both arms, lying and standing; peripheral pulses; carotid bruits; heart murmurs, arrhythmias).

2. Examine ears with otoscope looking for impacted cerumen, evidence of infection.

3. Have the patient *hyperventilate* to see if the symptoms are reproduced. The sitting patient should take a deep breath every 2 seconds for 3 to 5 minutes. At the end of this time, ask the patient if this is the same sensation as the presenting complaint.

4. Cerebellar function can be tested by having the patient tandem-walk and perform rapid alternating movements and the finger-to-nose test.

5. Cranial nerves should be examined carefully. Pay particular attention to nystagmus when testing extraocular movements. Nystagmus is a rhythmic, involuntary eye movement, present at rest or induced by eye movement but persisting after eye movements cease. Usually there is a slow deviation of the eye in one direction with a quick jerk in the opposite direction. Nystagmus is named for the quick

TABLE 4–1.
Differentiating Labyrinthine and CNS Nystagmus

Labyrinthine (Peripheral) Nystagmus	CNS Nystagmus
Horizontal or horizontal-rotary	Often vertical or rotary
Fatigable	Persistent
Suppressed by visual fixation	May increase with visual fixation
Latency of onset after head motion	Occurs immediately after head motion
Associated with vertigo	Not directly associated with dizziness
Always conjugate	May be dysconjugate

component. Table 4–1 may be helpful in differentiating peripheral (labyrinthine) from central nervous system (CNS) nystagmus. Specific types of nystagmus include:

a. *End-point* nystagmus will result if the normal patient gazes too far laterally. Therefore, the examiner should have the patient gaze laterally only to the point where in the adducting eye the limbus meets the lacrimal punctum (Fig 4–1).

b. *Toxic-metabolic nystagmus* is symmetric in both eyes, equal in both directions of gaze, and primarily horizontal.

c. *Asymmetric lateral nystagmus* (absent or reduced in one direction of gaze compared with the opposite direction of gaze) could indicate either CNS or peripheral dysfunction.

d. *Dysconjugate nystagmus:* The abnormal movement is greater in one eye than the other. This always indicates CNS disease.

e. *Upward-gaze, downward-gaze, or rotatory nystagmus* usually indicates CNS disease.

f. *Positional nystagmus* induced by the Nylen-Bárány maneuver often indicates peripheral vestibular disease. The Nylen-Bárány maneuver is performed by seating the patient on the examining table and suddenly lowering the patient to a supine position with the head held 45 degrees backward over the end of the table and turned 45 degrees to one side (see Fig 4–2).

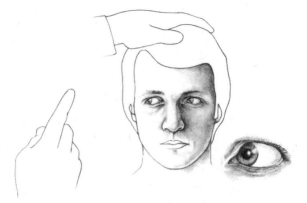

FIG 4–1. When testing for lateral-gaze nystagmus, to avoid end-point nystagmus do not force the limbus of the iris beyond the lacrimal punctum. Nystagmus at this point is usually abnormal.

6. Evaluation of trigeminal nerve (cranial nerve V) function: *Corneal reflex* is a sensitive index of fifth cranial nerve function, and an abnormality may suggest a lesion such as acoustic neuroma.

   Caveat: Be sure to touch only the cornea and not the sclera and also avoid producing a blink by threat reflex (Fig 4–3).

7. Evaluation of the function of the auditory and vestibular portions of the eighth cranial nerve:
   a. *Auditory acuity* is quickly tested by rubbing the fingers lightly several inches from the patient's ear. If an abnormality is present, perform the Weber's and Rinne tests.
   b. *Weber's test:* Place the base of a vibrating tuning fork on the patient's forehead. Ideally, a 512-Hz tuning fork should be used, but often only a 256-Hz tuning

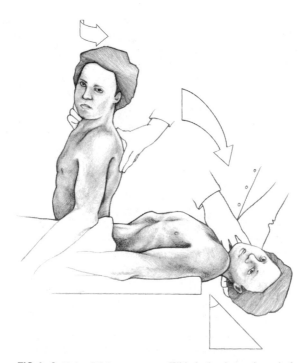

FIG 4–2. Nylen-Bárány maneuver: With the head over the end of the table and turned 45 degrees, observe the eyes for nystagmus. The patient is instructed to keep the eyes open. The onset and direction of nystagmus is noted. Note also whether the patient experiences vertigo. This maneuver is repeated with the head turned to the opposite side.

fork is readily available. Normally the sound from the tuning fork is heard nearly equally in both ears. With eighth nerve or cochlear destruction (sensorineural deafness), the sound is heard best on the side of normal acuity. With middle ear or outer ear disease (con-

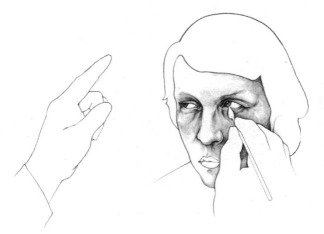

FIG 4–3. Testing the corneal reflex: With the patient looking to one side, bring a wisp of cotton (a few strands pulled out from a cotton-tipped applicator) from the opposite side and touch the *cornea*. The patient should blink.

      duction deafness), sound lateralizes to the involved ear (Fig 4–4).

  c. *Rinne test:* Hold a vibrating tuning fork first in front of the external auditory meatus (air conduction) and then place the base of the vibrating tuning fork firmly against the mastoid process (bone conduction). Ask the patient in which position the sound is loudest (Fig 4–5). Middle ear disease or plugging of the external canal should be suspected when bone conduction is greater than air conduction. In partial sensorineural loss, air conduction remains louder than bone conduction, but both are diminished. In total unilateral sensorineural loss, air conduction may be absent, while bone conduction is heard by the opposite ear.

  d. *Caloric test:* Examine the auditory canal to check that the eardrum is intact and that there is no blood or im-

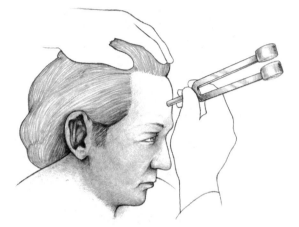

FIG 4–4. Weber's test: Place a tuning fork on the forehead and ask, "Is the sound the same in both ears?"

pacted cerumen. With the patient sitting, tilt the head to one side and inject approximately 2 mL cold water from a syringe equipped with a small-caliber soft polyethylene catheter directed at the posterior wall of the external canal. Start a stopwatch at the beginning of the injection. After 20 seconds, evacuate the water from the ear, tilt the patient's head backward 60 degrees, and have the patient look at the examiner's finger from a distance of approximately 3 ft (Fig 4–6). An ophthalmoscope can also be used to observe the nystagmus: in a darkened room visualizing a small-caliber retinal blood vessel permits detection of subtle nystagmus (with a slight rotatory component). In the alert patient, the eyes normally drift slowly toward the ear irrigated with cold water followed by the quick corrective component of the nystagmus back toward the primary position. (Nystagmus is named for the quick component which occurs in a direction away from the

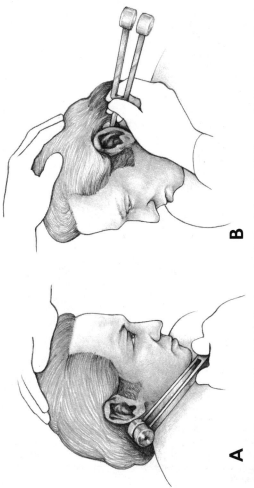

FIG 4–5. Rinne test: With a lightly vibrating tuning fork, ask the patient if the sound is loudest in position **A** or position **B**.

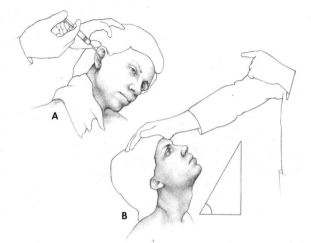

FIG 4–6. Caloric test: **A,** with the patient sitting in a chair with the head tilted to one side, inject 2 mL of water into the external canal. **B,** remove the water, tilt the head backward 60 degrees, and observe and time the nystagmus. Quick movements will be directed away from the cold ear.

cooled ear.) Abnormal responses include the absence of nystagmus or a marked difference in nystagmus between the two ears. (*Note:* Wait 15 minutes after irrigation of one ear before irrigating the other ear.) Instillation of warm water into the ear produces the opposite findings, but is ordinarily not necessary. (For caloric testing in the comatose patient, see Chapter 13, section I. B. 1.e. ii).

D. Laboratory investigations. Because the causes of dizziness are so varied, we cannot suggest a standard laboratory investigation of all dizzy patients. The choice of laboratory procedures should be guided by the history and physical examination.

1. A complete blood count, erythrocyte sedimentation rate (ESR), and analysis of electrolytes and blood components is necessary because dizziness is so often equated with "unwellness."
2. Audiometry should be performed in all patients with significant hearing loss or tinnitus.
3. Glucose tolerance test: if hypoglycemia is considered in the differential diagnosis.
4. Electrocardiogram (ECG): When the patient reports palpitations, consider performing carotid sinus massage during an ECG.
5. Electroencephalography (EEG) (sleep-deprived, with nasopharyngeal electrodes): when there is a suspicion of complex partial seizures.
6. Brainstem evoked responses are an inexpensive screening test in identififying acoustic neuromas and brainstem abnormalities.
7. Magnetic resonance imaging (MRI) identifies virtually all acoustic neuromas and cases of multiple sclerosis.

II. DIZZINESS OF PSYCHOLOGICAL ORIGIN.
A. Hyperventilation syndrome.
1. Diagnosis.
   a. Hyperventilation is a very common cause of dizziness (lightheadedness).
   b. It may be associated with circumoral paresthesias, paresthesias of the fingers, and carpopedal spasm (muscle cramps in the hands and feet).
   c. Patients with this syndrome frequently are anxious.
   d. The diagnosis is usually confirmed when the symptoms are reproduced by having the patient hyperventilate.
2. Treatment.
   a. Explain the cause of the dizziness and reassure the patient. Have the patient breathe into a paper bag (rebreathing) during attacks.
   b. Psychologic or psychiatric evaluation is not necessary in most cases.
B. Psychogenic dizziness.
1. Diagnosis.
   a. In psychogenic dizziness the patient is inconsistent in regard to history, description of the dizziness, and fac-

tors affecting the dizziness; if the dizziness is injury-related or event-related, the circumstances of the injury or events are described in explicit detail.

b. The patient may note dizziness in all body positions.

c. The history may be misleading if the patient has had previous exposure to leading questions by other examiners; sometimes the patient may consciously mislead the examiner.

d. There may be associated symptoms of anxiety or depression; hyperventilation is common.

e. During the examination, there are inconsistencies in many of the tests and often all of the test maneuvers reproduce the symptoms.

f. The sensation of acrophobia or claustrophobia is described by many patients as dizziness.

2. Treatment: A psychologic or psychiatric evaluation is indicated.

III. DIZZINESS AND VERTIGO OF VESTIBULAR ORIGIN.

A. **Symptomatic treatment** of dizziness of vestibular origin involves the following drugs (remember that all of these drugs may cause excessive drowsiness):

1. Transderm Scōp (a disc impregnated with scopolamine 1.5 mg and placed behind the ear) is the drug of choice for motion sickness and other peripheral labyrinthine disorders. Each disc lasts 3 days.

2. Promethazine hydrochloride (Phenergan) 50 to 100 mg daily in divided doses for adults and 12.5 to 25 mg bid for children.

3. Meclizine hydrochloride (Antivert) 25 to 100 mg daily in divided doses.

4. Dimenhydrinate (Dramamine) 50 mg q4h may be effective for adults.

5. Trimethobenzamide hydrochloride (Tigan) 100 to 250 mg tid or qid is usually effective for controlling nausea.

B. **Benign positional vertigo.**

1. Diagnosis and clincal features.

▶ a. *The most important diagnostic clue is* recurrent transient vertigo precipitated by head motion whether the patient is standing or lying.

    b. Vertigo is often associated with nausea; auditory symptoms are absent.

    c. Examination shows the following:

       1) Nystagmus in the Nylen-Bárány maneuver occurring after a latency period of a few seconds and disappearing after approximately 1 minute. The phenomenon is less apparent on repetition of the maneuver (fatigable). This finding is virtually diagnostic of benign positional vertigo.

       Caveat: If there is no latency period before onset of nystagmus and if the phenomenon does not become less apparent on repetition, suspect posterior fossa tumor.

       2) Caloric tests are normal in 50% of patients.

       3) This is a self-limited benign syndrome, initially severe, but gradually improving over days to weeks.

  2. Treatment: Symptomatic drug treatment.

C. Posttraumatic vertigo.

  1. Skull fractures.

    a. A lengthwise fracture through the petrous pyramid usually involves structures of the middle ear. The patient often presents with bleeding from the ear.

    b. Transverse fractures through the petrous pyramid involve the bony and membranous labyrinth; the patient presents with facial paralysis, vertigo, and spontaneous nystagmus.

  2. Acceleration-deceleration injuries.

    a. Severe positional vertigo, especially with the involved ear pointing downward, caused by an inorganic deposit in the semicircular canal (cupulolithiasis).

    b. Persistent leak of perilymph from oval window to middle ear space.

    c. Whiplash injuries may result in dizziness with objective findings referable to the vestibular system.

  3. Treatment: MRI of the posterior fossa and brainstem evoked responses may localize the lesion. A thorough otolaryngologic examination is indicated because of the possibility of surgical correction and because these cases so often involve litigation.

D. Ménière's disease.
1. Clinical features.
   ▶ a. *The most important diagnostic clues are* severe, dramatic (explosive onset), episodic vertigo lasting from hours to days associated with tinnitus (like a seashell held to the ear), and decreased hearing in the affected ear.
   b. Often preceded by an aura consisting of a fullness or pressure in the affected ear.
   c. This is a disease primarily of middle age, affecting one side in 75% of cases.
   d. Although hearing loss may fluctuate, it is progressive.
   e. Some patients note that an attack may be precipitated by heavy salt intake.
   f. The disease runs a prolonged course over many years and the vertiginous attacks tend to decrease as the deafness increases. Ultimately the patient becomes deaf and the vertiginous attacks cease.
   g. Examination shows the following:
      1) Decreased caloric response on affected side.
      2) Loss of hearing, especially low tones.
      3) Spontaneous nystagmus toward the affected side may be present during the attack.
      4) Definitive diagnosis should be made with an audiologic examination requiring specialized equipment.
2. Treatment
   a. The armamentarium of vasodilators, diuretics, low salt diets, vitamins, antihistamines, and tranquilizers suggests that no treatment is really effective.
   b. When the patient is severely incapacitated, some otolaryngologists suggest a shunt procedure (between the membranous labyrinth and the subarachnoid space).

   Note: There is a tendency to overdiagnose Ménière's disease. Other causes of severe acute vertigo include occlusion of the vestibular artery or the posterior inferior cerebellar artery, acute toxic labyrinthitis, and vestibular neuronitis. However, these causes of dramatic vertigo are usually not recurrent.

E. **Acute toxic labyrinthitis.**
1. Diagnosis.
   a. Acute toxic labyrinthitis is characterized by acute onset of vertigo that peaks in 24 hours and subsides in 7 to 10 days.
   b. It is often associated with a nose or throat infection. Other associations include allergy or ototoxic medication.
   c. Vertigo is exacerbated by head motion.
   d. Examination shows:
      1) Caloric tests are abnormal in 50% of patients.
      2) Examination of nose or throat may show evidence of infection.
      3) Spontaneous nystagmus may be present.
2. Treatment.
   a. Throat culture if clinically indicated.
   b. Limitation of movement (bed rest).
   c. Symptomatic drug treatment.
   d. Discontinuing drugs that may be vestibulotoxic.

F. **Postinfectious vestibular neuronitis.**
1. Postinfectious vestibular neuronitis is symptomatically very similar to acute labyrinthitis. The differentiating feature is that it is associated with the influenza syndrome and may occur epidemically.
2. This disease may have a longer recovery period (2–6 weeks) than acute labyrinthitis.

G. **Motion Sickness.** Some normal persons have an increased sensitivity to the stimulus of motion.

Note: Adults with migraine frequently have a history of motion sickness in childhood.

1. Treatment: Application of Transderm Scōp before the patient is in a situation in which motion sickness is likely to occur is especially effective.

IV. **DIZZINESS OR VERTIGO OF CENTRAL ORIGIN.**
A. **Cerebrovascular disorders (especially those involving the posterior fossa).** Dizziness or vertigo of central origin is a common complaint of patients with many types of cerebro-

vascular disease. The symptom of vertigo is related specifically to cerebrovascular diseases affecting the blood supply to the brainstem. The diagnosis is rarely easy, unless there are focal neurologic signs during or after the attacks. In many cases of vertebrobasilar transient ischemic attacks (TIAs) the patient is normal between attacks. A four-vessel cerebral angiogram performed by an experienced neuroradiologist may be necessary for confirmation of the diagnosis.

1. Vertebrobasilar insufficiency: The onset is abrupt and often associated with loss of consciousness. Initial neurologic symptoms may include diplopia, slurred speech, numbness, dysphagia, visual field defects, or motor or sensory losses.

2. The subclavian steal syndrome may include attacks of vertigo, especially upon exercising the arm on the affected side. A clue to the diagnosis is asymmetric blood pressure in the arms. This is a particular type of vertebrobasilar insufficiency in which there is an occlusion proximal to the origin of the vertebral artery.

   a. Treatment: If an occlusion is demonstrated, surgical correction can be considered, but in many cases the symptoms subside spontaneously.

3. Ischemic damage to vestibular nuclei or their connections often includes damage to other parts of the brainstem. Elderly hypertensive patients with diabetes, heart disease, or hyperlipidemia are likely candidates. Focal neurologic signs are present; caloric response is absent or asymmetric.

4. Lateral medullary syndrome: This is a specific type of ischemic damage to vestibular connections due to brainstem infarction in the distribution of the posterior inferior cerebellar artery. The patient presents with vertigo, nausea, hiccups, and dysarthria. Abnormal neurologic signs include ipsilateral loss of pain and temperature sensation in the face, contralateral loss of pain and temperature sensation in the body, ipsilateral cerebellar ataxia, and ipsilateral Horner's syndrome. Note that there is no paralysis of arms or legs. Prognosis for complete recovery is especially good with this type of infarction. These patients usually have a history of hypertension.

   a. Treatment: See Chapter 12.

B. **Acoustic neuroma (cerebellopontine angle tumor).**
   1. Diagnosis.
      ▶ a. Suspect acoustic neuroma (schwannoma, neurilemmoma) in any patient who develops insidious unilateral hearing loss unless clearly associated with trauma or infection. This tumor accounts for 10% of all primary intracranial tumors. High-pitched unilateral tinnitus may be an initial symptom.
      b. Most common vestibular symptom is unsteadiness; true vertigo is rare. Occasionally symptoms are episodic.
      c. As the disease progresses patients develop other neurologic complaints such as facial numbness, facial weakness, clumsiness, and headache.
      d. Examination shows one or more of the following:
         1) On the same side as the tumor:
            a) Sensorineural hearing loss (air conduction greater than bone conduction; tuning fork on forehead louder in normal ear).
            b) Decreased caloric response on affected side.
            c) Loss of corneal reflex and sensory disturbance over the face.
            d) Facial weakness involving forehead.
            e) Decreased sensation in external auditory canal.
            f) Ipsilateral cerebellar findings.
         2) Café au lait spots with or without cutaneous neurofibromas suggest neurofibromatosis. This disease has an association with bilateral cerebellopontine angle tumors.
         3) Papilledema may be seen with large tumors.
      e. Diagnostic studies. MRI with contrast should identify virtually all tumors.
   2. Treatment: When diagnosis is confirmed, surgical exploration is necessary.
C. **Other posterior fossa tumors.** Posterior fossa tumors are especially common in children, and although vertigo may be present, cerebellar and brainstem signs, cranial nerve abnormalities, and signs of increased intracranial pressure are usually more prominent. If suspected, referral to a neurologist or neurosurgeon is indicated.

D. Complex partial seizures. Vertigo, dizziness, or a feeling of unsteadiness may be an aura for complex partial seizures. For further diagnostic information and treatment, see Chapter 11, section VII. C. 3.

> *Note:* This type of seizure disorder is not necessarily associated with loss of consciousness or tonic-clonic movements.

E. Basilar migraine. Basilar migraine usually occurs in children and young women and lasts minutes. Symptoms may include attacks of vertigo, which can be associated with visual disturbance (diplopia, ataxia, tinnitus, and sometimes sudden loss of consciousness accompanying occipital throbbing headache).

F. Multiple sclerosis. Patients who later are diagnosed as having multiple sclerosis may present with altered sensation of balance, but this is seldom true vertigo. Dizziness may also be the result of multiple sensory deficits. For further diagnostic information. (see Chapter 10, section I).

G. Multiple sensory deficits (Aging balance system syndrome).

1. Elderly patients often have altered sensory input: visual (cataracts) and proprioceptive, touch, pressure (from peripheral neuropathy, often diabetic, or cervical cord involvement in cervical spondylosis). Vestibular abnormalities may occur secondary to basilar artery insufficiency or premature aging of the vestibular nuclei.

2. The diminished sensory input causes dizziness (out of touch with environment), especially when walking or turning.

3. Additional sensory cues, sometimes as simple as carrying a cane during maneuvers that produce dizziness, usually reduce the symptoms.

4. Treatment: Medications often make this condition worse. If possible, devise ways of increasing sensory input, e.g., cataract operation, moving slowly.

V. DRUGS AS A CAUSE OF DIZZINESS.

A. The vestibular nerve and the vestibular apparatus can be damaged by commonly used drugs. Some drugs produce reversible dysfunction, whereas others produce irreversible destruction. If the patient is taking one of the following drugs, it

should be considered as a possible cause of the dizziness:
1. Antibiotics.
    a. Aminoglycosides (e.g., streptomycin).
    b. Polypeptides (polymyxin B).
    c. Semisynthetic penicillin (ampicillin).
    d. Sulfonamides.
    e. Synthetics (chloramphenicol).
2. Diuretics (furosemide).
3. Salicylates (aspirin).
4. Anti-inflammatory drugs (phenylbutazone).
5. Antimalarials (quinine).
6. Anticonvulsants (phenytoin).
7. Antihistamines.

VI. **SYSTEMIC DISORDERS CAUSING FAINTNESS, DIZ-ZINESS, AND SYNCOPE.**
A. **Cardiovascular disturbances.**
    1. Orthostatic (postural) hypotension: Upon standing, the patient experiences faintness from a fall in blood pressure; the magnitude of the drop in blood pressure is less important than the association of the faintness in moving from a lying to a standing position. The differential diagnosis of possible causes is lengthy but includes the following:
        a. Hypovolemic states.
        b. Peripheral neuropathy (especially if the autonomic nervous system is affected as in diabetes).
        c. Lower extremity venous pooling (as in severe varicose veins).
        d. Antihypertensive drugs.
    2. Cardiac arrhythmias may be recognized by auscultation or routine ECG, but 24-hour Holter monitoring may be required.
    3. Carotid sinus hypersensitivity.
        a. The patient may relate a history of faintness or syncope with neck motion or pressure on the neck; examples include faintness while backing a car out of a driveway or faintness associated with shaving the neck. This syndrome is most common in children and adolescents and in older patients with atherosclerotic disease involving the carotid bifurcation.

b. The faintness or dizziness disappears rapidly (lasting about 15 seconds).

c. The diagnosis is confirmed by reproducing symptoms by lightly massaging the carotid sinus (do not occlude the carotid artery) and monitoring both the blood pressure and the heart rate (ECG). A pause of more than 3 seconds in the heart rate or a decrease in systolic blood pressure greater than 50 mm Hg (torr) is considered abnormal. Valsalva maneuvers may also precipitate cardiac slowing and a fall in blood pressure (micturition syncope); this can be checked at the same time as the carotid massage.

Caveat: Do not massage the carotid artery of patients with known carotid artery or intracranial cerebrovascular disease because of the risk of precipitating stroke. Cardiac arrest may also occur.

4. Hypertension: Patients with severe hypertension in the early phases of hypertensive encephalopathy may experience faintness and dizziness.

Caveat: The patient with symptoms of dizziness and rapidly elevating blood pressure may have an expanding mass lesion in the posterior fossa (see Chapter 13, section II. C).

B. Vasovagal phenomena.
1. *Common vasovagal syncope:* This is the common fainting that occurs in normal persons that is often precipitated by emotional stress or warm, crowded conditions. It is preceded by an aura of nausea and sweating. The loss of consciousness may be prevented by assuming a supine position and elevating the legs.
2. *Reflex vasovagal syncope:* This is similar to the common vasovagal syncope, but the fainting spell is precipitated by a stimulus, e.g., venipuncture. There may be a family history of similar stimulus-precipitated syncope, breath-holding spells, or migraine. This syndrome must be differentiated from a seizure by lack of either postictal sleepiness or tonic-clonic movements.

3. *Breath-holding spells:*
   a. A form of vasovagal syncope in children aged 6 months to 6 years. It may be of two types:
      1) Begins with crying; the child holds his or her breath and turns blue (cyanotic type).
      2) After minor startle or sudden painful stimulus, the child turns white and loses consciousness (pallid type).
   b. The period from onset through loss of consciousness usually lasts less than 60 seconds. There may be a few seconds of tonic stiffening at the end of the period of unconsciousness, which may be mistaken for a seizure.
   c. At the termination of the breath-holding spell, the child immediately awakens, usually with no apparent postictal symptoms (no headache, confusion, or lethargy).
   d. If the physician thinks an EEG is necessary, the EEG should be done with monitoring of respiration and ECG to differentiate seizures from breath-holding spells.
   e. Treatment: This condition is benign with the child outgrowing the disorder. Breath-holding spells do not lead to epilepsy. Parents should be reassured of the benign prognosis.

VII. OTHER MEDICAL CONDITIONS ASSOCIATED WITH FAINTNESS AND DIZZINESS.

A. Almost any medical condition may be associated with dizziness; this chapter assumes that the general health of the patient is good.
   1. Anemia causes dizziness due to hypovolemia or decreased oxygen-carrying capacity of the blood.
   2. Hypoglycemia, especially common in people with diabetes.
   3. Endocrine disorders, especially thyroid and adrenal insufficiency.
   4. Visual disorders, especially after a change in prescription for lenses, during diplopia, or after cataract surgery.
   5. Allergies: allergic reactions may cause a sensation of fullness in the head, lightheadedness, or faintness. This di-

agnosis should be pursued in patients with a strong allergy history. Remember that many of the drugs used to treat allergies also cause dizziness.

BIBLIOGRAPHY

Bucy PG: Vertigo with diseases of the central nervous system. *Arch Otolaryngol* 1967; 85:535–536.

Drachman DA, Hart CW: An approach to the dizzy patient. *Neurology* 1972; 22:323–334.

Harner SG, Laws ER: Clinical findings in patients with acoustic neuroma. *Mayo Clin Proc* 1983; 58:721–728.

Healy GB: Hearing loss and vertigo secondary to head injury. *N Engl J Med* 1982; 306:1029–1031.

Lipsitz LA: Orthostatic hypotension in the elderly. *N Engl J Med* 1989; 321:952–957.

Schumacher GA: Demyelinating diseases as a cause for vertigo. *Arch Otolaryngol* 1967; 85:537–538.

Sloane PD: Dizziness in primary care. *J Fam Pract* 1989; 29:33–38.

Sugrue DD, Wood DL, McGoon MD: Carotid sinus hypersensitivity and syncope. *Mayo Clin Proc* 1984; 59:637–640.

Wolfson RJ, Silverstein H, Marlowe F, et al: Vertigo. *Ciba Found Symp* 1986; 38:2–32.

SLEEP DISORDERS

It has been estimated that each year, almost 10 million Americans consult their physicians for sleep problems. In order to diagnose and treat sleep disorders successfully, the physician needs to have an understanding of the normal sleep cycle, the pharmacology of hypnotics and related medications, and the various disorders of sleep and arousal.

I. NORMAL SLEEP PATTERN.

A. Sleep stages.

1. On the basis of electroencephalographic (EEG) and other physiologic parameters, two categories of sleep can be recognized: non-rapid eye movement (NREM, slow wave, or spindle sleep) and rapid eye movement (REM, active, paradoxical) sleep. NREM sleep can be further divided into four stages on the basis of the EEG pattern (Table 5–1).

2. Certain sleep stages may affect underlying medical disorders adversely: e.g., during REM sleep, angina of coronary heart disease and the pain of duodenal ulcer may be exacerbated; stage I sleep (the transition between wakefulness and sleep) is most prone to enhance abnormal EEG activity or clinical seizures in patients with seizure disorders.

B. Sleep cycle.

1. In the young adult the normal sleep cycle is made up of 20% to 25% REM, 5% to 10% stage I, 50% stage II, and 20% stages III and IV. Typically, sleep begins with stage I and progresses through stages II, III, and IV and back through stages II and III. Then, about 70 to 100

TABLE 5–1.
Sleep Cycle*

Category	Stage	Patient Appearance	Physiologic Characteristics	Pathologic Disturbances
REM	REM	Very still, deep sleep; body apparently paralyzed; REM	Bursts of REM: irregular respiration; high BMR; inhibited peripheral muscle activity (except diaphragm); dreaming; penile tumescence; bursts of sympathetic nervous system activity	Narcolepsy; nightmares; REM behavior disorder
NREM	I	Drowsiness	Sleep myoclonus	Excessive sleep myoclonus; seizure activity
	II	Light sleep	Sleep spindles	
	III	Deep sleep	EEG slow waves	
	IV	Deep sleep	EEG slow waves	Decreased body temperature, pulse, and respirations; peripheral muscle activity present; increased vagal tone
				Sleepwalking; night terrors; enuresis

*REM = rapid eye movement; NREM = non-rapid eye movement; BMR = basal metabolic rate.

minutes after the onset of sleep, the first REM period occurs.

2. This cycle is repeated approximately every 90 minutes with a total of four to six cycles every night. Toward morning the REM periods lengthen and NREM sleep progresses only to stages II and III.

C. **Normal variations.**

1. There are specific variations in the sleep cycle with age. Thus a newborn may spend as much as 50% of sleep in REM, with the child reaching adult proportions by the third year. Children have a high percentage of stages III and IV sleep, while the elderly have virtually no stage IV sleep. The elderly also often have frequent and lengthy awakenings.

2. There is also considerable amount of individual variation in the sleep cycle and total duration of sleep. Some people can function with very little sleep, whereas others need much more than the suggested 8 hours.

II. **APPROACH TO THE PATIENT WITH SLEEP DISORDERS.**

A large number of clinical conditions affect sleep. The major categories include patients with disorders of initiation and maintenance of sleep and those with excessive daytime sleepiness.

A. **Clinical evaluation.**

1. Interview: The first and most important step in evaluating a patient with a sleep disorder is the interview.

   a. It is important to determine whether the sleep-related complaints are real or subjective. Patients tend to overestimate sleep complaints. A bed partner can give valuable information during the interview. A sleep log (written record kept by the patient and the patient's bed partner that charts bedtime, time of onset of sleep, awakenings during sleep, time of awakening, and other sleep habits like snoring, apnea, bruxism, myoclonus, etc.) could offer further insight into the sleep pattern of the patient.

    b. Obtain the following information without asking leading questions:

      1) Sleep habits: when, where, how long, naps.

      2) Sleep problems: difficulty in falling asleep, use of sleep aids; awakening during night, frequency and length; cause of awakenings—dreams, movement, pain, anxiety.

      3) Daytime somnolence: how often, duration, history suggestive of cataplexy (sudden loss of power in limbs while laughing or when emotionally upset).

      4) Medications and drug history: sedatives, stimulants, street drugs, alcohol.

      5) History suggestive of seizure disorders, anxiety neurosis, depression, affective disorders.

      6) Medical history: any medical condition that may lead to disturbances in sleep (e.g., cluster headache, asthma, cardiac failure, hyperthyroidism, etc.).

2. Physical examination: obesity, hypertension, cardiac abnormalities, neurologic deficits, evidence of endocrine dysfunction, such as thyrotoxicosis or hypothyroidism.

3. Investigations.

    a. A decision regarding investigations should only be taken after detailed consideration of the history and physical findings. Patients with transient sleep problems do not need costly investigations such as polysomnography.

    b. If an underlying medical disorder such as intracranial disease or endocrinopathy is suspected, perform the relevant investigations (e.g., computed tomography [CT] scan, magnetic resonance imaging [MRI], EEG, biochemical tests for endocrine disorders).

    c. Patients with persistent sleep disorders often need polysomnography (recording of EEG along with other physiologic parameters such as respiration, electromyography [EMG], ECG, electrooculography [EOG], etc.). This requires referral to a sleep disorders laboratory (Table 5–2).

TABLE 5–2.
Laboratory Investigations in Sleep Disorders

Test	Procedure	Indications
Multiple sleep latency test (MSLT)	During an 8 to 9-hour period the patient is allowed to sleep for five 20-min periods; the average sleep latency and any REM-onset sleep are documented	Excessive daytime sleepiness, particularly narcolepsy
Polysomnography	Simultaneous recording of EEG, EOG, EMG, respirations, ECG, and oxygen tension during all-night sleep readings; may also be combined with video recording	Sleep apnea syndrome, sleep myoclonus, and other sleep-related disorders; differentiation of nocturnal seizures from night terrors, nightmares, sleepwalking, and apneic spells

III. DISORDERS OF INITIATING AND MAINTAINING SLEEP (DIMS, INSOMNIAS).

A. **In evaluating a patient with insomnia,** one should take into account the normal variations as well as the effects of age on the architecture of sleep stages and cycle. Remember that there is significant variation from person to person regarding the optimal duration of sleep; it is important to ascertain whether the patient feels alert and is performing well despite a shorter duration of sleep, since this may simply be the normal pattern for that person.

B. **Transient insomnias.**
▶ 1. The characteristic features are: insomnia lasting less than 3 weeks and the presence of a clear precipitating cause such as emotional shock (e.g., the death of a loved one, divorce), depression, or anxiety provoked by circumstances such as change of job, tests, interviews, or sleeping in unfamiliar surroundings (e.g., the hospital).

2. Treatment.
    a. Reassurance and, if necessary, crisis intervention and counseling
    b. Temporary use of hypnotics, mainly to assure rest and to prevent chronic insomnia.

C. Persistent or chronic insomnia.
▶ 1. When insomnia persists for more than 3 weeks it is considered chronic insomnia.
2. May evolve from situational insomnia, or there may be no obvious factors.
3. Characterized by difficulty in falling asleep, frequent awakenings, or early-morning awakenings.
4. Somatization of anxiety and negative conditioning to sleep have been considered possible underlying factors, but it is necessary to exclude insomnia caused by an underlying neurologic disorder, major psychiatric illness, chronic sedative or alcohol use, or periodic leg movements.
5. Treatment.
    a. General measures for sleep hygiene include establishing regular schedules for bedtime and rising, improving sleep environment, late-afternoon or early-evening exercises, avoidance of alcohol and caffeine-containing drinks in the evening, and stress management.
    b. Hypnotics: Continual use of hypnotics should be avoided because they can be addictive, usually lose their effect within a few days (leading to escalation of dosage), tend to produce rebound insomnia when withdrawn, and may be dangerous if taken in larger than prescribed doses. Occasional use of hypnotics may be permissible to avoid panic and other psychological problems in patients experiencing a run of sleepless nights. Of the hypnotics, benzodiazepine derivatives are considered the drugs of choice. Table 5.3 lists the benzodiazepines currently approved as hypnotics. The non-benzodiazepine agent zolpidem tartrate (Ambien) 5–10 mg has rapid onset and short duration of action, is well-tolerated, and has few reported side effects.

TABLE 5-3.
Benzodiazepine Hypnotic Agents

Drug	Usual Dose (mg)	Duration of Sedative Effect (hr)	Remarks
Estazolam (Prosom)	1-2	6-8	Useful for sleep-onset and sleep maintenance insomnia
Flurazepam (Dalmane)	15-30	≥ 12	Useful for insomnia and daytime anxiety; metabolite has long elimination half-life resulting in tendency to accumulate with prolonged use; daytime sedation is a major problem.
Quazepam (Doral)	7.5-15	≥ 12	Useful for insomnia and daytime anxiety; metabolite has long elimination half life, resulting in tendency to accumulate with prolonged use; daytime sedation is a major problem.
Temazepam (Restoril)	15-30	6-8	Useful for frequent nocturnal awakenings; slow onset of action
Triazolam (Halcion)	0.125-0.25	4-6	Useful for sleep-onset insomnia owing to rapid onset and short duration of action; can cause early-morning rebound insomnia; with higher doses anterograde amnesia may occur

D. Insomnia associated with psychiatric disorders. Psychiatric disturbances are major causes of insomnia. The underlying condition may be excessive tension with somatization of symptoms, anxiety neurosis, depression, or major psychiatric disorders such as schizophrenia.

1. Treatment: Treatment should be directed toward the underlying cause (see Chapter 9).

   Caveat: Do not simply prescribe sedatives or hypnotics without adequate treatment of the underlying psychiatric disorder.

E. **Medical insomnia.** Underlying medical problems that disturb sleep may account for insomnia in about 20% of patients. Such conditions include chronic pain from cancer, arthritis, peripheral neuropathy, metabolic disorders such as uremia, and endocrine disorders such as hyperthyroidism.
   1. Treatment: The underlying medical problem should be identified and appropriately treated. Sedatives can be used as an adjunctive treatment if necessary.

F. **Insomnia associated with use of drugs or alcohol.**
   1. When sedatives or hypnotics such as barbiturates, glutethimide, chloral hydrate, or methaqualone are taken regularly they lose their effectiveness in about 2 weeks, leading to need for increased dosage. Later, tolerance develops and sleep becomes disturbed with frequent awakenings. Abrupt withdrawal leads to more marked insomnia.
   2. Use of central nervous system (CNS) stimulants: Excessive intake of caffeine-containing beverages, excessive use of weight-reducing agents, drug abuse (amphetamines, cocaine), or ingestion of other stimulants (pemoline, ephedrine, etc.) can lead to insomnia.
   3. Chronic alcohol abuse leads to insomnia, especially during withdrawal.

G. Insomnias associated with nocturnal myoclonus, restless leg syndrome, and sleep apnea syndrome are discussed next in section IV.

IV. DAYTIME SOMNOLENCE.

A. **Daytime somnolence** manifests as inappropriate sleepiness while awake, frequent naps, incomplete arousal in the morning, and sometimes cognitive dysfunction. Any condition that impairs nocturnal sleep may lead to daytime sleepiness. In addition, there are a number of disorders that lead to peri-

odic or persistent daytime somnolence. The two most important causes of persistent daytime somnolence are sleep apnea
syndrome and narcolepsy.

1. Narcolepsy.
   a. The manifestation of an imbalance between wakeful-
      ness and sleep in which the REM stage appears to be
      dominating over wakefulness.
   b. Irresistible "sleep attacks" occur at any time and usu-
      ally last less than 15 minutes.
   c. As part of the narcolepsy syndrome, the patient may
      also experience one or more of the following (11%–
      14% may show all the features):
      1) Cataplexy: A sudden loss of muscle tone (may
         fall down without warning) is often precipitated
         by laughter or any strong emotion. If cataplexy
         persists for more than 60 seconds the patient may
         go into actual REM sleep.
      2) Sleep paralysis occurs during the transition be-
         tween sleep and waking, most frequently at the
         time of falling asleep, and is characterized by an
         inability to move even though awake.
      3) Hypnagogic hallucinations (vivid visual or audi-
         tory perceptions) occur at the time of falling
         asleep.
   d. Onset is usually in adolescence or young adulthood.
   e. There may be a family history of similar problems.
   f. Diagnosis is confirmed by special studies such as the
      multiple sleep latency test (MSLT) which shows a re-
      duced sleep latency and REM-onset sleep.
   g. There is a close relationship between narcolepsy and
      HLA loci DQW1 and DR2.
   h. Treatment.
      1) Explain the nature of the symptoms to the pa-
         tient. This is crucial in the long-term manage-
         ment.
      2) Impress upon the patient the need to exercise ex-
         treme caution while driving an automobile or op-
         erating heavy machinery.
      3) Scheduled naps of 15 minutes in the morning and

afternoon may reduce the number of sleep attacks.

4) Pemoline (Cylert) 18.75 to 75 mg/day or methylphenidate hydrochloride (Ritalin) 5 to 60 mg/day in divided morning and early-afternoon doses may control the irresistible sleepiness. Start with a small dose, e.g., methylphenidate 10 mg once or twice a day, and find the smallest effective dose for the particular patient.

5) Imipramine hydrochloride (Tofranil) 50 to 200 mg/day may benefit cataplexy, sleep paralysis, and hypnagogic hallucinations, but it has minimal effect on irresistible sleep attacks. Protriptyline hydrochloride (Vivactil) 15 to 30 mg/day is an alternative.

6) Patient information materials may be obtained from the American Narcolepsy Association, P.O. Box 5846, Stanford, CA 94305.

2. Sleep apnea syndrome.

a. Sleep apnea may result from problems with neural control of respiration (central apnea), from obstruction of the upper airway (obstructive apnea), or from a combination of the two (mixed apnea). Apnea is defined as cessation of airflow at the nose and mouth lasting 10 seconds or more. A considerable number of such episodes occur in patients with sleep apnea syndrome.

b. Obstructive apnea is due to sleep-related upper airway obstruction (relaxation of muscles around the upper airway during sleep leads to the obstruction). It occurs predominantly in older males. It is characterized by extreme restlessness during the night with severe snoring, snorting, and frequent respiratory pauses and excessive daytime sleepiness. Once asleep, arousal may be difficult and accompanied by confusion, disorientation, and ataxia. Predisposing factors for sleep-related upper airway obstruction include enlarged tonsils and adenoids, micrognathia, retrognathia, macroglossia, and endocrinopathies (such as hypothyroidism and acromegaly).

Note: Sleep apnea syndrome may cause both insomnia and excessive daytime sleepiness.

c. A number of associated symptoms and complications are reported with sleep apnea syndrome: cardiac arrhythmias, right heart failure, hypertension, obesity, night sweats, and morning headache. A drop in oxygen tension may lead to cardiac arrhythmia and arousals. In children, nocturnal enuresis, learning difficulties, and hyperactivity interrupted by hypersomnolence may be seen.

d. CNS dysfunction that occurs only during sleep leads to lack of respiratory drive in patients with central apnea. Such patients experience frequent nocturnal awakenings. The syndrome may have some overlap with sudden infant death syndrome (SIDS).

e. Consider in the differential diagnosis: intracranial lesions (e.g., diencephalic tumor), nocturnal seizures, hypothyroidism, acromegaly, and drug dependence.

f. Confirmation of diagnosis should be done by night-long polysomnographic recording (see Table 5–3).

g. Treatment
   1) Factors such as the degree of daytime sleepiness, level of oxygen desaturation during the apneic spells, cardiac status, and the type of apnea (central or obstructive) should be taken into consideration in charting the treatment plan.
   2) Weight reduction, alcohol withdrawal, and sleeping in a position other than supine may prove helpful in mild cases.
   3) Respiratory stimulants such as theophylline, protriptyline, and progesterone have been tried with varying results.
   4) Nasal continuous positive airway pressure (CPAP) is being used extensively in obstructive and mixed apnea. The positive pressure tends to splint the upper airway, keeping it open during sleep. Dramatic improvement in the daytime functioning of the patient is often seen after using CPAP.

5) Some patients with airway obstruction are helped by surgery (i.e., tonsillectomy, adenoidectomy, uvulopalatopharyngoplasty, or removal of an intrathoracic goiter).

6) Permanent tracheostomy, which can be kept closed during the day and open at night, gives relief in severe cases with marked upper airway obstruction and cardiac decompensation.

7) No effective treatment has been found for central sleep apnea, although acetazolamide (Diamox) has been used in some cases. In severe cases the feasibility of pacing the diaphragm by electrophrenic stimulation is being evaluated.

Caveat: Do not prescribe hypnotics in sleep apnea. They will aggravate the apnea and the daytime sleepiness.

3. Sleep-related abnormal movements.
   a. Sleep-related (nocturnal) myoclonus (periodic leg movement syndrome) is characterized by abrupt jerking of feet and legs, which may be frequent enough to cause symptoms.
      1) The myoclonic jerks may be violent enough to awaken the individual fully or partially. Sometimes the patient may not be aware of the movements and the complaint may come from the bed partner.
      2) Both insomnia and excessive daytime sleepiness can result from this disorder.
      3) Treatment: Clonazepam (Klonopin) 0.5 to 1.0 mg at bedtime has been found to be helpful, particularly when troublesome insomnia accompanies abnormal movements.
   b. Restless legs syndrome is characterized by an indescribable, unpleasant sensation in the legs with an irresistible urge to move the legs.
      1) Movement seems to relieve the discomfort.
      2) Sleep-related myoclonus may also be present; insomnia may be a prominent complaint.

3) There may be a family history of similar complaints.
4) Sometimes associated with peripheral neuropathy (e.g., uremic neuropathy, diabetes, etc.).
5) Treatment.
    a) Phenytoin (Dilantin) 300 to 700 mg/day or carbamazepine (Tegretol) 400 to 1,200 mg/day may be useful in some patients.
    b) Clonazepam 0.5 to 1.0 mg at bedtime has been tried with varying success.
    c) Patients with nocturnal myoclonus or restless legs syndrome may also benefit from a bedtime dose of levodopa-carbidopa (Sinemet), beginning with a small dose and gradually adjusting the dosage depending on clinical response.
    d) Treatment should be directed at the underlying condition, e.g., diabetes, uremia.

4. Kleine-Levin syndrome. This syndrome of periodic daytime hypersomnia is very rare and is characterized by recurrent episodes of markedly prolonged sleep (several weeks) with intervening periods of normal sleep and wakefulness. It may also be associated with periodic increase in appetite for food and sex. It occurs in adolescence and young adulthood, more commonly in males. Consider lesions (inflammatory and neoplastic) involving the diencephalon or limbic system in the differential diagnosis.

V. DISORDERS OF SLEEP-WAKE SCHEDULE
A. These are disorders of the circadian or 24-hour biological clock.

1. Rapid time zone change (jet lag) syndrome: The patient's sleep-wake schedule does not adjust immediately to the new time zone and hence sleepiness and fatigue occur during wakefulness while insomnia occurs during the new sleep period. Symptoms last an average of 2 days.
    a. Treatment: Morning awakening time is a strong cue to reset the biological clock. Hence, the wake-up time should be adjusted to suit the new environment. Use

of a hypnotic for the first two nights may also be helpful.

2. Shift work change: When the work period is shifted to normal sleeping hours, the person is sleepy, performance is suboptimal, and the new sleep period disrupted.

3. Delayed and advanced sleep-phase syndromes: These are conditions in which the patient's biological clock is set differently from the norm, such that the circadian rhythm is out of phase with socially prescribed bedtime.

   a. Treatment: Chronotherapy, which involves "resetting the biological clock," consists of going to bed 3 hours later each day, e.g., functioning on a 27-hour "day," until the patient has advanced to the normal 10 or 11 P.M. bedtime.

B. Timed exposure to very bright light (phototherapy) has been used to treat disorders of the sleep-wake schedule, as well as seasonal affective disorder.

VI. PARASOMNIAS.

A. **The parasomnias** include a number of conditions which occur either exclusively during sleep or are exacerbated by sleep.

1. Bed-wetting (enuresis).

   a. Primary enuresis (child never toilet-trained):

      1) Often due to maturational lag.

      2) Ten percent to 15% of children 4 to 5 years of age continue to wet the bed; this rarely continues into adulthood.

      3) There is often a family history of this disorder. Enuresis occurs in all sleep stages.

      4) Treatment:

         a) Advise parents against overreacting to the situation, and reassure them that children usually outgrow it. Patience and understanding are important.

         b) Rewarding the child for a dry bed is helpful.

         c) Various behavior modification methods can be applied in difficult cases with the aid of experienced child psychologists.

         d) Imipramine (Tofranil), 10 to 75 mg at bedtime, is often effective in preventing bed-wetting but is not recommended for prolonged usage. Recently the antidiuretic hormone (ADH) analogue desmopressin administered intranasally in doses of 5 to 10 µg/day has been found to be useful.

b. Secondary enuresis (relapse to bed-wetting after a dry period of several months to years):

    1) Often due to psychological factors such as childhood depression.

    2) Organic disease must be ruled out, even if a psychological cause is obvious.

    3) Treatment.

        a) Psychological evaluation and family counseling are often necessary.

        b) Imipramine hydrochloride, a tricyclic antidepressant, in doses of 0.5 to 2.0 mg/kg/day at bedtime has been shown to be effective in reducing the frequency of bed-wetting. It is most effective when childhood depression is associated with the enuresis; with other causes the response is not as good. There is a tendency to relapse when the drug is withdrawn, and it is not recommended for prolonged use.

        c) Behavioral techniques, such as bladder control exercises, rewards for dry beds, and wetting alarms frequently improve the enuresis.

        Remember: An important organic cause of enuresis is urinary tract infection, and all children with enuresis should have urinalysis and a culture done. Other rare possibilities to consider include seizures in sleep, diabetes, congenital anomalies of the bladder, urethral obstruction, or ectopic ureter.

2. Sleepwalking (somnambulism).

a. The prevalence of sleepwalking is estimated at 1% to 6%.

b. It occurs mostly in children and usually disappears by 14 to 15 years of age.

    c. There is often a family history of sleepwalking.

    d. Episodes last several minutes with total amnesia for the incident.

    e. Episodes occur during stages III and IV sleep.

    f. Sleepwalkers have a high incidence of enuresis.

    g. The onset of sleepwalking in older age groups should arouse suspicion of a psychiatric disorder or medication effect. Nocturnal delirium ("sundown syndrome") may manifest as sleepwalking in the demented elderly.

    h. Treatment.

        1) Protect the patient from injury by locking doors and windows and avoiding other dangerous situations. Advise parents that children usually outgrow sleepwalking.

        2) Benzodiazepines, such as diazepam (Valium) 2 to 5 mg at bedtime, which suppress sleep stages III and IV, may be helpful for chronic and frequent sleepwalking.

        3) In adult sleepwalkers, psychological disturbances are frequent, unless there is a strong family history. Thorough psychological evaluation and treatment are recommended.

3. Night terrors.

    a. Night terrors occur early in the night during slow-wave sleep, most frequently at ages 4 to 6 years.

    b. Sudden apparent awakening is accompanied by extreme physiologic arousal (increased heart rate, respiratory rate, and sweating), and the child will scream and cry, but cannot be awakened.

    c. The incident is usually not remembered, although the child may recall a single frightening image or a sense of doom.

    d. Treatment.

        1) Advise the parents that children usually outgrow night terrors, and medication is generally not necessary.

        2) Night terrors may be abolished by diazepam 2 to 5 mg for children or 5 to 20 mg for adults. Long-term use is not recommended.

        3) Other medical conditions causing distress and

disturbing stage IV sleep may result in night terrors. Correction of this condition may decrease the frequency of night terrors.
   4) Psychiatric referral is indicated for night terrors past age 14 years.
4. Nightmares (dream anxiety attacks).
   a. Nightmares are frightening dreams occurring in REM sleep, more frequently toward morning.
   b. The degree of physiologic arousal is much lower than in night terrors.
   c. Patients often have detailed recall of dream content.
   d. Treatment.
      1) Usually reassurance is all that is necessary.
      2) In cases where nightmares are frequent and disabling to the patient, psychotherapy and behavioral treatment may be effective.
5. Sleep-related epileptic seizures.
   a. While seizures may occur predominantly or exclusively during sleep in epileptic patients, conditions such as enuresis, night terrors, and sleepwalking may be triggered by seizures originating in the temporal lobe.
   b. Nightlong EEG recording along with observation of the clinical phenomena (split-screen video recording) may be necessary to confirm the diagnosis.
   c. Treatment: Anticonvulsant therapy (see Chapter 11, section IX).
6. REM behavior disorder: This is a rare condition in which the normal loss of muscle tone fails to occur during REM sleep, such that the patient may actually act out dreams resulting in injury to self or to bed partner.
   a. Treatment: Responds readily to clonazepam 0.5 to 1.5 mg qhs.

VII. OTHER MEDICAL CONDITIONS AFFECTING SLEEP.

A. **Patients secrete 3 to 20 times more gastric acid during REM sleep.**
   1. Treatment.
      a. Treatment for sleep problems must not interfere with primary therapy of the underlying medical condition.

      b. Try to minimize sleep disruptions.

      c. Antidepressants, e.g., amitriptyline and doxepin, in low dosage may prove helpful for both the sleep disturbance and hyperacidity.

B.   **Angina** is more likely to occur during REM sleep.

C.   **Bronchial asthma attacks** often occur during REM sleep.

Caveat: Do not prescribe hypnotics to patients with bronchial asthma.

D.   **Hypo- and hyperthyroidism** may cause excessive sleepiness or insomnia, which are treated by correcting the thyroid dysfunction.

E.   **Pregnancy:** Sleep time is increased in early pregnancy and decreased in later pregnancy, but normal sleep patterns should be recovered a few weeks after delivery. Drugs should be avoided during pregnancy.

F.   **Alcohol** depresses REM sleep and results in REM rebound during withdrawal. Chronic alcoholics show fragmented shallow sleep. Insomnia is also associated with alcohol withdrawal.

BIBLIOGRAPHY

Coleman RM, et al: Sleep-wake disorders based on a polysomnographic diagnosis. *JAMA* 1982; 247:997–1003.

Czeisler CA, Johnson MP, Duffy JF, et al: Exposure to bright light and darkness to treat physiologic maladaption to night work. *N Engl J Med* 1990; 322:1253–1259.

Gillin JC, Byerley WF: The diagnosis and management of insomnia. *N Engl J Med* 1990; 322:239–247.

Hauri P, Esther MS: Insomnia. *Mayo Clin Proc* 1990;65:869–882.

Kryger MH: Management of obstructive apnea. *Clin Chest Med* 1992; 13:481–492.

Miller K, Atkin B, Moody ML: Drug therapy for nocturnal enuresis: *Drugs* 1992; 44:41–46.

Reite ML, Nagel KE, Ruddy JR: The evaluation and Management of Sleep Disorders. Washington, American Psychiatric Press, 1990.

Scharf MB, Flexcher KA, Jennings SW: Current pharmacologic treatments of narcolepsy. *Am Fam Physician* 1988; 38:1–6.

Treatment of Sleep Disorders in Older People: NIH Consensus Development Conference Statement, 1990.

DIMINISHED MENTAL CAPACITY AND DEMENTIA

6

Dementia is a general term for mental deterioration; stupid people are not necessarily demented (they may have been born that way) and people with apparently normal intelligence may be demented (at one time they may have been brilliant). The task of a physician caring for a demented patient is twofold: (1)identify those dementias that are treatable; (2)educate and provide support for the family of the patient with incurable dementia.

I. DIAGNOSIS OF DIMINISHED MENTAL CAPACITY.

A. **Suspect dementia** when the patient presents with any of the following:
   1. Confusion as a result of slight provocation such as a change in schedule or surroundings.
   2. A tendency toward repetition during the process of history taking.
   3. Slowness in following commands during physical examination (e.g., the examiner may have to demonstrate the tasks of station and gait).
   4. Emotional lability, irritability.

B. **If dementia is suspected,** or if the patient or the family complain of mental deterioration, a mental status evaluation *must* be performed. It should be conducted so that the patient does not become defensive. Usually, it can be worked in during the history and presented in an easy conversational style: "I'm going to ask you some questions that may sound silly, but it's part of my examination." We suggest three options (see Appendix B):

1. The mental status evaluation that has been used by neurologists for many years. The experienced physician gains considerable insight into brain function with this format, but it is not quantified.

2. The Six-Item Orientation Memory Concentration Test: This deceptively simple questionnaire is quantitative and is sensitive to mild dementing processes.

3. Formal neuropsychological evaluation: This must be administered by a trained person, takes 3 to 4 hours to complete, and is relatively expensive.

C. **In addition to the formal mental status examination,** specific notation of the following should also be made:

1. Appearance and behavior.
   a. Dress and grooming: Clean? Neat? Appropriate?
   b. Attention: Alert? Dull? Apathetic? Distracted?
   c. Movements: Slow? Hyperactive? Restless? Tremor?
   d. Discretion: Inhibited? Discusses intimate topics without restraint?

2. Language abnormalities.
   a. Quantity: Talkative? Noncommunicative?
   b. Content: Simple or complex sentence structure? Trouble finding words?
   c. Perseveration: Trouble changing topics? Words from earlier sentence used inappropriately in a new sentence?
   d. Appropriateness: Irrelevant? Illogical?
   e. Comprehension: Follows commands? Answers questions directly?

   Caveat: Aphasic or schizophrenic patients may appear to be demented. Patients with a motor aphasia have a paucity of speech and difficulty finding words and are aware of their problem. Patients with a sensory aphasia or schizophrenia may produce many words which make no sense (see Chapter 12, section VII. B).

3. Mood
   a. Depression: "I-don't-know" responses. (Degree is important, because many patients with neurologic abnormalities also have depression; see Chapter 9, section I.)
   b. Euphoria: Demented patients seem unconcerned about their problems.

II. ABNORMALITIES SOMETIMES SEEN IN DEMENTED PATIENTS.
A. Diagnostic considerations.

Caveat: These abnormalities do *not* diagnose dementia; but one or more of them are often seen in demented patients. The diagnosis is made on the basis of a *global* decline in intellectual function.

1. Expressionless or masklike facies; facial grimacing.
2. Bruns ataxia: a broad-based gait with short steps and feet placed flat on the ground as if on ice; a tendency to retropulsion increases the risk of falling; occurs in patients with frontal lobe deficits.
3. Athetoid posturing and tremors as seen in chronic or progressive diseases of the basal ganglia (see Chapter 7).
4. Grasp reflex: lightly stroking the palm of the patient's hand elicits a grasp response and reluctance to let go (Fig 6–1).

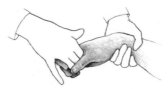

FIG 6–1. Grasp reflex: the patient will squeeze the examiner's fingers as the examiner rubs his or her fingers along the patient's palm from the hypothenar eminence toward the thenar eminence (normal response in infants).

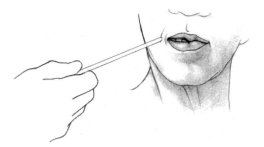

FIG 6–2. Rooting (suck) reflex: stroking away from the corner of the patient's mouth elicits lip movements and movement of the mouth toward the stimulus (normal response in infants).

5. Rooting reflex (sometimes incorrectly called suck reflex): patient turns lips toward a stroking stimulus at the corner of the mouth (Fig 6–2).
6. Snout reflex: patient puckers lips in response to gentle percussion of the lips (Fig 6–3).
7. Active jaw reflex (Fig 6–4).
8. Paratonic rigidity (gegenhalten): Advise the patient to relax his or her limbs. With passive manipulation of the patient's arm in unpredictable directions the examiner feels that the patient is consciously resisting every movement (Fig 6–5).

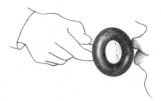

FIG 6–3. Snout response: lightly tapping the patient's closed lips causes the lips to pucker.

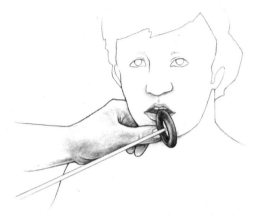

FIG 6–4. Jaw reflex: with the patient's mouth slightly open, striking the examiner's finger placed on the patient's chin causes the jaw to close momentarily.

9. Motor perseveration: When asked to perform a task such as rapid alternating movements, the patient continues for an inappropriate length of time.
10. Motor impersistence (inability to persist in a motor task):
    a. Keeping eyes closed.
    b. Keeping tongue out.
    c. Fixating gaze.
    d. Sustaining "ah" or "ee" sound.
    e. Maintaining hand grip.

Note: For example, in position sense testing, demented patents tend to peek (they are unable to sustain eye closure).

III. TREATABLE DEMENTIAS.

A. Table 6–1 is a list of some of those disease processes which present as diminished mental capacity and which may either

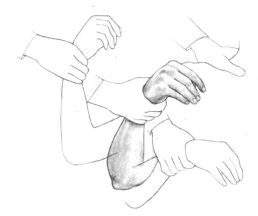

FIG 6–5. Gegenhalten: after instructing the patient to relax the arm "like a rag doll," the examiner moves the patient's arm in unpredictable directions. With gegenhalten, the examiner notes resistance as though the patient is actively attempting to prevent movement.

be cured or the progression stopped. The table suggests that the following laboratory studies should be considered in every demented patient:

1. Magnetic resonance imaging (MRI), with and without contrast (the computed tomography [CT] scan is less sensitive): MRI shows mass lesions, multiple infarcts, normal-pressure hydrocephalus, cerebral atrophy, white matter disease.

2. Electroencephalogram (EEG): generalized slowing is seen in toxic-metabolic encephalopathies, a periodic complexes pattern in Creutzfeldt-Jakob disease.

3. Endocrine studies: Since hypothyroidism is the most common endocrine cause of dementia, determination of triiodothyronine (T_3), thyroxine (T_4) and thyroid stimulating hormone (TSH) levels is recommended. Other studies should be ordered as suggested by the history and physical examination.

TABLE 6-1.
Selected Treatable Causes
of Dementia

Toxins and drugs
Nutritional deficiency states
Metabolic or endocrine disorders
Hypoxia
Normal-pressure hydrocephalus
Intracranial mass lesions
Central nervous system infections
Atherosclerotic cerebrovascular disease

4. Lumbar puncture (LP): LP is the only sure way to diagnose indolent infections and neurosyphilis.
5. Blood chemistry is essential in diagnosing secondary metabolic encephalopathies.
6. Complete blood count and erythrocyte sedimentation rate (ESR): Abnormalities may suggest infection, vitamin deficiency, or autoimmune disease.
7. Serum vitamin B_{12} and folate levels are especially important in patients with chronic ulcer disease or postgastrectomy. Serum methylmalonic acid levels are more accurate than serum vitamin B_{12} levels.
8. Urinary toxicology screen (including heavy metals).
9. Human immunodeficiency virus (HIV) titer: All HIV patients sooner or later become demented.

B. **Cerebrovascular disease.**
   1. Multi-infarct dementia (Binswanger's disease):
      a. Patients always have a history of chronic hypertension.
   ▶ b. History is of a "stepwise" progression—periods of stability with sudden decompensation.
      c. MRI shows multiple small infarcts just beneath the cortical gray matter.
      d. Treatment: Progression can be halted by controlling hypertension.
   2. Pseudobulbar palsy:
      a. Patients almost always have a history of chronic hypertension.

▶ b. Patients present with emotional lability: they may burst into tears at a trivial incident, but, when asked, deny they are sad. Neurologic examination shows generalized hyperreflexia, including a hyperactive jaw reflex.

   c. MRI shows multiple small infarcts in or near the internal capsule.

   d. Treatment: Control hypertension; some patients may be helped with tricyclic antidepressants.

3. Multiple cerebral emboli: The most common source of emboli is from the heart: atrial fibrillation, mural thrombosis, postmyocardial infarct, and mitral valve prolapse are common associated conditions.

4. Occlusive disease of large vessels in the neck: There are scattered reports of improvement in mental status after carotid endarterectomy, presumably because ischemic neurons function improperly. Selection of patients for surgery should be conservative.

C. Mass lesions.

1. Patients with large brain tumors sometimes may have no symptoms or signs other than dementia, especially if the tumor is slow-growing (e.g., meningioma).

2. CT scan or MRI easily diagnoses these conditions.

D. Alcoholism.

1. These patients usually have a history of consuming more than the equivalent of 150 mL/day of absolute alcohol for many years.

2. Lability of mood is common.

3. Recovery of mental faculties is surprisingly good if alcohol consumption can be stopped.

   Caveat: This dementia should be differentiated from Korsakoff's psychosis which is a specific defect in acquiring new information, not a global defect (see Chapter 8, sections II. B. 2 and III. B).

E. Drugs.

1. Many drugs, even when prescribed in conservative therapeutic doses, may result in diminished mental capacity. Examples include phenobarbital and phenytoin.

    2. All demented patients should be given a drug-free period if at all possible.

    3. Elderly patients are especially sensitive to medications; tranquilizers and sleep medication should be prescribed with great caution.

F. Subacute combined degeneration (combined system disease; vitamin B$_{12}$ deficiency).

    1. Patients commonly have a history of ulcer disease or gastrectomy; older patients may develop gastric achlorhydria and fail to produce intrinsic factor.

    2. Although the patients have four neurologic abnormalities (dementia, corticospinal tract signs, posterior column abnormalities, and peripheral neuropathy), the dementia may be the most prominent finding (see Chapter 15, section II. A. 2. a).

    3. Other vitamin deficiencies may produce a dementia, but rarely do so in the presence of an adequate diet.

G. Endocrine abnormalities.

    1. Hypothyroidism: Neurologic abnormalities include dementia and slowed relaxation phase of the Achilles (ankle) reflex.

    2. Hypoglycemia: The usual clinical setting is repeated hypoglycemic attacks precipitated by inappropriate doses of insulin. Acute attacks should be treated with intravenous (IV) glucose. The dementia already incurred is permanent, but can be made worse if care is not taken to prevent further hypoglycemic attacks.

    3. Both hyperparathyroidism and hypoparathyroidism may present as dementia; three normal fasting calcium levels are necessary to exclude parathyroid disease.

    4. Any endocrine abnormality, if severe enough, may cause mental slowness; this includes Cushing's syndrome and panhypopituitarism.

H. Secondary metabolic encephalopathy: The abnormality is usually obvious on general physical examination, multichannel chemistries, and blood gas determinations. Common causes include chronic obstructive pulmonary disease, and hepatic and renal failure. The EEG often shows generalized slowing.

I. Chronic infection.

1. Acquired immunodeficiency syndrome (AIDS): HIV positive patients become demented from the virus itself or from opportunistic infections of the brain.

2. Tuberculous and fungal meningitis may produce dementia both by destroying the brain parenchyma and by thickening the posterior fossa meninges and causing an obstructive hydrocephalus. The patient may have no other signs of infection, such as fever, and diagnosis can be excluded only by examining cerebrospinal fluid (CSF) (see Chapter 14, section I. C).

3. Tertiary central nervous system (CNS) syphilis: The presence of typical pupillary abnormalities (Argyll Robertson pupil) may suggest the diagnosis. The blood VDRL (Venereal Disease Research Laboratory) test may be nonreactive; the diagnosis is made with certainty only with a CSF VDRL test.

J. Normal-pressure hydrocephalus.

1. Diagnosis.
   - ▶ a. The diagnosis of normal-pressure hydrocephalus should be entertained with a subacute (months) onset of dementia associated with ataxia and urinary incontinence.
   - b. Many patients have a history of a previous subarachnoid hemorrhage or meningitis.
   - c. The neurologic examination shows hyperactive reflexes in the lower extremities (sometimes with a Babinski reflex) and normal reflexes in the upper extremities.
   - d. The CT scan or MRI shows large ventricles with little or no space between the skull and the surface of the brain. The gyri are not prominent.

2. Treatment: If the patient shows improvement in mental status after repeatedly removing CSF by LPs, a permanent shunt should be seriously considered.

IV. PSEUDODEMENTIA.

A. Diagnostic considerations.

1. The term *pseudodementia* refers to a major depressive disorder (see Chapter 9, section I. A. 2) in the elderly.

2. Often mistaken for Alzheimer's disease (Table 9–2 may help in distinguishing the two).
3. Vegetative signs such as sleep disturbance (early-morning awakening), motor slowness, and lack of energy are often present.

B. **Treatment** Antidepressant or electroshock therapy often results in dramatic improvement.

V. PROGRESSIVE DEMENTIAS.
A. Alzheimer's disease (presenile and senile dementia).
1. Diagnostic considerations.
   a. Alzheimer's disease accounts for over 50% of all dementias in patients over the age of 40 years.
   ▶ b. The *probable* diagnosis is made on gradual, progressive global cognitive changes (language use, perception, acquisition of skills, judgment, problem solving, abstract thinking) with no disturbance of consciousness and the absence of systemic disorders or other brain diseases that cause dementia.

   Caveat: Definitive diagnosis of Alzheimer's disease can be made only by brain autopsy or biopsy. A wrong diagnosis of Alzheimer's disease may deprive that patient of treatment for a curable dementia.

   c. Associated symptoms sometimes include depression, sleep disturbances, paranoia, agitation, and aggression.
   d. Hereditary tendency, especially if mother or father had relatively early onset of the disease (before age 65 years).

   Note: All patients with Down syndrome past the age of 40 years develop Alzheimer's disease.

   e. Except for the dementia, the routine neurologic examination is normal: cranial nerves, reflexes, sensation, and station and gait.
   f. Most patients show "intrusion"—incorporation of a previous response in a later, irrelevant context. For example, after correctly naming the month of "January,"

the patient asked to name his or her children, might
say "Bill, January, Erik."

g. CT scan or MRI shows progressive atrophy, but this
is *nonspecific* and the atrophy does *not* correlate well
with the degree of dementia.

h. EEG is normal until very late in the disease.

2. Management.

a. After diagnosis, sympathy, support, listening, education, and referral to appropriate support agencies are
very important to both the family and the patient. The
book *The 36-Hour Day* (see Bibliography) may be
very helpful. More information may be obtained from:
Alzheimer's Association, 70 East Lake St., Chicago,
IL 60601, telephone (312) 853-3060 or 800-621-0379.

b. Protect the patient from unproven and often expensive
therapies (lecithin, megavitamins, etc.).

c. If depression is present, low-dose antidepressant
medication, such as imipramine 25 mg qhs, may be
useful.

d. Use psychotropic medications in very low doses, if at
all; Alzheimer's disease patients seem to be more sensitive than the average patient to side effects.

e. Drugs that enhance CNS cholinergic neurotransmis-
sion are being evaluated. Tacrine (Cognex) has recently been approved for use, but it has serious hepatotoxicity and provides little benefit in most patients.

B. **Creutzfeldt-Jakob disease (Jakob's disease, Jakob-
Creutzfeldt disease).**

1. Diagnostic considerations.

a. Any patient with dementia and generalized myoclonus has a high probability of Creutzfeldt-Jakob disease.

b. The course is generally more rapid than Alzheimer's
disease, and death usually occurs in 1 to 2 years.

c. The infectious agent is related to the agent of sheep
scrapie and transmissible mink encephalopathy and
has been called a prion; the only proven mode of transmission is direct contact between the nerve tissue of
an infected patient and an open wound of a recipient.

> *Note:* Transmission has occurred through use of incompletely decontaminated neurosurgical equipment, corneal transplants, human pituitary-derived growth hormone injections, and patch grafts prepared from human dura.

   d. The EEG often shows characteristic periodic complexes.
   e. Brain biopsy is rarely necessary, but will show typical spongiform alterations.

> *Caveat:* Formaldehyde does not inactivate the responsible infectious agent. Pathologists and neurosurgeons are at particularly high risk for infection. A correct diagnosis is important for protection of these physicians, as well as for epidemiologic studies. Organ donations should not be permitted from affected persons.

C. Huntington's disease. Dementia may precede the choreoathetosis and psychosis by many years. The correct diagnosis is most strongly suggested by a family history of dominantly inherited psychosis or dementia (see Chapter 7, section III. A).

D. Pick's disease.
   1. Diagnostic considerations.
      a. Pick's disease may be difficult to distinguish from Alzheimer's disease.
      b. Initial symptoms include prominent alterations in emotion, affect, and behavior.
      c. Pick's disease progresses to death within several years, whereas Alzheimer's disease generally progresses at a slower rate.
      d. CT scan or MRI may show frontal and temporal lobe atrophy which is out of proportion to the atrophy in the rest of the brain.
      e. Twenty percent of cases have a pattern of autosomal dominant inheritance.
   2. Management: Same as for Alzheimer's disease (see section V. A. 2).

BIBLIOGRAPHY

Benson DF, Blumer D: *Psychiatric Aspects of Neurologic Disease.* New York, Grune & Stratton, 1975, pp 123–147.

Duckett S (ed): *The Pathology of the Aging Nervous System.* Philadelphia, Lea & Febiger, 1991.

Gajdusek DC, Gibbs CJ Jr, Asher DM, et al: Precautions in medical care and in handling materials from patients with transmissible virus dementia (Creutzfeldt-Jakob disease). *N Engl J Med* 1977; 297:1253–1258.

Heston LL, White JA: *Dementia: A Practical Guide to Alzheimer's Disease and Related Illnesses.* New York, WH Freeman, 1983.

Jenike MA: Alzheimer's disease: Clinical care and management. *Psychosomatics* 1985; 27:407–416.

Katzman R: Validation of a short orientation-memory concentration test of cognitive impairment. *Am J Psychiatry* 1983; 140:734–739.

Katzman R: Alzheimer's disease. *N Engl J Med* 1986; 314:964–973.

Katzman R, Rowe JW (eds): *Principles of Geriatric Neurology.* Philadelphia, FA Davis, 1992.

Khachaturian ZS: Diagnosis of Alzheimer's disease. *Arch Neurol* 1985; 42:1097–1105.

More NL, Robins PO: *The 36-Hour Day: A Family Guide to Caring for Persons with Alzheimer's Disease.* Baltimore, Johns Hopkins Press, 1982.

Prusiner SB: Prions and neurodegenerative disease. *N Engl J Med* 1987; 317:1571–1581.

Selkoe DJ: Aging, amyloid and Alzheimer's disease. *N Engl J Med* 1989: 320:1484–1487.

Rappaport EB: Iatrogenic Creutzfeldt-Jakob disease. *Neurology* 1987; 37:1520–1522.

Whitehouse PJ (ed): *Dementia.* Philadelphia, FA Davis, 1993.

MOVEMENT DISORDERS

7

Accurate observation and description are essential for classifying movement disorders. The patient's abnormal movements and postures can often be observed during the interview—one look is worth a thousand words.

I. **TYPES OF ABNORMAL MOVEMENTS.**

A. **Tremor:** Involuntary, rhythmic oscillating sinusoidal movement across a joint. The movement may be present at rest (static or repose tremor) or only apparent with motion (kinetic tremor) or a specific posture (postural tremor).

B. **Chorea and athetosis:** *Chorea* is irregular, arrhythmic, unpredictable, brief jerky movement which usually involves the extremities and the face in continuous, random sequence; *athetosis* is a slow, sinuous usually more proximal movement. In some cases the distinction between these two types of movement is unclear and the term *choreoathetosis* is used. When chorea is seen in slow motion on a videotape, it often closely resembles athetosis.

C. **Myoclonus:** Spontaneous, brief, shocklike contractions of one or more muscles, causing movement across a joint (think of the jerklike movements often seen in dogs, cats, or people as they go to sleep).

D. **Tics:** Repetitive, rapid, usually brief, purposeful stereotyped movements. The movements, commonly are complex and may involve the face, axial muscles, and proximal limbs. They seldom involve fingers or toes.

E. **Focal motor seizures:** Relatively rhythmic movements, usually involving multiple joints and often persisting in sleep (tremors, choreoathetosis, and tics commonly disappear during sleep).

F. **Clonus:** Rhythmic movement precipitated by sudden stretching of a tendon. This is most commonly seen at the ankle, and is associated with upper motor neuron lesions.

G. **Fasciculations:** Very brief twitches of a group of muscle fibers, all innervated by the same anterior horn cell. Best seen where subcutaneous fat is thinnest, e.g., the back or the tongue. Generally, fasciculations do *not* cause movement across a joint, but they may occasionally cause slight movement of the fingers.

H. **Dystonia:** Sustained muscle contractions frequently causing twisting and repetitive movement or abnormal postures.

II. **HISTORY AND EXAMINATION OF THE PATIENT WITH A MOVEMENT DISORDER.**

A. **History.**

1. Many movement disorders are *familial*.

2. Drug and alcohol history: e.g., alcoholism may cause cerebellar degeneration and alleviate familial tremor; phenothiazines may cause Parkinson's syndrome or tardive dyskinesia; excess thyroid hormone (endogenous or exogenously administered) may result in a metabolic tremor.

3. Medical history: Liver disease may cause asterixis; Sydenham's chorea is associated with streptococcal infections.

4. A description of the movement disorder should include age at onset, rate of progression, symmetry, and exacerbating or alleviating factors (stress, drugs, sleep).

B. **Neurologic examination.**

1. Have the patient draw a spiral or connect dots as a permanent record of the motor dysfunction; later this can be used to monitor the efficacy of treatment.

2. Muscle tone: *Hypotonia* may be seen as floppiness of joints or an excessive number of swings after the patellar reflex is elicited when the patient is sitting on the examining table (Fig 7–1). *Hypertonia* may be appreciated by passive movement of the arm, especially when the patient is distracted, as when the contralateral arm is engaged in some activity such as drawing an imaginary figure eight in the air.

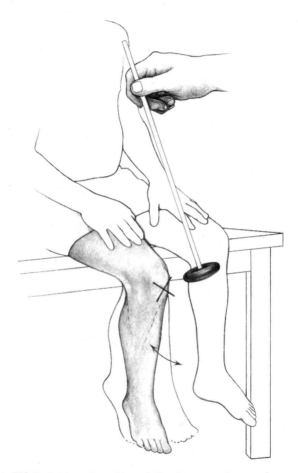

FIG 7–1. The patient with cerebellar disease may have an abnormal number of swings of the leg when the patellar reflex is tested.

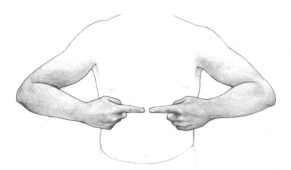

FIG 7–2. Having the patient point (but not touch) the index fingers as illustrated may differentiate between a proximal and distal tremor. With a proximal tremor there is flapping of the arms; with a distal tremor the fingers are constantly in misalignment.

3. Instruct the patient to approximate the tips of his or her index fingers (Fig 7–2) to bring out some tremors and to differentiate proximal and distal tremors.
4. Abnormal postures are most often appreciated during station and gait testing.

Caveat: Never make the diagnosis of a movement disorder on the basis of a single finding. Table 7–1 illustrates this point by showing the overlapping fea-

TABLE 7–1.
Overlapping Features of Various Types of Tremor

Feature	Parkinson's Syndrome	Cerebellar Tremor	Essential Tremor
Present at rest	Yes	No	Yes
Increased tone	Yes	No	No
Decreased tone	No	Yes	No
Postural abnormality	Yes	Yes	No
Head involvement	Yes	Yes	Yes
Intentional component	No	Yes	Yes
Incoordination	No	Yes	No

tures of Parkinson's syndrome, cerebellar tremor, and essential tremor. Also note that on the finger-to-nose test, both cerebellar tremor and essential tremor have an intentional component (Fig 7–3).

III. PARKINSONISM.

A. **Parkinson's disease is an idiopathic disorder** associated with a progressive loss of neurons in the midbrain substantia nigra; Parkinson's *syndrome* involves entirely different

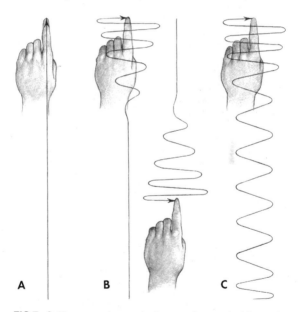

FIG 7–3. Finger-to-nose test. **A,** the normal person is able to point to a target accurately and smoothly. **B,** the patient with cerebellar hemispheric disease shows a tremor that increases in amplitude as the target is approached. **C,** the patient with essential tremor shows a tremor throughout the range of motion. Note the increase in amplitude as the target is approached. **B** and **C** are easily confused.

pathophysiologic processes and is associated with dozens of other neurologic diseases, including repeated head trauma, Alzheimer's disease, and the acute effect of neuroleptics such chlorpromazine (Thorazine), haloperidol (Haldol), promethazine (Phenergan), prochloperazine (Compazine), or metoclopramide (Reglan). In a relatively mild case of parkinsonism, suspect Parkinson's *syndrome* (and refer to a neurologist) if:

1. Reflexes are abnormal (hyperactive, in amyotrophic lateral sclerosis [ALS]-dementia-parkinsonism complex or olivopontocerebellar degeneration).
2. Significant dementia is present (Alzheimer's disease).
3. Downward or lateral gaze is impaired (progressive supranuclear palsy).
4. Postural hypotension is present (Shy-Drager syndrome).
5. The patient does not respond to combination carbidopa-levodopa (repeated head trauma).

B. **Early symptoms.**
1. Voice changes (decrease in volume and loss of melody): These are often not apparent to the examiner but are quite obvious to the family and close friends of the patient.
2. Sleep disturbances: frequent nocturnal awakenings, possibly secondary to loss of automatic motor movements during sleep; considerable relief may be obtained from sleeping on satin sheets.
3. Wet pillows: Saliva often is not swallowed during sleep even if there is no such problem during waking.

C. **Late signs and symptoms (Fig 7–4).**
1. Tremor.
   a. Present at rest, worse with emotional stress or when the examiner calls attention to it.
   b. A "pill-rolling" motion with the index finger flexing and extending in contact with the thumb, at approximately 4 to 10 Hz. May involve the arm with rhythmic flexion-extension, abduction-adduction, pronation-supination, or a combination thereof.
   c. Present most commonly in the hands and fingers; often begins unilaterally and distally and spreads

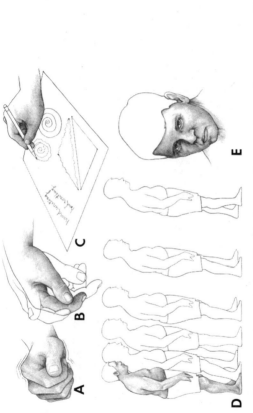

FIG 7–4. The parkinsonian syndrome. **A,** the "pill-rolling" tremor. **B,** tremor that may become worse with emotional stress. **C,** handwriting abnormalities, which include micrographia. **D,** typical posture and gait, which becomes faster (festination). **E,** lack of facial expression as well as "stare" from decreased blinking.

proximally and to the other side over a period of months or years.

2. Rigidity: Passively move the extremities; instruct the patient to relax the arm ("like a rag doll") and then passively move the arm. Increased tone (rigidity) is appreciated as increased resistance throughout the range of movement (the so-called lead pipe rigidity); tremor may also be felt during this movement (the so-called cogwheel phenomenon).

3. *Postural changes* are observed during testing of station and gait. These include stooping of shoulders and slight flexion of back, hips, and knees. In starting to walk, steps at first are slow and small (the *marche à petit pas*) and then rapidly increase. In turning, the motion is not fluid but is done in a rigid whole-body fashion (en bloc), and is seemingly accomplished by "walking" rather than "pivoting."

4. *Bradykinesia* is a major problem manifested as difficulty in initiating movements (including bowel), and as slowed movements and slowed thought processes (sometimes referred to as a "constipated mind"). Typically the family will notice the patient's lack of interest or involvement in many usual activities (this may be confused with depression or dementia).

5. Handwriting is slow and small with letters tightly bunched together (micrographia).

6. The basal ganglia are a center for automatic motor functions such as walking, maintenance of posture, maintenance of facial expression, clearing of saliva from the mouth, swallowing, arising from a chair, regaining balance; most of the symptoms of Parkinson's syndrome can be explained in this context (i.e., a dysfunction of automatic motor behavior).

D. Treatment.

1. Treatment is directed toward relieving the symptoms of tremor and rigidity; none of the drugs is a "cure." Initial doses should always be small and built up slowly.

2. Patient education materials may be obtained from the

United Parkinson Foundation, 360 West Superior St., Chicago, IL 60610, telephone (312) 664-2344; or the National Parkinson Foundation, 1501 NW 9th Ave., Miami, FL 33136, telephone (305) 547-6666 or 800-327-4545.

3. Drug therapy.
   a. General principles.
      1) Begin selegiline (Eldepryl) as soon as the diagnosis is established (a short course of carbidopa-levodopa may be necessary to establish the diagnosis).
      2) Avoid dopamine-blocking agents in a patient with Parkinson's disease.
      3) Delay administration of carbidopa or levodopa until symptoms are truly bothersome.
      4) Always start drugs at a low dose and titrate slowly.
   b. Selegiline (Eldepryl): monamine oxidase-B (MAO-B) enzyme inhibitor that seems to retard Parkinson's disease possibly by decreasing free radical formation in neurons. Recommended dose is 5 mg bid (given upon awakening and at midday), but a single morning dose may be just as effective (a single dose of selegiline 5 mg inhibits MAO-B in platelets for 2 months).
   c. Bromocriptine mesylate (Parlodel): direct dopamine receptor agonist, which may also retard progression of the disease. Starting dose is 1.25 mg (half-tablet) tid. Dosage may be increased slowly (weekly changes in dosing) as needed to 10 mg tid.
   d. Pergolide (Permax): direct dopamine receptor agonist with similar action to bromocriptine. Beginning dose is 0.05 mg tid, which may also be slowly increased.
   e. Carbidopa-levodopa therapy.
      1) Sinemet comes as a single tablet containing 25 mg of carbidopa and 100 mg of levodopa; initial dosage is one tablet tid, but can be increased to one tablet five times per day.

2) Sinemet CR: long-acting form of Sinemet, supplied in tablets containing 50 mg of carbidopa and 200 mg of levodopa. Usual dosage is one tablet bid or tid. May be useful in patients with advanced disease.

3) If cost is a major factor, generic carbidopa 25 mg tid and levodopa 100 mg tid can be prescribed separately.

f. Adjunct medications:

1) Anticholinergics such as benztropine mesylate (Cogentin) may be helpful in controlling the tremor. Start at a dose of 0.5 mg/day and increase until tremor is subdued or until intolerable side effects occur.

Caveat: Anticholinergic drugs may exacerbate constipation and result in urinary retention.

2) Amantadine hydrochloride (Symmetrel) is a mild dopamine agonist. Start with a dose of 50 mg qd and gradually increase to 100 mg bid. (Although capsules are only available in 100 mg size, a syrup is available which contains 10 mg/mL.)

4. Complications of drug therapy.

a. Patients with advanced Parkinson's disease respond poorly to levodopa, because there are no longer sufficient cells in the substantia nigra to convert it to dopamine. Patients with Parkinson's syndrome respond poorly or not at all to levodopa, because the defect is at the postsynaptic receptor or in the continuity of nigrostriatal fibers.

b. Toxic amounts of dopamine cause abnormal movements most frequently involving the tongue (buccolingual dyskinesia). In this circumstance the dosage of dopaminergic agents should be reduced.

c. The "on/off" phenomenon: Some patients, especially those receiving levodopa for a long period of time, may have symptoms which change dramatically from hour to hour. One moment they may be virtually immobile and unable to walk, while the next they may be mobile but suffer from abnormal movements. The measures to combat this disabling condition include using direct dopamine receptor agonists, increasing the time period at night when no dopaminergic medicines are used, and using multiple different dopaminergic agents in combination.

5. Exercise is an extremely important part of therapy; walking or water aerobics are critical in order to keep patients mobile as the disease progresses.

IV. ESSENTIAL TREMOR (BENIGN, FAMILIAL, HEREDITARY, OR SENILE TREMOR).

A. Diagnostic considerations.

1. Coarse, rhythmic, usually symmetric, movement which may be present at rest, most noticeable in the fingers, usually beginning in the hands, and which may also involve the head, but seldom affects the legs.

2. Persists throughout the range of voluntary activity and often (like a cerebellar tremor) increases in amplitude as the limb approaches an object (finger-to-nose test) (Fig 7–1).

3. Characteristically increases with attempts to write or to bring liquids to mouth to drink.

4. Increases markedly under stress (like a parkinsonian tremor).

5. Often attenuates or disappears with a small amount of alcohol. (This feature, if present, is almost diagnostic.)

6. Onset may be in adolescence or early adult years; often called senile tremor if it develops late in life.

7. Autosomal dominant inheritance can be identified in most families.

8. Tremor increases in amplitude with age and may eventually interfere with fine movements.

9. Neurologic examination is normal except for tremor. Distinguish from parkinsonism by lack of rigidity and bradykinesia; distinguish from cerebellar lesion by lack of hypotonia and ataxia.

10. Cerebellar and parkinsonian tremors rarely involve the head. Tremor similar to essential tremor may be seen in persons with thyrotoxicosis and patients receiving lithium, epinephrine, or terbutaline sulfate. Fatigue and anxiety may cause a similar fine rapid tremor.

B. Treatment.

1. Reassurance is often all that is necessary. If the tremor interferes with social adjustment or activities of daily living, drug treatment may be necessary.

2. Propranolol hydrochloride (Inderal) is often effective. The long-acting form at an initial dose of 80 mg is convenient.

3. Some patients respond to primidone (Mysoline). The initial dose should be 50 mg qhs increased by 50 mg weekly until the tremor is controlled.

Caveat: Primidone may occasionally cause nausea, vomiting, drowsiness, and ataxia even in small doses.

4. Alcohol is often the most effective agent, but is not recommended for chronic use. In fact, chronic alcoholism may occur in patients with essential tremor who attempt this form of treatment. Wine with dinner or about 20 minutes prior to a stressful event occasionally may be used for elderly patients with symptomatic senile tremor.

V. CEREBELLAR TREMOR.

A. Diagnostic considerations.

1. Cerebellar tremor is noted only during movement. It may be unilateral or bilateral and indicates disease of the cerebellar hemisphere.

2. In the finger-to-nose test, tremor increases as the finger reaches the target and is less noticeable between targets (Fig 7–3).

3. Other signs of cerebellar hemispheric disease include the following:

a. Ipsilateral (same side) difficulty with rapid alternating movements (have patient rapidly alternate pronation and supination of hand against the thigh or other hand).

   b. Hypotonia manifested as a limp "rag doll" arm with passive motion and as a pendular patellar reflex (see Fig 7–1). Hypotonia may also be manifested by hyperextension of the fingers (Fig 7–5).

   c. Rebound is commonly elicited by having the patient flex his or her arm against resistance from the examiner, and then having the examiner suddenly let go of the arm; normally the arm remains relatively stationary, but with cerebellar disease, the arm will rebound and tend to strike the patient's face.

     Caveat: The examiner must place his or her arm or hand so as to guard the patient's face (Fig 7–6).

   d. Occasionally speech abnormalities occur, which consist of loss of normal speech melody. Speech tends to have an explosive quality (ataxic dysarthria or scanning speech). This can be demonstrated by having the patient vocalize a sustained "Ah," which will have markedly variable volume and pitch.

Note: Disease of midline cerebellar structures may cause only difficulty in tandem walking (gait ataxia) with no abnormalities of finger-to-nose testing and no tremor or other signs of cerebellar hemispheric disease. Commonly this is seen in chronic alcoholism, as a remote effect of carcinoma, or with phenytoin or carbamazepine intoxication. In chil-

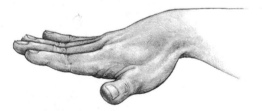

FIG 7–5. "Spooning" of hands is occasionally seen in cerebellar disease. Hyperextension of fingers in this manner may also exacerbate an essential tremor.

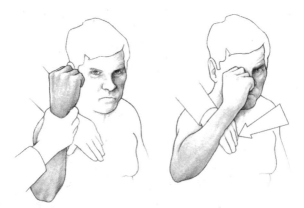

FIG 7–6. Testing for rebound. Request the patient to pull against resistance, then suddenly release the arm without warning. *CAVEAT:* If not protected by the examiner's arm, patients with cerebellar disease will strike themselves.

dren, medulloblastoma or a midline cerebellar tumor can cause similar abnormalities.

B. **Treatment:** Therapy must be directed at the underlying cerebellar disorder. Lesions of the cerebellum including cerebellar atrophy may be demonstrated with computed tomography (CT) scans or, magnetic resonance imaging (MRI). Cerebellar tremor is commonly seen in patients with multiple sclerosis or brainstem strokes.

VI. **HUNTINGTON'S DISEASE (HUNTINGTON'S CHOREA).**
A. **Diagnostic considerations.**
▶ 1. Huntington's disease is a dominantly inherited disorder with abnormal involuntary movements and progressive dementia, with symptomatic onset usually after age 30 years.
   2. Initial symptoms may include clumsiness of move-

ment, slowness of finger movements, or a tendency to drop objects. Abnormal movements at first may be converted to seemingly purposeful movements in order to conceal the abnormality.

3. The abnormal movements are irregular, rapid jerky movements of the fingers and wrists associated with slower dystonic movements of the upper limbs.

4. The gait is unsteady with a tendency to bob and weave.

5. Facial grimacing with involuntary movements of the tongue are common; this produces a dysarthria.

6. The abnormal movements can be exaggerated by sustained activity such as clenching a fist (milkmaid grip) or protruding the tongue (darting tongue).

7. Patients may present with subtle signs of intellectual deterioration, personality change, or frank psychosis (depression and suicide attempts are frequent), with the movement disorder not being evident until many years later.

8. Family history is a very important diagnostic clue but may be exceptionally difficult to elicit; the family history may include mental deficiency, alcoholism, suicide, psychosis, and behavior disorders.

B. **Treatment.**

1. There is no cure for Huntington's disease; genetic counseling is necessary. The genetic locus of this disease has been identified on the short arm of chromosome 4. Both in utero and presymptomatic diagnosis are available but their use is controversial.

2. For improvement of the abnormal movements or treatment of the associated psychoses:

a. Haloperidol 3 to 6 mg/day may initially be effective for the movement disorder and for behavior control.

b. Phenothiazines such as chlorpromazine (up to 150 mg/day), perphenazine (10–16 mg tid), or trifluoperazine hydrochloride (2 mg tid) are alternative treatments.

3. If serious depression is present, suicide precautions may need to be taken.

4. Educational materials for patients and information

about local support groups may be obtained from Huntington's Disease Society of America, 140 West 22nd St., New York, NY 10011, telephone (212) 242-1968 or 800-345-HDSA.

VII. SYDENHAM'S CHOREA (INFECTIOUS OR RHEUMATIC CHOREA).

A. Diagnostic considerations.

▶ 1. Begins as an apparent restlessness, clumsiness, and behavior disorder characterized by involuntary movements, incoordination, and weakness in children and adolescents (more common in girls) aged 5 to 15 years. It is often associated with rheumatic fever and a β-hemolytic streptococcal infection, which may precede the onset of chorea by days to months, and is important to recognize because Sydenham's chorea has the same cardiac implications as rheumatic fever.

2. Choreic movements are nonrepetitive, abrupt, jerky, and purposeless; present at rest and accentuated by posturing; usually seen in the face and hands; and may involve only one side of the body (hemichorea).

3. Facial grimacing, dysarthria, and explosive speech are common.

4. When asked to sustain a grip on the examiner's fingers, the patient will exhibit a "milking grip"; the patient cannot maintain a protruded tongue ("darting tongue sign").

5. There may be decreased resistance to passive movements; reflexes may be hypoactive, delayed, or pendular.

6. Duration is usually 4 to 6 weeks; complete recovery is usual, but residua may be evident.

7. The patient may have an elevated erythrocyte sedimentation rate (ESR). Serum calcium and phosphorous levels should be obtained to rule out hypocalcemia. Electrocardiographic (ECG) changes or other features consistent with the Jones criteria for rheumatic fever should be sought, including throat culture for β-hemolytic streptococcal infection and serum antistreptolysin O (ASO) titers.

B. **Treatment.**
1. Bed rest with a tranquil environment.
2. Haloperidol at an initial dose of 0.5 mg, gradually increased until movements are controlled. When movements are controlled for 3 to 4 weeks, the medication can be slowly discontinued.
3. Streptococcal infections should be treated with penicillin.
4. Prevent rheumatic complications by prophylactic *lifelong* antibiotics (additional antibiotics may be necessary in situations where there may be bacteremia, e.g., dental work). Penicillin G benzathine is the recommended drug at the following dosages:

Age (yr)	Penicillin G Dosage (units/mo)
<6	600,000
6–12	900,000
>12	1,200,000

5. Frequent examinations are necessary to detect early signs of cardiac involvement.

VIII. CHOREA GRAVIDARUM.
A. **Incidence and course.**
▶ 1. Chorea gravidarum occurs in approximately 1 in every 2,000 to 3,000 pregnancies. It occurs more commonly in first pregnancies and may recur in subsequent pregnancies. The cause is unknown, but it is often preceded by thyrotoxic chorea or Sydenham's chorea.
2. The average duration is 1 to 2 months; chorea usually subsides spontaneously during pregnancy or shortly after delivery.
B. **Treatment:** Termination of pregnancy is rarely required. If the chorea is incapacitating, sedatives or phenothiazines may be used to control the movements, but use of such medications may pose a risk to the fetus.

IX. SPASMUS NUTANS.
A. **Diagnostic considerations.**
▶ 1. Rhythmic nodding or rotatory tremor of the head associated with pendular nystagmus.

2. It occurs in infants between ages 4 and 18 months.
3. It must be differentiated from the head tremor associated with congenital nystagmus (due to reduced visual acuity).
4. The tremor disappears when the infant is lying down.

B. **Treatment:** This disorder is rare, but is important to recognize because it is self-limited and disappears by age 2 years. Further workup is not necessary. The parents need reassurance.

X. KERNICTERUS.
A. **Diagnostic and clinical considerations.**
▶ 1. Jaundiced newborn at 2 or 3 days of age may show symptoms such as listlessness, poor sucking, fever, hypotonia, weak cry, and Moro's and deep tendon reflexes that are difficult to elicit. Permanent symptoms appear after 18 months of age and may include choreoathetosis, dystonia, rigidity, tremor, upward gaze paralysis, mental retardation, spasticity, and hearing impairment.
2. Related to the combination of hyperbilirubinemia and cerebral ischemia and hypoxia in the newborn with resultant deposition of unconjugated bilirubin in the brain (primarily the basal ganglia). This form of "cerebral palsy" is now rare because most infants are effectively treated early for hyperbilirubinemia, and good prenatal care prevents most causes of perinatal hypoxia.

B. **Treatment:** An attempt should be made to prevent kernicterus by treating newborn hyperbilirubinemia using techniques such as phototherapy and exchange transfusion.

XI. GILLES de la TOURETTE SYNDROME.
A. **Diagnostic considerations.**
▶ 1. Syndrome of axial (trunk, neck, and face) tics with onset usually between 6 and 15 years of age; more common in males. Childhood hyperactivity may precede the onset of tics.
2. Initial symptoms include eye blinks, facial tics, and facial grimaces followed (in months and years) by sud-

den involuntary movements of the head, neck, shoulders, trunk, or legs. These movements may be repeated several times a minute and become worse with stress.

3. Frequently movements are accompanied by phonic (vocal, respiratory) tics which initially are grunts, snorts, or yells, but eventually may develop into repeated obscenities yelled in a loud voice with no provocation (coprolalia). Phonic tics are a hallmark of the disease.

4. The character of the abnormal movements may change over the years.

B.   Treatment.

1. Patients seem to be able to gain some voluntary control of the tics, but must, from time to time, "let it out." It should be emphasized that this is purely a social disability, and has not prevented many patients with this disease from leading productive lives.

2. Haloperidol, at a recommended dose of 0.25 to 10.0 mg daily, may result in improvement. Careful dose adjustment is important for long-term therapy.

    Caveat: Long-term use of a neuroleptic such as haloperidol may result in tardive dyskinesia.

3. Another dopamine receptor blocking drug, pimozide, has been found to be effective in suppressing the phonic and motor tics. Initial dose is 1 to 2 mg/day, which can be gradually increased to achieve a maintenance dose of less than 0.2 mg/kg/day.

    Caveat: Electrocardiographic (ECG) study should be done periodically, since the drug prolongs the QT interval.

4. Clonidine, 0.05 mg/kg/day, increased by 0.05 mg/kg every 2 weeks to a therapeutic dose ranging from 0.1 to 0.9 mg/kg/day, is often effective in controlling the behavior disorder sometimes associated with the syndrome. Clonidine patches (TTS) are a convenient form of treatment.

5. Educational material for patients and information about local support groups may be obtained from the Tourette Syndrome Association, Inc, 4240 Bell Blvd., Bayside, NY 11361, telephone (718) 224-2999 or 800-237-0717.

XII. HEMIBALLISMUS.
A. Clinical features.
▶ 1. Rare disorder characterized by sudden onset of violent involuntary movement (unilaterally and contralateral to the lesion), mainly of the arm; the appearance is similar to a baseball pitcher's windup.
2. Movement is worsened by stress.
3. Caused by a lesion of the subthalamic nucleus, usually as a result of hemorrhage or infarction. The patient frequently suffers from chronic hypertension.
B. Treatment.
1. There is usually spontaneous recovery.
2. For long-term control of movement, oral diazepam alone or diazepam supplemented with reserpine or haloperidol has been used with variable success.

Caveat: This disorder should not be confused with focal motor seizures (see Chapter 11, section VII. B).

XIII. MYOCLONUS.
A.
Myoclonus resembles the muscular twitching seen in dogs and cats as they drop off to sleep. Causes of myoclonus include central nervous system (CNS) degenerative disorders, benign hereditary myoclonus, cerebral anoxia, and metabolic disorders. The movement is indicative of a CNS disorder, but from a neurologic point of view, has poor localizing value. For severe persistent myoclonus, pharmacotherapy (as with clonazepam or valproic acid) may be helpful.

Caveat: A demented patient with myoclonus very likely has Creutzfeldt-Jakob disease (see Chapter 6, section V. B). The brains of such patients harbor an infectious agent.

XIV. ASTERIXIS.
A. **Clinical features.**
▶ 1. A movement disorder brought out primarily when the patient extends the arm forward with the wrist also extended. Irregular sudden flexion at the wrist (from gravitational pull) is followed by extension of the wrist back to the original position (Fig 7–7). This movement has also been called "negative myoclonus."
  2. Although originally described in hepatic disease ("liver flap"), it occurs in patients with a wide variety of metabolic disorders (such as renal failure, pulmonary insufficiency, malabsorption syndromes).

B. **Treatment:** Treatment of the underlying metabolic disorder is indicated.

XV. DYSTONIA.
A. Dystonia is a sustained abnormal posture. The most common form is spasmodic torticollis with persistent contraction of the sternocleidomastoid. Patients may also have sustained closure of the eyes (blepharospasm). Medical treatment for dystonia is often ineffective, but botulinum

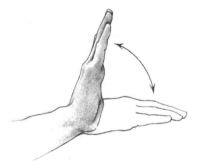

FIG 7–7. Asterixis. The patient is unable to maintain wrist extension; intermittently there is a sudden loss of tone, causing the hand to flap in a "bye-bye" gesture.

toxin A (Botox) injected into an affected muscle may give relief for several months. This should be done under electromyographic (EMG) control by an experienced practitioner. Causes of dystonia include cerebral anoxia, birth injury, head trauma, or the rare syndromes of dystonia musculorum deformans and hepatolenticular degeneration (Wilson's disease).

XVI. **MOVEMENT DISORDERS ASSOCIATED WITH NEUROLEPTICS.**

A. **Acute parkinsonism.** The symptoms of acute parkinsonism often are dramatically relieved with diphenhydramine hydrochloride (Benadryl) 50 mg intravenously (IV).

B. **Tardive dyskinesias.**
   1. Tardive dyskinesia develops in a significant number of patients receiving long-term treatment with neuroleptic drugs (especially the more potent phenothiazines or haloperidol).
   2. Symptoms include an oral-buccal-lingual stereotypy involving tongue protrusion, lip smacking, and facial grimacing. Abnormal movements of limbs and trunk may be seen.
   3. Treatment.
      a. In many patients, tardive dyskinesia remains refractory to all forms of treatment. Symptoms may be relieved by titrating reserpine slowly until movements are relieved. After control for 1 to 3 months slow weaning may be possible.
      b. A therapeutic trial of reserpine at an initial dose of 0.25 mg bid increased to 2 to 8 mg/day may relieve symptoms in some patients.
      c. Clozapine (Clozaril) is sometimes effective in controlling tardive dyskinesia, but should only be prescribed by a clinician thoroughly experienced in its use.
      d. The best treatment is preventive, i.e., prescribing neuroleptics only for serious psychiatric disorders and monitoring patients carefully for the side effects.

C. **Akathisia.** Akathisia is a *reversible* motor restlessness which is often confused with psychotic agitation. It is seen acutely with treatment with neuroleptics and with some antihistamines or as part of the tardive dyskinesia syndrome.

XVII. **OTHER MEDICATIONS ASSOCIATED WITH MOVEMENT DISORDERS.**

A. **CNS stimulants** (amphetamine or methylphenidate) may produce tics.

B. **Antihistamines, oral contraceptives (similar to chorea gravidarum of natural pregnancy), anticonvulsants, and chloroquine** occasionally produce involuntary choreoathetosis, dystonia, or myoclonus.

C. **The meperidine analogue MPTP** (1-methyl-4-phenyl-1,2,3,6-tetrahydropyridine), an illicit "designer" drug, damages the substantia nigra and produces parkinsonism.

BIBLIOGRAPHY

Carter CO, Evans KA, Baraitser M: Effect of genetic counseling on the prevalence of Huntington's chorea. *Br Med J* 1983; 286:281–283.

Elble RJ, Koller WC: *Tremor*. Baltimore, Johns Hopkins University Press, 1990.

Elizan TS, Moros DA, Yahr MD: Early combination of selegiline and low dose levodopa as initial symptomatic therapy in Parkinson's disease. *Arch Neurol* 1991; 48:31–34.

Fahn S, Jankovic J: Practical management of dystonia. *Neurol Clin* 1984; 2:555–569.

Fahn S, Marsden CD, Van Woert MH: *Myoclonus*. New York, Raven Press, 1986.

Harding AE, Deufel T: *Inherited Ataxias*. New York, Raven Press, 1993.

Harper PS: *Huntington's Disease*. Philadephia, WB Saunders, 1991.

Jankovic JJ, Brin MF: Therapeutic uses of botulinum toxin. *N Engl J Med* 1991; 324:1186–1194.

Joseph AB, Young RR: *Movement Disorders in Neurology and Neuropsychiatry*. Boston, Blackwell Scientific, 1992.

Kennedy RH, et al: Treatment of blepharospasm with botulinum toxin. *Mayo Clin Proc* 1989; 64:1085–1090.

Koller WC: *Handbook of Parkinson's Disease*, ed 2. Basel, Marcel Dekker, 1992.

Marsden CD, Schachter M: Assessment of extrapyramidal disorders. *Br J Clin Pharmacol* 1981; 11:129–151.

Muenter MD: Should levodopa therapy be started early or late? *Can J Neurol Sci* 1984; 11:195–199.

Muenter MD, Daube JR, Caviness JN, Miller PM: Treatment of essential tremor with methazolamide. *Mayo Clin Proc* 1991; 66:991–997.

Nutt J: Effect of cholinergic agents in Huntington's disease: A reappraisal. *Neurology* 1983; 33:932–935.

Shapiro AK, Shapiro ES, Young JG, et al: *Gilles de la Tourette Syndrome*, ed 2. New York, Raven Press, 1988.

Snyder SH: Parkinson's disease: Fresh factors to consider. *Nature* 1991; 350:195–196.

Swaiman KF: Myoclonus. *Neurol Clin* 1985; 3:197–208.

Weiner WJ, Lang AE: *Movement Disorders: A Comprehensive Survey*. Mount Kisco, NY, Futura, 1989.

NEUROLOGIC COMPLICATIONS OF ALCOHOLISM

8

In the United States, alcohol abuse accounts for a substantial percentage of hospital admissions, highway deaths, and psychiatric disturbances, yet alcoholic beverages are readily available and accepted by many Americans as a routine adjunct to social interaction. Identifying a pathologic user is one of the most common and difficult challenges facing the physician.

I. ALCOHOL ABUSE.

A. Establishing the diagnosis.

1. Table 8–1 may be used as a basis for the patient interview. Positive responses in several categories make it likely that the patient is alcohol-dependent.

2. The CAGE questionnaire consists of four questions, and has proved to be a specific and sensitive tool in the diagnosis of alcoholism. The acronym comes from *c*utting down, *a*nnoyance by criticism, *g*uilty feelings, and *e*ye openers. Positive answers to two or more of these four questions correlates highly with alcoholism:
   a. Ever felt the need to cut down drinking?
   b. Ever felt annoyed by criticism of drinking?
   c. Ever had guilty feelings about drinking?
   d. Ever take morning eye openers?

3. The diagnosis of alcoholism is associated with social stigmata: patients from lower socioeconomic classes more often (unfairly) have the diagnosis on their medical chart than do more affluent patients from higher socioeconomic classes. A clear medical diagnosis of alcoholism may be a powerful incentive to reform.

TABLE 8-1. Suggested Questions for Use in Establishing the Diagnosis of Alcohol Dependence

Preoccupation

　　What are the occasions on which you have had a drink this past week (month)?

　　When do you think about drinking?

　　When during the day do you sometimes feel you need a drink?

　　How often during the past week (month) did you crave a drink in the morning?

Increased tolerance

　　How often during the past week (month) have you been able to drink more than others and not show it?

　　Has anyone ever commented on your ability to hold your liquor?

　　Why do you think you are able to do this?

　　How does this make you feel?

Gulping drinks

　　What strength drinks do you prefer?

　　How long does it take you to finish your first drink?

　　How many drinks do you usually have before going out to dinner or to a party?

Drinking alone

　　When in the past week (month) did you have a drink alone?

　　Where were you when you had a drink alone? (At home? In a bar?)

Use as a medicine

　　What are some of the reasons you drink? (Calm nerves? Reduce tension? As a nightcap to get to sleep? Relieve physical discomfort? Relieve feelings of inadequacy or depression?)

　　Do you enjoy parties or dances if there is nothing to drink?

Blackout

　　When during the past week (month) have you been unable to remember what happened the night before?

　　When during the past week (month) have you been unable to remember how you got home after a night's drinking?

Physical

　　What reasons have doctors given you to cut down or stop drinking?

　　Where have you been hospitalized for drinking or a complication from drinking?

Social

　　How many of your friends drink?

　　How has your group of friends changed since you began drinking?

　　How have your hobbies and interests changed since you began drinking?

　　How often in the past week (month) have you been ashamed of what you did while you were drinking?

　　What kinds of things have you done that you were ashamed of while you were drinking?

　　How do you act while you are drinking?

Family

　　Is there anyone in the family who is or was an alcoholic?

4. Many alcoholics are extremely skillful (consciously or subconsciously) in camouflaging their addiction.

5. Any patient with a physical disability secondary to alcohol *is* an alcoholic (peripheral neuropathy, cirrhosis, dementia, cerebellar degeneration).

6. Any patient with withdrawal symptoms from alcohol abstinence *is* an alcoholic.

7. The quantity of alcohol consumed does not necessarily define an alcoholic; body weight, nutrition, ethnic background, medical condition, and medical therapy all influence a patient's sensitivity to the acute and chronic effects of alcohol.

8. In making a diagnosis of alcoholism, the physician must make every effort to be *objective;* the alcoholic physician makes the diagnosis too seldom, and the teetotaler makes it too often.

B. Clinical clues to alcohol abuse.

1. Physical examination: On the general physical examination the following signs may indicate a diagnosis of alcoholism:

   a. Excessive sweating, tachycardia, flushed face (withdrawal syndrome).

   b. Bruises, cigarette burns, or other trauma often incurred with severe drunkenness.

   c. Signs of liver disease: palmar erythema, vascular spiders, jaundice.

   d. Neurologic abnormalities: coarse hand tremor, peripheral neuropathy, forgetfulness, emotional lability.

   e. Poor hygiene, dehydration, poor nutrition.

   f. Persistent or recurrent infections.

   g. Odor of alcohol on breath at the time of examination.

2. Laboratory findings: On the laboratory profile the following abnormalities may indicate a diagnosis of alcoholism:

   a. A blood alcohol level of 150 mg/dL in a rational patient strongly suggests tolerance to alcohol, implying heavy and persistent alcohol ingestion.

   b. Blood count showing a mean corpuscular volume (MCV) greater than 97 with round macrocytosis.

   c. Elevated serum uric acid levels without history of gout.

   d. Elevation of serum alanine aminotransferase (glutamic-pyruvic transaminase, or SGPT), serum aspartate aminotransferase (glutamic-oxaloacetic transaminase, or SGOT), and γ-glutamyltransferase (GGT, or glutamyl transpeptidase).

C. **Stupor and coma in alcoholic intoxication.** This diagnosis should *only* be made with a blood alcohol level greater than 300 mg/dL and *without* other cause for coma. *Most* comatose patients with an "odor of alcohol" on their breath will have some other cause for coma, such as diabetic ketoacidosis or another drug. Subdural hematoma, particularly bilateral subdural hematomas without localizing signs, must be suspected or ruled out in all cases of stupor or coma in an alcoholic.

1. Treatment
   a. The physician must look for some other cause of coma and treat that cause appropriately.
   b. Immediate measures as in treatment of any coma: Assure clear airway, treat shock, check blood glucose levels, administer glucose and thiamine (see Chapter 13, section I. A).
   c. Gastric lavage is unnecessary; the bladder should be emptied and drainage instituted.
   d. Check vital signs frequently; mechanical ventilation may be necessary.
   e. In addition to blood levels for blood alcohol, obtain blood levels for other sedative drugs.

D. **Alcoholic blackouts:** Alcoholic patients with blackouts may be suffering from seizures or may be having *simple alcoholic blackouts.*

1. Alcoholic blackouts are periods of amnesia during which the patient apparently functions normally but later has no recall for that period; they are related to the acute effect of alcohol.
2. Blackouts are not necessarily correlated with blood alcohol level.
3. They are usually of short duration.
4. Blackouts often are an early neurologic symptom of potential alcoholism.
5. They may rarely occur paradoxically in the nonalcoholic person who consumes a large quantity of alcohol.
6. A related phenomenon is pathologic intoxication in which

relatively small amounts of alcohol produce irrational and combative behavior for which the patient may later be amnesic.

E. Alcohol withdrawal syndromes.
1. Chronic consumption of alcohol results in physical dependence. There are at least four withdrawal syndromes:
   a. Tremulousness.
   b. Alcoholic hallucinosis.
   c. Withdrawal seizures.
   d. Delirium tremens.
2. Withdrawal symptoms (listed separately here but often occurring in various combinations) usually begin at any time during which there is a falling blood alcohol level, and may occur as late as 7 days after cessation of alcohol intake. Prolonged or late withdrawal syndromes may occur in patients who abuse other drugs along with alcohol, or in patients who are receiving tranquilizers or sedatives in a treatment program. The severity of the syndrome is affected by a variety of factors including associated illness, other drug use or abuse, and environmental factors, as well as the amount of alcohol consumed and the duration of alcohol abuse.
3. In all of the withdrawal syndromes, treatment with atenolol is recommended in addition to the other therapy. The maximum dose is atenolol 100 mg/day, with no drug given if the heart rate is less than 50 beats/min and 50 mg given when the heart rate is 50 to 70 beats/min. This regimen significantly reduces the duration of the withdrawal syndrome.
   a. Tremulousness.
      1) The "shakes" or "jitters" often occur in the morning following a few days of excessive alcohol consumption and are frequently responsible for early-morning alcohol consumption to relieve symptoms.
      ▶ 2) Tremulousness is associated with general irritability and gastrointestinal problems (especially nausea and vomiting). There may also be overalertness, flushed facies, tachycardia, anorexia, or insomnia.
      3) A tendency to startle, uneasiness, jerkiness of movement, and insomnia may persist for as long as 2 weeks.

4) Treatment: In severe reactions benzodiazepines (such as diazepam 5–10 mg PO q2h prn) may be instituted and can be withdrawn over several days.

b. Alcoholic hallucinosis.

▶ 1) The patient complains of terrifying hallucinations with no disorientation. Generally these are auditory hallucinations, lasting a brief period of time. Visual hallucinations are less common.

2) May be related to rapid eye movement (REM) rebound, since alcohol is known to suppress REM sleep.

3) Treatment.

a) Hospitalization is usually necessary; if the patient is not hospitalized, close supervision is necessary.

b) Diazepam (Valium) 5 to 10 mg PO q2h prn may be used for sedation. Alternative drugs are lorazepam 1 to 2 mg or chlordiazepoxide 50 to 100 mg.

c) Institute a high-protein diet, supplemented with multiple vitamin therapy including thiamine 50 mg bid PO.

d) Make every attempt to keep the patient oriented to reality by having a sympathetic person present who can reassure the patient that the hallucinations are not real.

e) Occasionally, patients with alcoholic hallucinosis may enter a chronic stage of hallucinosis following the clearing of the alcohol withdrawal process. Such a condition may require neuroleptic treatment.

f) During the phase of acute and remitting alcoholic hallucinosis, the patient may need treatment with a neuroleptic, which can be discontinued following remission of symptoms and a successful withdrawal regimen.

c. *Withdrawal seizures* ("rum fits").

▶ 1) Withdrawal seizures are characteristically brief generalized convulsions with loss of consciousness.

2) They may be preceded by an aura of "fear" (anticipation of doom).

3) About one third of patients with alcohol withdrawal seizures develop delirium tremens.

4) In patients with preexisting epilepsy, alcohol withdrawal may increase the frequency and intensity of seizures.

5) Alcoholics frequently have cortical scars from repeated head trauma, and these scars may trigger seizures during alcohol withdrawal.

6) Treatment.

a) Usually anticonvulsant medication is *not* necessary since seizures cease before medication becomes effective; diazepam 5 to 10 mg PO q2h prn for treatment of other associated withdrawal symptoms may be preventive.

b) Rarely, a withdrawal seizure may result in status epilepticus, which should be handled as described in Chapter 11, section X.

c) An alcoholic with epilepsy who continues to consume alcoholic beverages should probably not be given anticonvulsants, since compliance is usually poor. If compelled to use long-term anticonvulsants because of frequent seizures, phenytoin is the drug of choice. Phenobarbital should not be used since abrupt withdrawal may cause seizures even in patients who are not epileptic.

d. Delirium tremens.

▶ 1) Delirium tremens is characterized by profound confusion, delusions, extremely vivid visual hallucinations, tremor, agitation, and insomnia, as well as signs of increased autonomic nervous system activation (i.e., fever, tachycardia, profuse sweating).

2) The patient is suspicious, restless, very disoriented, and difficult to distract; he or she carries on imaginary conversations or activities and may shout for hours or mutter inaudibly.

3) The peak incidence is between 72 and 96 hours following cessation of alcohol consumption.

4) Treatment.

a) *This is a medical emergency, since mortality may reach 15% in the untreated state.*

b) Maintenance of fluid and electrolyte balance is the most important consideration.

c) Treat with diazepam 5 to 20 mg PO q2h prn or diazepam 10 mg intravenously (IV) immediately, then 5 mg IV q15 minutes until the patient is quiet, but not asleep. Alternatively, lorazepam 1 to 2 mg (or 0.07 mg/kg) IV can be given.

d) Carefully record all intake and output.

e) Administration of large quantities of IV fluids are necessary. Usually 6 L of IV fluids are required per day:
   i) Glucose (at least 5%) must be included in each IV solution.
   ii) Thiamine 50 mg must be included in each liter of IV solution.
   iii) A therapeutic multivitamin preparation must be included in the first IV solution.
   iv) Potassium, sodium, calcium, and magnesium must be added to the IV solutions based on the patient's laboratory determinations.

f) Restraints are almost always necessary, but a patient adequately sedated with diazepam may need less restraint.

g) Search for associated injury or infection (especially cerebral laceration, subdural hematoma, pneumonia, and meningitis).

h) Seizures require treatment *if* they are repeated, continuous, or life-threatening. Anticonvulsants need not be continued past the withdrawal period, unless there was a preexisting seizure disorder.

i) Pancreatitis, cirrhosis, and renal disease frequently complicate the course of delirium tremens.

Caveat: The symptoms of delirium tremens resemble those of carbon dioxide narcosis. Carbon dioxide narcosis may occur in patients with delirium tremens who also have chronic obstructive pulmonary disease and have been given sedatives that can depress respirations.

II. NUTRITIONAL DISEASES SECONDARY TO ALCOHOLISM.

A. **Wernicke-Korsakoff syndrome:** This is an acute, subacute, or chronic disease of central nervous system (CNS) injury related to thiamine deficiency.

1. Wernicke's syndrome is the *acute* disorder.
   a. Clinical features.
      ▶ 1) Nystagmus associated with ataxia and a confusional state.
      2) Followed by paralysis of extraocular muscles in any combination.
   b. Treatment: *This is a neurologic emergency* and should be treated *immediately* with thiamine 100 mg IV. Prompt treatment will reverse the neurologic deficit.

2. Korsakoff's psychosis results if Wernicke's syndrome is not treated.
   a. Clinical features.
      1) The outstanding feature of the mental disturbance is the inability to form new memories despite relatively intact immediate recall and relatively preserved remote memory. In effect, it is as though the patient's intellectual life was arrested at the moment of the onset of the pathologic condition.
      2) In conversation, the patient may discuss situations or give answers which sound very plausible but have little basis in reality (part of the mental aberration known as confabulation). For example, when asked what was served for breakfast, the patient may describe a sumptuous feast when in reality there was no meal that day.
   b. Treatment: Thiamine 50 mg bid should be administered to patients with Korsakoff's psychosis even though the disease is generally considered irreversible.

III. OTHER ALCOHOL-ASSOCIATED DISORDERS.

A. **Peripheral neuropathy associated with alcohol.**

1. Diagnostic considerations.
   a. Peripheral neuropathy is usually the earliest neurologic symptom of chronic alcoholism.
   b. The disorder is primarily a sensory neuropathy with the

patient complaining of burning or painful feet (see Chapter 15, section II. A).

c. Very hypoactive or absent ankle reflexes are usually evident on examination before the patient notes any symptoms, and should alert the physician to the diagnosis of alcoholism. Evidence of summation on sensory examination (see Chapter 1, section I. G) as well as subjective symptoms of sensory loss are apparent later.

d. The patient's feet may have thin, atrophic skin devoid of hair.

e. Peripheral neuropathy is often seen in association with the Wernicke-Korsakoff syndrome.

2. Treatment: May respond to thiamine 50 mg bid, as well as abstinence from alcohol.

B. Alcoholic dementia.

1. Cerebral atrophy by computed tomography (CT) scan or magnetic resonance imaging (MRI) and deterioration of intellectual function are well documented in chronic alcoholics.

2. Alcohol abuse is one of the common causes of dementia. Fortunately, *substantial recovery* of function may occur if the patient ceases alcohol consumption.

C. Alcoholic cerebellar degeneration.

1. Clinicopathologic features.

a. Alcoholic cerebellar degeneration is characterized primarily by truncal ataxia and difficulty in tandem walking with lesser degrees of abnormality seen on finger-to-nose testing (see Fig 7–3).

b. Subacute onset is over several weeks or months

c. Pathologic finding is degeneration of midline cerebellar structures.

d. Not clearly related to thiamine deficiency.

2. Treatment: Abstinence from alcohol and oral thiamine 50 mg bid supplementation is recommended but is of no clear benefit.

D. Alcoholic myopathy.

1. Diagnostic considerations.

a. The chronic form of alcoholic myopathy presents with proximal muscle wasting and weakness; creatine phosphokinase (CPK) is mildly elevated; muscle biopsy shows type II muscle fiber atrophy, necrosis, and other anatomic abnormalities.

b. The acute form presents with severe weakness, myoglobinuria, and rhabdomyolysis. This constitutes a medical emergency and should be treated with vigorous diuresis to prevent renal failure from the myoglobinuria; additionally, serum potassium levels must be closely monitored to prevent hyperkalemia.

2. Treatment: Alcoholic myopathy is potentially reversible if the patient abstains from alcohol.

E. **Neurologic disorders due to liver dysfunction.**

1. There are two syndromes of hepatic encephalopathy:

a. *Acute hepatic encephalopathy* is a progressive state of altered consciousness, ataxia, dysarthria, asterixis, lethargy, and finally coma. During this progression, characteristic electroencephalographic (EEG) abnormalities can be detected. This syndrome is reversible with appropriate treatment of the liver disease. The degree of coma does not necessarily correlate with the degree of hyperammonemia.

b. *Chronic hepatic encephalopathy:* After repeated episodes of hepatic coma with recovery, a chronic progressive dementia develops.

2. Treatment: Treatment should be directed at the underlying liver disease.

F. **Chronic alcoholism:** The treatment of alcohol abuse (chronic alcoholism) has the goals of sobriety and amelioration of the psychological problems underlying the alcohol abuse. The "cure" rate is low, but no worse than that of bronchogenic carcinoma. Sadly, many physicians treat only the complications of alcoholism, not the disease itself.

1. Alcoholics Anonymous (AA), a worldwide informal fellowship of recovering alcohol abusers, has been shown to be the most effective therapy. The philosophy is embodied in a series of steps to guide the person to recovery. There are also associated groups for the spouses (Al-Anon) and for teenage children (Al-Ateen). It is generally agreed that alcoholic patients should be encouraged to attend AA meetings on a regular basis. Each physician should identify a local resource person in AA to contact should the

need arise. Alcoholics Anonymous information may also be obtained from the General Service Office of AA, Box 459, Grand Central Station, New York, NY 10017, telephone (212) 870-3400.

2. Some alcoholic patients may need supportive individual therapy. For others, group therapy or family therapy, or both, may be more effective. It is very important to encourage family support and employment when appropriate and realistic. When a mental disorder is associated with alcoholism, the most likely condition is an affective disorder, either bipolar or unipolar depression, and referral to a psychiatrist is necessary.

3. If there is lack of social support, or if it is deemed necessary by a psychiatrist, live-in programs, such as in halfway houses, may be appropriate. The physician must be aware of the facilities available in the community, such as programs administered by local mental health centers and other local agencies.

4. A source of information on alcohol for both physicians and patients is the National Clearinghouse for Alcohol, P.O. Box 2345, Rockville, MD 20852, telephone (301) 468-2600.

BIBLIOGRAPHY

Alldredge BK, Lowenstein DH, Simon RP: Placebo-controlled trial of IV diphenylhydantoin for short-term treatment of alcohol withdrawal seizures. *Am J Med* 1989; 87:645.

Berowitz NL: CNS manifestations of toxic disorders, in Avieff AJ, Griggs RC (eds): *Metabolic Brain Dysfunctions in Systemic Disorders.* Boston, Little, Brown, 1992, pp. 409–436.

Charness ME, Simon RP, Greenberg DA: Ethanol and the nervous system. *N Engl J Med* 1989; 321:442–454.

Ewing JA: Detecting alcoholism. The CAGE questionnaire. *JAMA* 1984; 252:1905–1907.

Kraus ML, Gottlieb LD, Horwitz RI, et al: Randomized clinical trial of atenolol in patients with alcohol withdrawal. *N Engl J Med* 1985; 313:905–909.

Martin F, Ward K, Slavin J, et al: Alcoholic skeletal myopathy, a clinical and pathological study. *Q J Med* 1985; 55:233–251.

McMicken DB: Alcohol withdrawal syndrome. *Emerg Med Clin North Am* 1990; 8:805–820.

Ng SKC, Hauser WA, Brust JCM, et al: Alcohol consumption and withdrawal in new-onset seizures. *N Engl J Med* 1988; 319:666.

Noori SS, Adelstein J: Evaluating and treating chronic alcoholism. *Pa Med* 1978; 81:33–36.

Reuler JB, Girard DE, Cooney TG: Wernicke's encephalopathy. *N Engl J Med* 1985; 312:1035–1039.

Victor M: Alcoholism, in Baker AB, Joynt RJ (eds): *Clinical Neurology*. Hagerstown, Md, Harper & Row, 1986.

Victor M, Adams RD, Collins GH: *The Wernicke-Korsakoff Syndrome*, ed 2. Philadelphia, FA Davis, 1989.

Young GP: Seizures in the alcholic patient. *Emerg Med Clin North Am* 1990; 8:821–834.

PSYCHIATRIC DISORDERS IN NEUROLOGIC DISEASE

9

Psychiatric and neurologic abnormalities often occur concomitantly in the same patient. Diseases once thought to be "emotional" now unquestionably have an organic basis: these include schizophrenia and manic-depressive psychosis. The boundary between psychiatry and neurology is becoming less and less distinct. If a physician is able to recognize the common psychiatric disturbances, diagnosis of many "neurologic" problems is facilitated and unnecessary diagnostic tests and referrals may be avoided. Psychiatric conditions should never be diagnosed by exclusion. Positive evidence must be gathered from the history and physical examination, and inconsistencies with known patterns of anatomy and physiology are major diagnostic clues. Unfortunately for the diagnostician, the presence of mental, emotional, or behavior disturbances does not preclude the existence of another underlying organic abnormality. In order to convince a physician of the seriousness of the presenting complaint, patients sometimes considerably embellish symptoms. Psychiatric diagnosis should not be made lightly, because such labels may preclude investigation of organic symptoms at a later date. The intent of this chapter is to illuminate the interrelationship between common neurologic and psychiatric disorders, not to be a definitive psychiatric text.

I. DEPRESSION.

A. **Depression** is so pervasive in the population of ill adults that physicians may unwittingly accept it as the norm. This depression may be the basic underlying illness, the result of a chronic disease process or disability, or drug-induced.

1. Grief reaction (bereavement, reactive depression): This is the sadness which is a natural human emotion following personal loss. It is especially common in patients who have chronic diseases which in some way result in the loss of normal functional abilities and activities. It may also result from the death of, or separation from, a loved one. This type of depression does not usually respond to drug therapy.

   a. Treatment.

      1) Grief reaction is potentially a life-threatening situation, e.g., the man who has just lost his wife and children in an automobile accident may commit suicide.

      2) The patient needs the opportunity to discuss feelings and requires sympathetic support; this may be accomplished through a pastor, close friend, or professional counselor. If the family physician assumes this counseling responsibility, the physician must be available to the patient whenever things are not going well.

      3) Drugs are not indicated; the disorder is self-limited and will gradually fade with time.

2. Major depression (endogenous depression).

   a. Description.

      1) The depressed patient has an "emptiness" that is out of proportion to any life crises experienced. If questioned carefully, such patients reveal a mood alteration that is different in quality from the sadness experienced after personal misfortunes, bereavements, and tragedies.

      2) Major depressions may seem to be precipitated by some life event, but this is coincidence and not causation. In addition, positive changes in life circumstances do not improve the depression.

      3) Although patients with either major depression or grief reaction may have a variety of psychological symptoms, it is the physiologic symptoms characteristic of major depression (see Table 9–1) that

TABLE 9–1.
Symptomatology of Depressive Illness

Physiologic (Biologic, Vegetative)	Psychological (Behavioral)
Sleep disturbance Delayed insomnia Frequent awakening	Dysphoric mood, unhappiness, sadness, crying spells
Somatic complaints Headaches Abdominal pain Dizziness Vague aches and pains Blurred vision	Cognitive negatives Negative feelings about self (low self-esteem, self-deprecation) Negative feelings about relationships or friendships (or paranoia) Negative feelings about the future (pessimism, hopelessness)
Alimentary tract disturbance Eating disorder (increase in or loss of appetite) Constipation	Irritability, anger, poor frustration tolerance, temper outbursts
Weight change (loss or gain)	Social withdrawal
Fatigue	Guilt
	Loss of interest or pleasure in usual activities (including loss of interest in school)
Diminished sexual function (loss of libido)	Preoccupation with death; suicidal thoughts, threats, or attempts
Psychomotor disturbance Increased body activity (agitation or hyperactivity) or decreased body activity (retardation) Increased or decreased mental activity (including impaired concentration and confusion)	
Nonreactivity to surrounding events (including inconsolability or nonreactivity to cheering efforts)	
Diurnal variation in mood and symptoms (usually worse in the morning)	

often cause a patient to seek the physician's help. Common presentations include headaches, chronic pain, sleep disturbances, eating disturbances, confusion, and memory disturbances.

4) Major depression is the result of an alteration of central nervous system (CNS) biochemistry and thus responds to drug therapy. Usually the condition is idiopathic, but occasionally the major depression may have a demonstrable cause.

b. Treatment: The patient with major depression often may be successfully treated by the primary care physician, if the depression is not severe and if the following guidelines are followed:

1) Take time to form a supportive relationship with the patient. Explain the nature of the illness, the fact that the medication may not be effective immediately, and will probably not be magical. Schedule frequent return visits to discuss any problems, including troublesome side effects of the drugs and possible suicidal ideation.

2) Take suicidal thoughts and gestures seriously. Patients who talk about suicide will often attempt suicide. Clear suicidal ideation or attempts are stark testimony to the existence of a suicidal state. Such patients should be hospitalized with appropriate psychiatric evaluation and treatment.

3) Involve family members in the treatment; insist that they accompany the patient on office visits. The family may be very helpful in assessing the efficacy of the drug and may notice improvement in the patient's condition before the patient does. Families are an excellent source of information with regard to compliance, side effects, and suicidal thoughts.

4) Be familiar with the side effects of antidepressant medications. Patients will have a dry mouth, some grogginess, especially in the mornings, and some constipation. Orthostatic hypotension, blurring of vision, tachycardia, and minor memory difficulties

may also be troublesome. The patient should be told that the side effects often subside with time.

5) The most widely used antidepressant medications are amitriptyline hydrochloride, imipramine hydrochloride, and nortriptyline hydrochloride. One of these should be initiated at a single dose of 25 to 50 mg at bedtime, and the dosage gradually increased to a therapeutically effective level (150–200 mg/day) during the next week or so. Occasionally a patient who is unusually sensitive to side effects may require a smaller starting dose (10 or 20 mg/day). Serum drug levels may be obtained to monitor the dosage. Once remission is attained, the dosage may be gradually lowered to a maintenance level, which is usually about 10% to 20% lower than the maximum dosage reached. Remember that these drugs are potentially lethal when taken as an overdose and not more than 500 mg should be dispensed at any one time to a patient when there is any possibility of suicidal risk.

6) Fluoxetine (Prozac) 20 mg in the morning is an excellent alternative or initial drug for depression. Side effects are few and the therapeutic effect is often dramatic. Unwarranted adverse publicity, however, makes the drug unacceptable to a significant number of patients. However, it must be remembered that patients with behavior disturbances will often do bizarre or "crazy" things whether or not they are receiving medication, and the medication may not be the cause.

Caveat: Severely depressed patients are most apt to commit suicide as they improve; in such patients, hospital admission for medication administration and careful monitoring is preferable.

7) Encourage the patient to continue with usual activities, but to make as few important decisions as possible while in the depressed state. Irretrievable steps such as resigning from a job, divorcing a

spouse, or selling property should be expressly discouraged while the patient is depressed.

8) Discontinue the antidepressant medication gradually over a period of several weeks after the patient has been asymptomatic for at least 6 months.

9) Recognize anticholinergic psychosis characterized by restless agitation, confusion, disorientation, and perhaps seizures. The patient may have dry and sometimes flushed skin, tachycardia, dilated pupils, constipation, and urinary retention. This occurs especially in elderly patients who are taking other drugs such as benzodiazepines, antihistamines, and phenothiazines in addition to the tricyclic antidepressants.

3. Drug-induced depression. In otherwise normal persons (as well as persons susceptible to depression), the following drugs may induce depression: alcohol, reserpine, propranolol, α-methyldopa, benzodiazepines (such as diazepam), barbiturates, clonidine, corticosteroids, and oral contraceptives.

   a. Treatment: Withdrawal of the above drugs will often, but not always, result in remission of the depression. Concomitant pharmacotherapy for major depression is sometimes necessary.

4. Depression with neurologic disorders.

   a. Neurologic diseases commonly accompanied by depression are:
      1) Huntington's disease.
      2) Parkinson's disease.
      3) Multiple sclerosis.
      4) Stroke syndrome (especially involving the right hemisphere or bilateral frontal lobes).
      5) Myotonic dystrophy.

   b. Treatment: Physicians often identify with the depressed patient with neurologic disease ("I'd be depressed too, if I were that crippled"). However, if such patients have symptoms of major depression, a therapeutic drug trial is indicated and will often be successful. Antidepressant pharmacotherapy usually makes the neurologic disease more amenable to treatment.

5. Organic disease disguised as depression.
   a. *Dementia:* Especially in elderly patients, depression (depressive pseudodementia) may be virtually indistinguishable from dementia (see Chapter 6, section IV). Clinical clues for distinguishing these two entities are shown in Table 9–2.
   b. *"Silent" brain tumor:* With severe frontal or right parietal lobe involvement, the patient may present with only an alteration in mood. Paresis and alteration in reflexes may be subtle or absent. Such patients usually do not have a history of mood fluctuation; differentiation from dementia and depression may be made by:
      1) Focal neurologic findings.
      2) Abnormal neuropsychological test results.
      3) Magnetic resonance imaging (MRI) or computed tomography (CT) scan abnormality.
   c. *Pseudobulbar palsy:* Such patients will cry easily with minimal provocation, but will deny a feeling of sadness or emptiness. They have bilaterally increased deep tendon reflexes and an active jaw reflex. This is most frequently seen in elderly patients with a long history of hypertension (see Chapter 6, section III. B. 2).

II. ANXIETY.

A. **Anxiety** is a common accompaniment of many illnesses, but sometimes may be the underlying illness itself. When the anx-

TABLE 9–2.
Features Distinguishing Depression and Dementia

Feature	Dementia	Depression
Onset	Gradual	History of mood fluctuation
Appetite	Normal	Decreased
Constipation	Rare	Frequent
Motor activity	Relatively normal	Often decreased (may be agitated)
Mental status	Errors frequent	Tasks performed slowly but accurately

ious patient walks into the office, the following features may
be observed:
1. A hesitant or inappropriately hurried gait.
2. Rigid posture, often with excessive fidgeting.
3. Poor eye contact.
4. Excessive decoy activity (e.g., lighting a cigarette).

B. **The history** will often include the following:
1. Gastrointestinal disturbances (anorexia, nausea, vomiting, diarrhea, constipation).
2. Genitourinary dysfunction (urgency, frequency, dysmen-
orrhea, impotence).

C. **On examination,** the following may be noted:
1. Dilated pupils, tremulousness.
2. Excessive sweating.
3. Elevated blood pressure, rapid pulse.

D. **Recognition of anxiety symptoms** is important in the following conditions:
1. Headache: especially important with muscle contraction
headache (see Chapter 3, section IV).
2. Low back pain (see Chapter 17).
3. Alcohol and drug abuse: Anxiety may be an early symptom of alcohol withdrawal (see Chapter 8, section I. E),
or amphetamine or cocaine abuse.
4. Excessive use of coffee, caffeine-containing soft drinks,
and tobacco.
5. Vertigo: especially the hyperventilation syndrome (see
Chapter 4, section II. A).
6. May be one of the presenting symptoms of a serious depression.

Note: Prescription of benzodiazepines may aggravate
the underlying depression.

7. Patients receiving neuroleptic medication (such as haloperidol) may develop an inward restlessness and fidgety
legs and hands (akathisia). This is not a symptom of anxiety but a manifestation of neuroleptic toxicity and an increase in the neuroleptic dosage will only increase this
toxicity.
8. Symptoms resembling anxiety may be seen in the follow-

ing medical conditions: hypoglycemia, thyroid disorders, pheochromocytoma.

E. Treatment.

1. Identify the cause of anxiety, e.g., stressful occupation or home situation, phobias. A supportive physician-patient relationship is often sufficient treatment; occasionally psychological or psychiatric counseling is indicated.

2. Withdraw all drugs or toxic substances that may be related to anxiety, and diagnose and treat any underlying medical condition.

3. Pharmacologic treatment of anxiety.

   a. Pharmacologic treatment should be avoided if possible. Drugs should never be used as a substitute for a supportive physician-patient relationship. All antianxiety drugs become ineffective after a few months.

   b. Never prescribe barbiturates in anxiety states. The risk of dependency is too great, and overdosing is more lethal than with other drugs.

   c. Benzodiazepines are sometimes recommended in the treatment of anxiety, but a paradoxical reaction may worsen the anxiety in some patients and may cause drowsiness or ataxia. If benzodiazepines are used, the patient should be monitored closely and the length of treatment should be limited. Although alprazolam (Xanax) is commonly prescribed, we do not recommend it because of its highly addictive potential and a propensity to result in seizures on withdrawal.

   d. Never combine antianxiety drugs, and be sure to obtain a drug history before prescribing any medication. Patients with a history of heavy use of alcohol, tobacco, and nicotine should be given antianxiety agents with caution. The risk of dependency in such patients is high.

   e. The largest dose of an antianxiety drug may be given at bedtime to exploit its sedative properties. Diazepam (Valium) is the most frequently prescribed antianxiety drug: the dose is 5 to 10 mg PO tid.

   f. Buspirone hydrochloride (Buspar) is an antianxiety drug unrelated to the benzodiazepines; the usual dosage is 5 mg PO tid.

g. Propranolol hydrochloride (Inderal) 10 mg PO qid will alleviate many symptoms but should be prescribed with caution because it may induce or exacerbate a depression.

III. HYSTERICAL DISORDERS.

A. **There are two major categories** of hysterical disorders: 1) patients with factitious illness such as malingering or Munchausen's syndrome; 2) patients with signs and symptoms that have no organic basis, but the patient is not deliberately attempting to mislead the physician.

Caveat: The diagnosis of hysteria should be established on the basis of positive evidence, not the fact that all tests are negative. Also, even if the patient has an obvious hysterical disorder, a serious medical illness may still be present (**Remember:** Even hysterics sooner or later become ill and die.) However, many medical diagnostic tests carry serious risks, and hysterical patients should never be subjected to tests unnecessarily.

1. Factitious disorders (malingering; conscious, nonphysiologic disorder).
   a. The patient consciously feigns an illness in order to obtain something perceived as valuable.
   b. Often the examination is inconsistent with the complaint; e.g., weakness of an extremity or side of the body will not be associated with any change (increased, decreased, or pathologic) in tone or reflexes. When testing muscle strength, the patient may give way with a ratchet-like quality.
   c. Some patients make malingering a lifelong occupation. These persons feign illness with remarkably clever and complex histories, inflicting self-injury or administering drugs to produce abnormal signs consistent with the reported disease process. For example, such a patient will instill atropine into one eye to produce a fixed, dilated pupil, and then present with neurologic symptoms suggesting intracranial disease.

d. *Treatment.*
    1) The physician should attempt to determine the nature of the underlying gratification the patient obtains from the illness. Occasionally the patient will have had an organic disability that has resolved; however, because of the adverse social or legal repercussions of improvement, the patient must maintain the appearance of illness.
    2) Confrontation is usually of no benefit. A cure most frequently occurs when legal matters are settled or when the patient realizes that a secondary gain is not obtainable.
2. Conversion disorder (subconscious, nonphysiologic disorder with apparent neurologic dysfunction).
    a. Conversion symptoms have no physiologic or pathologic substrate. **Remember:** The patient is asking for help, but in an inappropriate way.
    b. Conversion symptoms often occur in mentally defective persons or in adolescents as a way of coping with the environment (albeit inadequately).
    c. Common presentations include blindness, deafness, paresis, sensory disturbances, ataxia, seizures, and unconsciousness.
    d. The following is a list of some conversion reactions with suggestions on how they may be recognized during the neurologic examination:
        1) *Bilateral blindness:* The patient will commonly avoid injury when walking and will blink to unexpected threat. Pupillary reactions are normal and opticokinetic nystagmus (nystagmus induced by rotating a striped drum in front of the patient's eyes) is normal. In organic blindness, pupillary reflexes and opticokinetic nystagmus are frequently abnormal. A hysterical visual field defect, when plotted out on a tangent screen, will not change with varying distance between the patient and the screen.
        2) *Unilateral blindness:* If there is an organic basis, the lesion must be anterior to the optic chiasm, and the pupillary reaction is usually abnormal. The

Marcus Gunn phenomenon is especially useful in evaluating unilateral blindness (see Chapter 10, Section I.B.2).

3) *Paralysis of the legs:* Reflexes are normal, and there is no atrophy. A useful test is as follows:
   a) With the patient supine, the examiner places both palms beneath the heels of the patient.
   b) The patient is then asked to lift the nonparalyzed leg. The patient will unconsciously increase the pressure in the palm of the hand in the paralyzed leg.
   c) The patient is then asked to press down with both heels. If pressure is not applied as it was when the patient lifted the nonparalyzed leg, a conversion reaction can be suspected (Fig 9–1).

4) *Hemiparesis:* A patient with a paralyzed leg and arm may incorrectly assume that there will also be difficulty in turning the head toward the paralyzed side (Fig 9–2). Pronation drift and hemiplegic posturing are also absent on station and gait.

5) *Reduced level of consciousness:* In a conversion reaction the pupillary and corneal reflexes and plantar responses will be normal. Often, when the patient's hand is held and dropped over the face, it will swerve to avoid striking the face. A patient with an organically caused reduced level of consciousness will usually have pupillary abnormalities and other positive neurologic signs (Fig 9–3).

6) *Deafness:* The patient with a conversion reaction may startle to loud noise and can be awakened from a sound sleep by a loud noise.

7) *Sensory disturbance:* Conversion reactions that involve only the sensory systems are difficult to prove. Organic sensory losses make anatomic sense, while conversion reaction sensory disturbances will follow the patient's perception of body anatomy:
   a) Patients with organic sensory disturbances are able to appreciate a vibrating tuning fork placed on either side of the head and on either side of

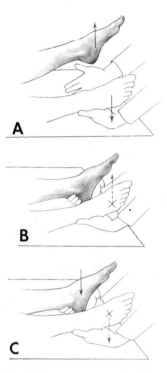

FIG 9–1. Distinguishing true paralysis from hysterical paralysis of the leg. Place both hands under the heels and ask the patient to raise the *good* leg: **A,** the examiner will feel increased downward pressure by the "paralyzed" leg. **B,** ask the patient to lift the paralyzed leg; there is little or no response. **C,** then ask the patient to bear down with both heels; if the same pressure noted in maneuver **A** cannot be exerted, "something is rotten in the state of Denmark."

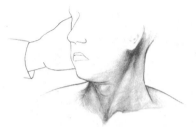

FIG 9–2. The *left* sternocleidomastoid muscle turns the head to the *right,* as illustrated. Patients with a psychogenic *left*-sided weakness will often show weakness when turning toward the left (or vice versa).

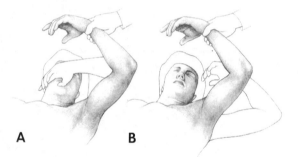

A   **B**

FIG 9–3. A, a hand dropped over the face of a comatose patient will strike the face. **B,** in psychogenic coma, a hand held over the face and then dropped often swerves to the side.

the sternum owing to the conduction of the vibration through the bone. In a conversion reaction, the sternum or head is split, i.e., vibration is perceived on one side of the midline of the forehead or sternum but not on the other (Fig 9–4).

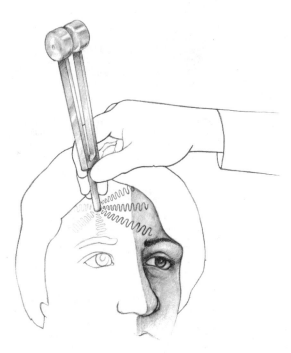

FIG 9–4. Even with an anesthetic face, the vibrations from a tuning fork will be transmitted via bone to the opposite side.

   b) If anesthesia is present, instruct the patient to close his or her eyes, and then instruct the patient to answer "yes" if the pinprick is felt or "no" if it is not. Obviously, the only appropriate answer is silence when the supposedly anesthetic area is touched. **Remember:** Many of these patients have limited intelligence.

c) If a sensory disturbance involves the hands, have the patient make a fist as illustrated in the diagram (Fig 9–5), and then quickly touch the fingers for differences in sensation. In this position, most hysterical patients cannot tell the difference between their right and left hands.

8) *Pain syndrome*. The conversion reaction patient has a very vivid description of the pain, but the pain usually does not interfere with the "pleasures of life." Analgesics, even narcotics, have little effect on the pain. Often the patient is addicted to narcotics. The patient with pain from an organic disorder will usually receive some relief from narcotics, and the pain will interfere with such pleasures of life as sleeping.

e. *Treatment*.
1) Confrontation of the patient is usually not helpful since the patient often develops other symptoms and will "doctor-shop." Such patients usually find psychiatrists very threatening, and often will refuse a psychiatric interview.

2) Rather than confront the conversion reaction patient, the physician should emphasize that the symptoms are not medically serious (e.g., "I'm so happy to be able to tell you that you do not have cancer or a brain tumor"). From that point on, try to substitute a discussion of life problems and interpersonal relations. It is important that the physician not reject or become angry with the hysterical patient. Limited, precisely scheduled visits and telephone calls on a regular basis are often helpful. With time, the physician may learn what goal or conflict is producing the conversion reaction. Administration of the Minnesota Multiphasic Personality Inventory (MMPI) and hypnosis in the hands of a skilled specialist may be helpful in this regard.

3) Once the diagnosis is made, the major goal is to avoid unnecessary hospitalization and surgery.

4) Drugs of any kind should be avoided in conversion states.

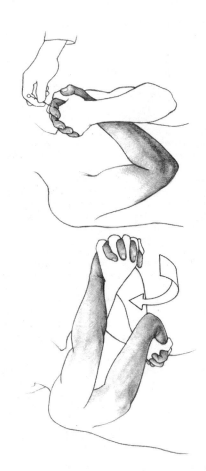

FIG 9–5. After having first demonstrated a sensory deficit in one hand, have the patient perform this maneuver and then quickly test sensation in the fingers again. This maneuver seriously distorts a person's sense of which hand is which, and accurate responses are extremely difficult unless sensation is truly disturbed.

IV. SCHIZOPHRENIA.

A. **Schizophrenia and the following neurologic problems occasionally cause diagnostic confusion:**

1. *Basal ganglia disease.* As a side effect of therapy with neuroleptics (phenothiazines and major tranquilizers), the schizophrenic patient may develop a restlessness, especially in the legs (akathisia). These patients are usually more "inwardly" restless than is immediately apparent. Neuroleptics may also produce a parkinsonian syndrome (see Chapter 7, section III).

2. *Dementia* (see Chapter 6, section I). Patients with catatonic schizophrenia may appear to be demented. However, schizophrenia causes a disorder of thought, while memory is spared.

3. *Aphasia* (see Chapter 12, section VII). The patient with parietal or temporal lobe damage (from tumor, infarct, hemorrhage, or trauma) may have a speech disturbance in which speech melody is normal, but the words make little sense. Specific testing for aphasia will distinguish aphasia from schizophrenia.

4. *Complex partial seizures* (see Chapter 11, section VII.C). With seizures, the onset of symptoms may begin and end abruptly. An electroencephalogram (EEG) using nasopharyngeal leads may reveal a spike focus in the temporal lobe. Patients with complex partial seizures have a distinctive personality profile, perhaps because of a disturbed limbic system, and this profile may be confused with schizophrenic personality profiles.

5. *Illicit drugs,* such as lysergic acid diethylamide (LSD), amphetamines, and phencyclidine (PCP) may produce states closely resembling schizophrenia. A history of drug abuse and a subacute onset will usually be distinguishing features. Prescribed medications such as thiazides, steroids, and disulfiram may also cause a disturbance of thinking resembling schizophrenia.

6. *Delirium tremens* may produce hallucinations and an agitated state (see Chapter 8, section I.E.3.d). The hallucinations with delirium tremens are usually visual, while those of schizophrenia are generally auditory.

7. *Wernicke-Korsakoff syndrome* (see Chapter 8, section II.A). This is an acute or subacute onset of extraocular muscle paralysis, ataxia, and mental changes that may resemble schizophrenia. When this is suspected, immediately give thiamine 100 mg intramuscularly (IM) or intravenously (IV). Schizophrenic patients do not have abnormal eye movements and ataxia.

8. *Diffuse CNS vascular disease,* such as that seen in hypertensive encephalopathy, tertiary syphilis (meningovascular syphilis), or collagen-vascular disease, may produce acute or chronic disturbances in thought processes that resemble schizophrenia.

9. *Endocrine dysfunctions,* especially those associated with thyroid and adrenal disorders, on occasion produce striking changes in mentation.

10. *Hereditary neurologic disease,* especially Huntington's disease, may produce schizophrenic symptoms years before the movement disorder becomes obvious.

B. **To differentiate true schizophrenia** from the preceding schizophrenic-like states, it is essential to take a careful history with special regard to:

1. Mode of onset (acute, subacute, or chronic).
2. Past history of similar disturbances.
3. Drugs, licit and illicit.
4. Alcohol intake.
5. Head trauma, seizures, or headache.
6. Temperature intolerance, weight change.
7. Family history.
8. History of viral encephalitis, especially herpes simplex encephalitis.

C. **On a screening neurologic examination,** pay particular attention to focal neurologic signs, abnormal movements, and posture.

D. **Minimal laboratory tests** that should be performed include the following:

1. Complete blood count (CBC) with erythrocyte sedimentation rate (ESR).
2. Serum sodium, potassium, blood urea nitrogen (BUN).
3. Serum test for syphilis.
4. Thyroid function tests.

     5. Consider also the following tests:
        a. Lumbar puncture.
        b. CT scan or MRI.

E. The following points may help the primary care physician recognize a schizophrenic patient. Florid schizophrenia is seldom seen, but borderline or subclinical schizophrenia, schizophrenia in remission, and schizophrenic patients being treated with neuroleptics are relatively common.

    1. Schizophrenic patients may be described as having "sunburned minds." That is to say, they are extremely sensitive to criticism, stress, emotional closeness, and rejection.

    2. Onset of symptoms is usually before the age of 40 years.

    3. The patient has a disorder of thought processes with an inappropriate rate, flow, or content of thinking, but the sensorium is clear. When a patient has delusions or hallucinations, there is no disorientation or memory disturbance.

      Caveat: The presence of delusions, hallucinations, paranoid ideation, or catatonia (disturbed psychomotor activity) should not automatically lead to the diagnosis of schizophrenia. These symptoms are also common among manic-depressive patients.

    4. Often there is a blunted, shallow, inappropriate affect or bizarre motor behavior, or both. Unfortunately, physicians often have little sympathy for emotional reactions in schizophrenic patients.

    5. Patients are often single and have poor premorbid social adjustments or work history.

    6. Frequently there is a family history of schizophrenia.

F. Treatment.

    1. Acutely disturbed schizophrenic patients are usually best treated with antipsychotic medications at inpatient mental health facilities.

    2. When the primary care physician is following a schizophrenic patient in remission on neuroleptics (phenothiazines or other major tranquilizers), it is important to recognize that akathisia may be a symptom of neuroleptic

TABLE 9–3. Characteristics of Common Personality Types

Personality Type	Description	Practical Suggestions
Passive-dependent	Chronic inability to adjust to life demands; completely dependent upon others; long-term hospitalization or institutionalization common	"I'll take care of you"
Passive-aggressive	Stubborn obstructionist who makes intentional errors; follows directions poorly; intolerant of authority; blames others for any bad outcomes	"I know you are tough enough to do it"
Antisocial	Selfish, callous, with no loyalty or trustworthiness; no sense of guilt; low frustration tolerance with frequent interpersonal difficulties; antisocial behavior	These are extremely difficult patients to treat (see Cleckley's *The Mask of Sanity*)
Obsessive-compulsive	Excessive concern about standards, morals, image; excessive inhibitions; frequently isolated and usually chronically unhappy	Give patient orders, lists, and schedules
Paranoid	Suspicious, blames others for all problems; frequently involved in lawsuits; feels self-important and entitled to better	Explain all procedures in a simple, straightforward manner
Hysterical	Immature behavior; sexually seductive in most interactions; dependent, but avoids meaningful interpersonal relationships	Avoid seduction; recognize dependency needs; do not become angry and punitive toward these patients
Schizoid	Isolated, secretive, eccentric; avoids interpersonal relationships of all kinds	These patients are threatened by the natural warmth and closeness of many physicians; on the other hand, the door to communication must be left open because these patients are also very sensitive to rejection.

toxicity; the symptoms of akathisia are often mistakenly interpreted as being due to anxiety and the dose of the neuroleptic may be increased, when actually the proper treatment is to decrease the dose or discontinue the medication.

V. RECOGNIZING PERSONALITY TYPES AS AN AID TO PATIENT MANAGEMENT.

A. The primary care physician should be able to recognize the common personality types and disorders in order to avoid letting the physician's own emotional reactions interfere with the physician-patient relationship.

Remember: Every patient has a personality! Different personality types often need different approaches to management. For example, if the therapeutic goal is to have a patient remain at bed rest, the independent, machismo young man should be told, "Staying in bed like this is a tough job, and a lot of my patients can't do it, but I know a person with your determination and will power certainly won't disappoint me." On the other hand, if the patient is passive-dependent, one would say, "Just lie there in bed, and don't worry about a thing because we will care for you completely." Some of the more common personality types are listed in Table 9–3.

BIBLIOGRAPHY

American Psychiatric Association: *Diagnostic and Statistical Manual of Mental Disorders,* ed 3, revised. Washington, DC, American Psychiatric Association, 1987.

Benson DF, Blumer D: *Psychiatric Aspects of Neurologic Disease*. New York, Grune & Stratton, 1975.

Black JL, Richelson E, Richardson JW: Antipsychotic agents: A clinical update. *Mayo Clin Proc* 1985; 60:777–789.

Cleckley H: *The Mask of Sanity*. St Louis, Mosby–Year Book, 1976.

Cooper GL: The safety of fluoxetine—an update. *Br J Psychiatry* 1988; 153:77–86.

Goodwin DW, Guze SB: *Psychiatric Diagnosis,* ed 3. New York, Oxford University Press, 1984.

Guze BH, Baxter LR: Neuroleptic malignant syndrome. *N Engl J Med* 1985; 313:163–169.

Herskowitz J, Rosman NP: *Pediatrics, Neurology, and Psychiatry—Common Ground.* New York, Macmillan, 1982.

Jacobs JW, Bernhard MR, Delgado A, et al: Screening for organic mental syndromes in the medically ill. *Ann Intern Med* 1977; 86:40–46.

McAlpine DE: Suicide: Recognition and management. *Mayo Clin Proc* 1987; 62:778–781.

Michels R, Marzuk PM: Progress in psychiatry. *N Engl J Med* 1993; 329:552–557, 628–637.

Miller R: Schizophrenia as a progressive disorder: Relations to EEG, CT, neuropathological and other evidence. *Prog Neurobiol* 1989; 33:17–43.

Richardson JW, Richelson E: Antidepressants: A clinical update for medical practitioners. *Mayo Clin Proc* 1984; 59:330–337.

Winokur G, Clayton P (eds): *The Medical Basis of Psychiatry.* Philadelphia, WB Saunders, 1986.

MULTIPLE SCLEROSIS

10

I. DIAGNOSIS.

Modern technology, particularly the invention of magnetic resonance imaging (MRI), has greatly improved the accuracy of diagnosis of multiple sclerosis (MS). Because the disease is common and because it is emphasized in medical school neuroscience curricula, it is often mistakenly listed as a presenting symptom in primary care surveys. In fact, it is a specific disease entity with protean manifestations.

A. History.

1. Transient blurring of vision in one eye (retrobulbar neuritis) is very common. Vision is often normal by the time the patient is examined by a physician.
2. Double vision.
3. Transient clumsiness of one arm (cerebellar involvement).
4. Urinary urgency or frequency and male impotence (spinal cord involvement).
5. Excessive fatigue unrelated to focal symptoms.
6. Paralysis of a leg or arm.
7. Symptoms usually begin in the third decade of life (but cases have been reported in children and in the sixth decade).
8. Patients often note that symptoms recur when they are overheated, e.g., after a hot shower, fever.

   Caveat: Most patients have repeated exacerbations and remissions of symptoms, but 10% of patients with MS may have a gradually progressive course without readily apparent exacerbations or remissions.

B. Examination:
Because any central nervous system (CNS) white matter may become demyelinated, almost *any* neurologic

abnormality is possible. The following are common findings in MS patients:

1. The optic nerve often shows temporal pallor as a residuum of retrobulbar neuritis. A Marcus Gunn pupil is frequently seen; this indicates damage to the optic nerve anterior to the chiasm from any cause (Fig 10–1).

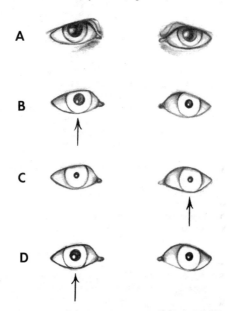

FIG 10–1. Marcus Gunn pupil: The pupil that paradoxically dilates with direct light. **A,** both pupils initially are equal. **B,** direct light into the affected eye *(arrow)* causes minimal constriction; the opposite pupil constricts equally because of consensual reflex. **C,** direct light into the normal eye causes significant constriction of both pupils, direct and consensual. **D,** swinging the flashlight back to the affected eye causes it "paradoxically" to dilate owing to removal of strong consensual reflex.

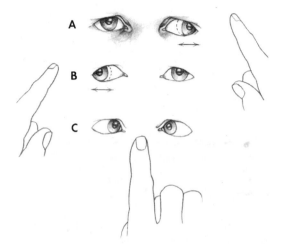

FIG 10–2. Bilateral internuclear ophthalmoplegia: When looking to either side, the adducting eye does not go beyond the midline, while the abducting eye shows nystagmus (**A** and **B**). This looks somewhat like a bilateral medial rectus palsy; however, the patient is able to converge and focus on a near object (**C**).

2. Internuclear ophthalmoplegia—especially if bilateral—is highly suggestive of MS (Fig 10–2). Incomplete forms exist such as pronounced nystagmus in the abducting eye and minimal nystagmus in the adducting eye. Rare causes of internuclear ophthalmoplegia include brainstem infarcts or tumors or myasthenia gravis.

3. Intention tremor and incoordinated rapid alternating movements are common because of cerebellar peduncle involvement.

4. Tingling or electric shock-like paresthesias on neck flexion (Lhermitte's sign).

5. Impaired recognition of objects by touch alone (astereognosis).

6. Motor involvement: increased or asymmetric reflexes, Babinski reflex.

Caveat: MS affects *only* the CNS; absent reflexes, muscle atrophy, and sensory loss in the distribution of a peripheral nerve make the diagnosis unlikely. The presence of significant dementia, papilledema, or symmetric proximal muscle weakness also makes the diagnosis unlikely.

C. **Laboratory studies:** In the modern era, the diagnosis of MS should be confirmed by laboratory studies:
   1. *Magnetic resonance imaging:* The presence of multiple, predominantly periventricular plaques in a young patient with exacerbations and remissions of neurologic symptoms strongly supports the diagnosis of MS and further tests probably need not be done. If no plaques are seen on MRI, the diagnosis of MS is unlikely.

   Caveat: The number of plaques seen does not correlate with the severity of the disease.

   2. *Evoked responses:* Visual, somatosensory, and brainstem auditory evoked responses are abnormal in a majority of patients.
   3. *Lumbar puncture* (see Chapter 2, section I): Routine studies show a normal or slightly increased cell count, normal or slightly increased protein, and an increased gamma-globulin level. Tests more specific for MS include:
      a. IgG synthesis calculated by the formula:

$$\frac{\text{CSF IgG/serum IgG}}{\text{CSF albumin/serum albumin}} = [\text{normal} < 0.7]$$

      b. Oligoclonal bands.
      c. Myelin basic protein (normal < 1.0 ng/mL).
         Computed tomography (CT) scans, electroencephalography (EEG), electromyography (EMG), myelography, and radionuclide scans are of little or no use in establishing a firm diagnosis of MS.

D. **Specific Treatment.**
   1. Experts agree that MS is associated with an altered immune response, possibly triggered by an unspecified viral agent.

Many centers are currently conducting clinical trials with a variety of agents that affect the immune system, and it can be reasonably expected that a number of products will, in the next few years, be available to prevent the development of new plagues. The only agent that is currently available and Federal Drug and Food Administration (FDA) approved is Betaseron (interferon β1b). Clinical benefit has been proven for only ambulatory patients with a relapsing-remitting course, but many neurologists suspect that the drug may be of some value in all patients with MS. The clinical trials clearly show there is a 30% reduction in exacerbation, although at the termination of the 3 year study there was no statistical difference in disability. This drug currently costs up to $10,000 per year, and most patients cannot afford to take the drug unless assisted by third-party payors. The recommended dosage is 0.25 mg (8 million IU) injected subcutaneously every other day. The major side effects are mild inflammation at the injection site and initial flu-like syndrome. This drug is far safer than steroids and other immunosuppressants that have been used in the past.

2. In severe cases, progression can sometimes be halted by high-dose intravenous (IV) cyclophosphamide and adrenocorticotropic hormone (ACTH), but this treatment should be reserved for severely ill patients in tertiary care centers.

3. Physician advice.

   a. Because of the exacerbations and remissions and chronicity of the disease, MS patients are particularly prone to quack treatments. Advise patients to use only Food and Drug Administration–approved medications or to participate only in drug trials sponsored by respectable scientific agencies.

   b. Most patients are initially upset with their diagnosis. The positive features of the disease should be emphasized: one third of patients have a relatively benign course and the recovery rate from individual attacks is 80% or more.

   c. Stress is generally recognized as a precipitating factor for attacks. This includes infections.

   d. Avoid situations where the body temperature is raised (hot baths, saunas, prolonged exposure to hot sun) as this may cause a temporary recurrence of old symptoms.

e. Bladder hygiene should be emphasized, and self-catheterization should be taught if residual urine is present.
4. Symptomatic drug therapy.
   a. Antispasticity agents.

   Caveat: In some patients, spasticity is beneficial for weightbearing, and treatment with antispasticity drugs will make such patients worse.

   i) Baclofen (Lioresal) at an initial dose of 5 mg bid up to 20 mg tid. Dose should be slowly titrated for maximal benefit.
   ii) Dantrolene sodium (Dantrium): Begin with 25 mg/day; every 3 or 4 days increase the dose by 25 mg until the therapeutic goal is obtained. Doses as high as 100 mg tid occasionally are necessary. If this drug is used, liver function tests should be performed at regular intervals since hepatitis and liver failure have been reported.
   b. Amantadine hydrochloride (Symmetrel): Fatigue is a most bothersome symptom to MS patients; some patients improve dramatically with 100 mg once or twice a day.
   c. Pemoline (Cylert) 18.75 mg bid, gradually titrated to a maximum of 75 mg/day, may also alleviate fatigability.
   d. Steroids (prednisone and ACTH): These drugs should never be used on a chronic basis. Steroids worsen the outcome in optic neuritis, and there is a suspicion that they do the same for other symptoms.
   e. Amitriptyline hydrochloride: In MS patients with major depression or with emotional lability, the tricyclic antidepressants, specifically amitriptyline 50 to 150 mg/day, may ameliorate the symptoms.

E. Rehabilitation.
1. Physical therapy is indicated for patients in remission with residual motor disability. Ideally, this is best carried out in a rehabilitation center.
2. Occupational therapy assists patients with a fixed disability in adjusting to the activities of daily living.
F. Patient education: The National Multiple Sclerosis Society is a good source of information: National Multiple Sclerosis So-

ciety, 205 East 42nd St., New York, NY 10017, telephone (212) 986-3240 or 800-637-6303. In addition, most cities have a local MS society and support groups which are invaluable sources of education and emotional support.

BIBLIOGRAPHY

Beck RW, Cleary PA, Anderson MM Jr, et al: A randomized controlled trial of corticosteroids in the treatment of optic neuritis. *N Engl J Med* 1992; 326:581–587.

Hauser SL, Dawson DM, Lehrich JR, et al: Intensive immunosuppression in progressive multiple sclerosis. *N Engl J Med* 1983; 308:173–180.

International Federation of Multiple Sclerosis Societies: *Minimal Record of Disability for Multiple Sclerosis*. New York, National Multiple Sclerosis Society, 1985.

Johnson KP, Belediuk G: Use of cyclosporine in neurological autoimmune disease? *Arch Neurol* 1985; 42:1043–1044.

Markowitz H, Kokmen E: Neurologic diseases and the cerebrospinal fluid immunoglobulin profile. *Mayo Clin Proc* 1983; 58:273–274.

McFarlin DE, McFarland HF: Multiple sclerosis. *N Engl J Med* 1982; 307:1183–1188,1246–1251.

Paty DW, Li DKB: Interferon beta-1b is effective in relapsing-remitting multiple sclerosis. *Neurology* 1993; 43:662–667.

Paty DW, Oger JJ, Kastrukoff LF, et al: MRI in the diagnosis of MS: a prospective study with comparison of clinical evaluation, evoked potentials, oligoclonal banding, and CT. *Neurology* 1988; 38:180–185.

Peterson RC, Kokmen E: Cognitive and psychiatric abnormalities in multiple sclerosis. *Mayo Clin Proc* 1989; 64:657–663.

Poser CM: *Diagnosis of Multiple Sclerosis*. New York, Thieme, 1984.

Rodriguez M: Multiple sclerosis: Basic concepts and hypothesis. *Mayo Clin Proc* 1989; 64:570–576.

Scheinberg LC (ed): *Multiple Sclerosis. A Guide for Patients and Their Families*. New York, Raven Press, 1983.

Stewart JM, Howser OW, Baker HL, et al: Magnetic resonance imaging and clinical relationships in multiple sclerosis. *Mayo Clin Proc* 1987; 62:174–184.

Weiner HL, Haffler DA: Immunotherapy of multiple sclerosis. *Ann Neurol* 1988; 23:211–222.

Wilson H, Olson WH, Gascon GG, et al: Personality characteristics and multiple sclerosis. *Psychol Rep* 1982; 51:791–806.

Wynn DR, Rodriguez M, O'Fallon WM, et al: Update on the epidemiology of multiple sclerosis. *Mayo Clin Proc* 1989; 64:570–576.

SEIZURES AND EPILEPSY

I. DEFINITION AND OVERVIEW.

A *seizure* is a sudden change in body functioning due to abnormal, excessive electrical discharges of neurons in the brain. *Epilepsy* is a symptom complex in which there is a tendency to have repeated seizures. It follows that not everyone who has seizures has epilepsy, but everyone who has epilepsy has seizures. Neither seizures nor epilepsy is a final diagnosis but a symptom complex requiring a search for underlying etiologic factors.

A. **Frequently, only generalized tonic-clonic movements** are recognized as seizures, but consideration of seizures should arise whenever a patient presents with loss of consciousness or any sudden brief change in functioning with or without loss of consciousness. Paroxysmal changes in consciousness, sensation, emotion, or thought processes all may be manifestations of a seizure disorder. A diagnosis of a seizure disorder is especially likely if such changes are repetitive, stereotyped, and preceded by a premonition or warning (aura) or followed by (postictal) confusion, exhaustion, or headache. The physician's initial task when a patient presents with what might be a seizure is to determine whether the episode was indeed a seizure, or some other episodic, periodic, or recurrent paroxysmal event that is nonepileptic, such as syncope, migraine, pseudoseizure, transient ischemic attack (TIA), or narcolepsy. When the diagnosis of a seizure is made, the patient should be evaluated for common toxic-metabolic or structural abnormalities. These commonly include hypoglycemia, infection, alcohol or drug withdrawal, stroke, or tumor. Patients with recurrent seizures over a long period of time (epilepsy syndrome) most likely have either no structural abnormality or a static abnormality such as a glial scar. Recurrent seizures with neurologic deterioration require evaluation for inborn errors of metabolism, chronic infection, or tumor.

B. **Patients with recurrent seizures** and an anatomically normal brain or a nonprogressive lesion require only symptomatic treatment with anticonvulsants (antiepileptic drugs). If the seizures are secondary to a generalized systemic medical condition or a progressive brain lesion, then the patient requires specific treatment in addition to symptomatic treatment with anticonvulsants.

C. **Summary:** The questions, then, are:
1. Seizure or nonseizure?
2. If seizure, what type?
3. Acute medical or neurologic condition or epilepsy?
4. Symptomatic or specific treatment, or both?

D. **In the primary epilepsies** no focal brain lesions are found, there is often a family history of epilepsy, and the neurologic examination is normal. They often begin in childhood, and the response to anticonvulsants is usually very good. In the secondary epilepsies neurologic abnormalities may be present, a family history of epilepsy is usually lacking, and the response to anticonvulsants is variable to poor.

II. HISTORY.

A. **The history** is the single most important part of the diagnostic evaluation and management of seizures. It should include:
1. An accurate description of the onset of the seizures. (If the patient cannot give a history, attempt to interview an eyewitness.)
   a. Bilaterally symmetric onset without warning (primary generalized seizure) vs. focal, partial, or unilateral. For example, arm jerking on one side suggests a lesion in the frontal lobe of the opposite hemisphere.
   b. Dynamic character of seizures (march of movement, focal movement becoming generalized, etc.).
   ▶ c. *An important diagnostic clue* to seizures is drowsiness or confusion that follows the seizure event; this does not occur following other episodic phenomena such as TIAs or migraine.

TABLE 11-1.
Age Correlation with Seizure Syndromes

Age	Seizures	Etiology
Newborn (0-3 wk)	Poorly defined seizures; generalized tonic, focal, and multifocal clonus, and myoclonus	Hypoxia, hemorrhage, congenital malformations, hypoglycemia, hypocalcemia
Infants and toddlers (3 wk-3 yr)	Simple febrile seizures, infantile spasms, Lennox-Gastaut syndrome	Inborn errors of metabolism, no specific cause (as in febrile seizures), hypoxic brain damage
Children (3-12 yr)	Petit mal, benign centrotemporal epilepsy, benign occipital epilepsy	Familial
Adolescents (13-20 yr)	Generalized tonic-clonic	Familial
Adults (21-60 yr)	Complex (and simple) partial or secondarily generalized	Head trauma, tumor
Elderly (>60 yr)	Partial or secondarily generalized	Postinfarction (vascular)

2. A review of symptoms suggesting seizures, e.g., loss of memory; strange, unexplained smells or other sensations; visual hallucinations; distortions in visual, auditory, or time sensation; feeling of having experienced events before; previous staring episodes (absences); previous undiagnosed nocturnal seizures with bed-wetting or rolling out of bed; awakening exhausted with muscle aches and pain.
3. A family history of seizures. (In primary generalized seizure disorders the familial incidence is as high as 25%.)
4. Previous head trauma or other central nervous system (CNS) damage.
5. Specific seizure syndromes tend to occur with highest frequency at certain ages (Table 11-1).

III. MINIMAL LABORATORY STUDIES.

A. **The laboratory examination** will be directly based on the clinical history and type of seizure and will be different for each type of seizure and each age group.

1. *Electroencephalogram* (EEG): The EEG measures the electrical activity of cortical surface neurons. The EEG is a finite sample of activity in time. Remember that the recording is often done between seizures (interictal) and may or may not reveal epileptiform abnormalities. The reliability of the EEG also depends on the competence of the EEG technologist doing the recording and the expertise of the electroencephalographer. Routine activation techniques such as hyperventilation, photic stimulation, and sleep deprivation, and use of nasopharyngeal leads may add more information. In specialized referral centers continuous monitoring by video-EEG techniques and ambulatory cassette recording are now available for refractory epilepsies or when diagnostic difficulties arise.

   Caveat   A normal EEG does not rule out the diagnosis of a seizure, and rarely patients may have abnormal EEGs with no clinical symptoms.

IV. SEIZURES.
A. **Neonatal seizures:** Newborns, unlike older infants, do not have well-organized, symmetric tonic-clonic seizures. Seizures in premature infants are even less organized. Suspect seizures when there are unexplained autonomic, respiratory, or motor changes.
   1. Subtle seizures: eye blinking, tonic eye deviation, sucking, lip-smacking, drooling, swimming movements, pedaling movements, apnea.
   2. Tonic seizures: usually extension of all limbs.
   3. Multifocal clonus: usually associated with perinatal asphyxia.
   4. Focal clonus: hypocalcemia, focal brain contusion.
   5. Myoclonus: multiple or single flexion jerks of upper or lower extremities.
   6. Generally there is an underlying cause, such as neonatal hypoxia-ischemia, trauma, intracranial hemorrhage, meningitis, hypocalcemia, or rarely, inborn errors of metabolism (pyridoxine dependency, phenylketonuria, maple syrup urine disease, galactosemia). Ultrasound

imaging or computed tomography (CT) scan of the head may demonstrate anatomic abnormalities (hemorrhage, developmental brain anomalies). Blood and urine chemical analysis may detect metabolic disturbances.

7. Generally, the best prognosis is seen with focal clonic jerking and the worst prognosis with fragmentary multifocal clonic seizures. Prognosis for normal neurologic development and recurrent seizures relates ultimately to the cause and response to treatment of the underlying cause. Reversible metabolic disorders (hypocalcemia) have the best prognosis.

8. Treatment.

 a. Prevention or early detection with adequate treatment of the underlying disorder(s) is the best approach to neonatal seizures.

 b. If seizures occur frequently, then do the following:

 1) Draw blood for glucose, calcium, magnesium, and electrolytes, and leave the needle in place for an intravenous (IV) line.

 2) Inject the following solutions (if there is an immediate response, the cause of the seizures will have been determined):

 a) 50% glucose 1 to 2 mL/kg.

 b) Calcium gluconate 200 mg/kg.

 c) Pyridoxine 50 mg.

 c. If the seizures still do not stop, then phenobarbital 15 to 20 mg/kg should be infused IV slowly over an hour. Subsequent IV phenobarbital dosages can then be ordered according to serial serum phenobarbital levels, attempting to keep the blood level between 20 and 30 μg/mL. If seizures continue, phenytoin 15 to 20 mg/kg IV (never intramuscularly [IM]) can also be used. Phenobarbital can be continued orally for long-term maintenance, but oral phenytoin is poorly absorbed in infants and is not recommended for long-term maintenance.

 d. If seizures stop in the neonatal period, it is accepted practice to continue anticonvulsants for 3 months and then discontinue them gradually.

B. Simple febrile seizures.
1. Simple febrile seizures are the most common seizures in infants and toddlers; the greatest incidence is between ages 18 and 36 months.
2. Onset with fever (often during rapidly rising or falling stage of temperature); fever is often not detected until after seizure occurs.
3. Brief (less than 10 minutes) generalized seizure; seizure has almost always stopped by the time the patient arrives at the physician's office.
4. EEG is normal by 2 weeks after the seizure.
5. Family history of simple febrile seizures in early childhood supports the diagnosis of simple febrile seizure.

   Caveat: If the seizure is focal or prolonged or if the neurologic examination shows focal abnormalities, it is *not* a simple febrile seizure and a search must be made for underlying pathologic changes, especially infection. It is also unusual for the *first* simple febrile seizure to occur before 6 months or after 3 years of age.

6. Treatment.
   a. If CNS infection is suspected, patients should have a lumbar puncture and cerebrospinal fluid (CSF) examination.
   b. Parents should be reassured that the condition is benign (not associated with brain damage and highly unlikely to develop into epilepsy).
   c. If the aim is to prevent future febrile convulsions, anticonvulsants are *not* beneficial if given intermittently, i.e., with fevers. *Phenobarbital* is effective (phenytoin is not) prophylactically, but enough must be given to produce therapeutic blood levels (15–30 µg/mL). The usual dosage of 3 to 5 mg/kg/day can be given as a single evening dose.
   d. Valproic acid is the only other effective prophylactic anticonvulsant for simple febrile seizures, but it is not recommended because of possible hepatotoxicity.
   e. Since simple febrile seizures are so benign and since anticonvulsants may have significant side effects,

many physicians do not treat them; however, the physician may find it difficult to resist pressure from parents to treat the child.

C. Complicated febrile seizures.

1. Fever lowers the seizure threshold, i.e., fever of any cause may trigger seizures in persons with underlying epilepsy, or fever and seizures may be associated with CNS infection such as meningitis or encephalitis.

2. These seizures occur in all age groups, but are a diagnostic problem especially in children under the age of 5 years.

3. Thorough neurologic evaluation is necessary if it is the patient's first seizure. The risk of febrile seizures developing into an epileptic disorder is increased by: neurologic abnormalities by history or examination, developmental delay, focality or long duration of the seizure, multiple seizures with each febrile episode, prolonged seizures (greater than 15 minutes), family history of epilepsy, and epileptiform abnormalities in the EEG.

4. Treatment.

   a. Diagnostic lumbar puncture and appropriate antibiotic treatment are necessary for meningitis or encephalitis (see also Chapter 14, sections I. C and II).

   b. Reducing or preventing the fever with antipyretics (aspirin or acetaminophen) will reduce the likelihood of seizures.

   Caveat: Although its role is still undetermined, aspirin has been associated with Reye's syndrome, particularly when the underlying cause of fever has been influenza or chickenpox.

   c. For maintenance give anticonvulsants to prevent further febrile or afebrile seizures: phenobarbital 3 to 5 mg/kg/day is the drug of choice; if seizures recur after adequate blood levels, phenytoin 5 to 7 mg/kg/day may be added. Once the phenytoin level is therapeutic, phenobarbital is gradually withdrawn. Blood levels of the anticonvulsants must be obtained to determine the adequacy of the dosage.

V. EPILEPTIC DISORDERS.

A. **Infantile spasms.** This epileptic syndrome, consisting of massive myoclonic seizures in the first year of life, developmental arrest, and a hypsarrhythmic EEG, is the most devastating seizure syndrome and should be treated with great concern.

1. Massive myoclonic seizures last a second or so and consist of sudden bending forward at the waist with the arms and legs extended in the posture of prayer (hence "salaam seizures"). A lesser number are extensor spasms, with arching of the back and extending of the neck. Rarely there are hemispasms, involving only one half of the body.

2. The spasms occur in flurries, usually upon awakening, many times daily.

3. Often misdiagnosed as "colic," particularly if noticed during feeding times.

4. Usual onset is between age 3 and 12 months.

5. Associated with developmental arrest and subsequent moderate to severe mental retardation in greater than 90% of these children.

6. The EEG shows a hypsarrhythmic pattern consisting of disorganized background activity, multiconfigurational and multifocal discharges during the waking state. Sleep tracings may mimic "burst-suppression" patterns.

7. Etiologies are:
   a. Symptomatic: previous static encephalopathies or (rarely) progressive CNS disease, or neurocutaneous syndromes, particularly tuberous sclerosis.
   b. Cryptogenic: normally developing babies suddenly have the syndrome, and no CNS disease is found.

8. Seizures may be difficult to control, and may evolve into other seizure syndromes (see Lennox-Gastaut syndrome, section V. B).

9. Treatment.
   a. Early treatment of the seizures alone is not sufficient. Search for an underlying cause with neurometabolic urine screen and CT scan or magnetic resonance imaging (MRI) (for developmental brain malformations, such as agenesis of the corpus callosum).

   b. After obtaining baseline EEGs, treat with adrenocorticotropic hormone (ACTH) 100 units/m^2/day (usually 80 units) for 3 to 4 weeks. Clinical improvement usually does not occur before 10 to 14 days, and may be preceded by EEG improvement.

   c. After this initial course, follow with ACTH gel IM every other day until the patient is spasm-free for 1 month. Monitor for steroid toxic side effects, the most important of which is hypertension.

   d. If spasms persist or evolve into other seizure types, clonazepam 0.5 mg bid can be started and then increased. Valproic acid can be substituted if clonazepam is only partially effective or ineffective.

   e. Genetic counseling is necessary if a genetic syndrome can be identified.

   f. Families should be offered assistance in managing the young retarded child (see Chapter 16).

B. Lennox-Gastaut syndrome.

   1. The Lennox-Gastaut syndrome is similar to infantile spasms but presents in a later age group, usually age 2 to 5 years; akinetic and myoclonic seizures (drop spells), absences, and generalized convulsions occur, often many times daily.

   2. Associated with mild to moderate mental retardation, hyperactivity, and behavior disturbances.

   3. Characteristic EEG changes consist of poorly developed background activity, and multifocal slow (less than 3 Hz) spike and wave complexes.

   4. Since both the infantile spasms and Lennox-Gastaut syndrome are clinically devastating, initial management is probably best handled by someone experienced with these disorders, such as a pediatric neurologist, epileptologist, or a pediatrician with specialized training and experience with epilepsies.

   5. Treatment.

     a. Total control of seizures is difficult to achieve. Management usually includes use of the major anticonvulsants such as barbiturates (be careful not to make a hyperactive child worse), clonazepam, and valproic acid (see Table 11–2), but might include ACTH and

TABLE 11–2.
Drugs Used in Treatment of Seizures

Drug	Dosage		Therapeutic Blood Level (μg/mL)	Plasma Half-Life (hr)
	Adults (mg)	Children (mg/kg)		
Phenobarbital	100–180	3–5	15–30	72–96
Phenytoin	300–400	4–7	10–20	12–24
Primidone (partially metabolized to phenobarbital)	750–1,500	10–25	6–12	3–12
Carbamazepine	800–1,600	20–30	4–12	7–18
Ethosuximide	750–2,000	20–30	40–100	24–48
Clonazepam	1.5–20	0.01–0.2	0.02–0.07	18–50
Valproic acid	1,000–3,000	15–30	50–100	7–15

a ketogenic diet. Protective helmets (football or hockey type) help prevent head injury from drop spells.

    b. If the subsequent course shows persistent myoclonic seizures, and persistent developmental arrest, or developmental regression, suspect a progressive CNS disease (such as a ganglioside storage disease) and refer the patient to a pediatric neurologist.

    c. Felbamate (Felbatrol) may be the most effective treatment for this disorder in a dosage of 45 mg/kg/day divided into 2 to 4 doses.

C. Benign centrotemporal epilepsy: Benign centrotemporal epilepsy (rolandic epilepsy, sylvian seizure syndrome, lingual seizures) is a relatively common, but often unrecognized and misdiagnosed epileptic disorder. Making the correct diagnosis is important because of the benign prognosis—excellent response to anticonvulsants and "outgrowing" the disorder by mid- or late adolescence.

    1. This is a focal or partial seizure syndrome not associated with focal structural CNS lesions.

    2. Often presents as nocturnal generalized convulsions in school-age children. These are actually secondarily generalized convulsions.

3. The partial onset, seen easily after institution of anticonvulsants and incomplete control of the seizures, consists of localized tongue or oral paresthesias, dysarthria, drooling, and facial twitching, with preservation of consciousness. A careful history for this initial onset of the seizures will give the diagnosis.
4. The EEG shows characteristic central and midtemporal spikes or sharp waves. These are best seen in a sleep EEG.
5. Treatment.
   a. The treatment of choice is phenytoin (keep blood level between 15 and 20 μg/mL) until adolescence.
   b. Phenobarbital is also effective (keep blood levels at 25 ± 5 μg/mL).

VI. PRIMARY GENERALIZED EPILEPSIES.

A. **The most common clinical types** of primary generalized epilepsies are *grand mal* and *petit mal*. The following features apply to all generalized seizures:
   1. Onset is almost always in childhood or adolescence.
   2. From the onset the seizures are generalized, with immediate alteration of consciousness. Motor manifestations are symmetric and bilateral.
   3. EEG discharges are generalized and bilaterally synchronous from the start of a recorded seizure.
   4. Neurologic examination and CT scan or MRI of brain are normal during the interictal period.
   5. The EEG background activity is normal, interrupted by generalized, bilaterally synchronous, symmetric spike and wave or poly-spike and wave complexes. These occur spontaneously, or are activated by hyperventilation, intermittent photic stimulation, or sleep.
   6. No previous history of brain injury.
   7. Family history of seizures is often positive.
   8. Good response to appropriate anticonvulsants (antiepileptic drugs).
   9. Relatively good prognosis. Next to the primary partial epilepsies just described (benign centrotemporal), the primary generalized epilepsies have the best long-term prognosis for seizure control, as well as for intellectual, cognitive, and emotional functioning.

10. Previous terms commonly used that are synonymous with primary generalized epilepsy are "idiopathic" or "centrencephalic" epilepsy.

B. Petit mal epilepsy: The term *petit mal* is probably the most misused term applied to seizures by the general physician. It does *not* denote any minor seizure that falls short of being a generalized convulsion. *Petit mal* epilepsy is a *specific* clinical and EEG syndrome and has a *specific* therapy.

1. Differential diagnosis.

   a. The usual onset is between age 3 and 10 years.

   b. Petit mal is characterized by *absences* lasting 2 to 30 seconds associated with a characteristic EEG abnormality (3-Hz spike and wave discharges activated by hyperventilation).

   c. Absences clinically appear as staring spells during which the patient is momentarily unresponsive; they may be associated with eyelid fluttering. Sometimes, the eyes roll upward or there may be automatisms of lip-smacking, chewing, or other purposeless repetitive mouth or hand movements.

   d. Absences occur frequently in flurries during the day; the child may be called a daydreamer, absent-minded, or inattentive; absences may be recognized as transient pauses during eating, speaking, or any other activity.

   e. Petit mal is distinguished from complex partial seizures (psychomotor, temporal lobe) by lack of aura, brief duration, and lack of postictal confusion, drowsiness, or headache.

   f. Absences can be brought out by hyperventilation, which can be done as an *office test:* Have the patient hyperventilate for 3 minutes under observation. During an absence, the hyperventilation will stop while the typical features of absence are observed, and then hyperventilation will resume immediately.

   g. Petit mal may be complicated by other seizure phenomena (petit mal triad): myoclonic jerks (sudden increase in muscle tone *throwing* patient forward or backward), and atonic-akinetic seizures (drop or *slumping* of head or body due to sudden decrease of muscle tone).

h. Petit mal responds readily to treatment unless complicated by other seizure phenomena, in which case there is a risk for later generalized convulsions.

i. Petit mal status consists of continuous absence seizures, and may appear as a confusional state. The EEG shows continuous 3-Hz spike and wave activity. It usually occurs:

1) As a withdrawal syndrome (sudden cessation of anticonvulsants).

2) As previously undiagnosed and untreated petit mal epilepsy occurring in adolescence or early adulthood.

3) Incorrectly treated petit mal (e.g., using phenobarbital or phenytoin, rather than valproate or ethosuximide).

2. Treatment.

a. The drug of choice is ethosuximide 20 to 30 mg/kg/day in two to three divided doses to maintain a blood level of 40 to 100 μg/mL.

b. Valproic acid in doses of 10 to 30 mg/kg/day to maintain a therapeutic blood level of 50 to 100 μg/mL is also effective. Valproate is probably preferable as a single drug in petit mal triad or if generalized convulsions occur concomitantly with absences.

c. Barbiturates or phenytoin or both may be necessary to control other associated seizure phenomena or generalized convulsions, but should not be used alone.

C. Grand mal epilepsy.

1. Differential diagnosis.

a. Onset is most frequent during childhood and adolescence.

b. Seizures, usually tonic-clonic seizures, are bilaterally symmetric from the onset. Typically the patient loses consciousness and the body becomes rigid (tonic phase) followed by jerky movements (clonic phase) and postictal confusion or prolonged sleep.

c. Interictal EEG may be normal in as many as one third of patients.

d. Mental retardation and psychiatric disturbances are *not* usually associated with this disorder.

       e. A family history of seizures is often elicited.

       f. Neurologic examination and CT scan or MRI normal.

   2. Treatment: See comments concerning anticonvulsants in section IX.

VII. SEIZURES OF FOCAL ORIGIN (PARTIAL EPILEPSY).

A. Clinical features.

1. Onset at any age.
2. The features of these partial seizures depend on the site and side of the lesion (and epileptogenic foci that result from the lesion) and the pattern of spread of the ictal electrical discharge. A partial seizure with impairment of consciousness is categorized as complex partial type; otherwise it is a simple partial type.
3. Seizures of focal origin may produce simple symptomatology (e.g., focal motor), a complex picture (e.g., complex partial), or a convulsion due to secondary generalization (the aura is the clue to focal onset).
4. A localized ictal EEG discharge is present at seizure onset, while the interictal EEG shows localized spikes or spike and wave activity with possible abnormalities of background activity focally or regionally.
5. An abnormal interictal CT scan or MRI and neurologic examination are obtained in many cases.

B. Focal motor seizures:
Focal motor seizures manifest as clonic movements usually involving the arms or the legs. Sometimes the seizure may start in the thumb or the big toe and spread to involve the more proximal parts (jacksonian seizure). A new-onset focal seizure suggests a structural lesion.

C. Complex partial seizures (psychomotor or temporal lobe seizures).

1. Most common form of seizures in adults.
2. Complex partial seizures consist of various automatisms—complex, coordinated but purposeless motor movements (e.g., lip-smacking or walking in a circle) with a blank stare or stereotyped verbal responses; any repeated stereotyped behavior may be a complex partial seizure.

3. Preceded by auras (these may be only some type of difficult-to-describe feeling of strangeness); typical auras include the following:
   a. Déjà vu—the feeling of having experienced an event previously.
   b. Jamais vu—the feeling of strangeness in familiar surroundings.
   c. Fugue state—lapses in time, e.g., shopping in one store and then finding oneself in another store without explanation of how or when one got there.
   d. Abdominal or epigastric sensations (often a rising sensation).
   e. Unexplained sudden fear with an urge to run.
   f. Visual, auditory, or olfactory hallucinations, which are usually complex, vivid and unpleasant.

   Note: Unpleasant olfactory hallucinations (called uncinate auras) are commonly associated with brain tumor.

4. Seizures last about 1 minute with a postictal state of confusion, headache, and exhaustion. Combativeness and violent behavior may occur during this postictal confusional period (especially if well-meaning observers attempt to help or restrain the individual).

5. Seizures may generalize secondarily with loss of consciousness and tonic-clonic convulsive activity.

6. Routine awake EEG shows abnormality in less than 50% of patients; optimal records (about 65% showing temporal lobe spike discharge) are obtained with nasopharyngeal leads (during sleep) performed after 24 hours of sleep deprivation. EEG-activating procedures and long-term monitoring further increase the yield of positive tracings.

7. Personality, behavior, and cognitive disorders frequently complicate the picture and may produce severe psychosocial disability.

8. Complex partial status epilepticus may present as a state of confusion or stupor. The EEG shows continuous 5- to 6-Hz high-voltage, rhythmic theta waves or temporal spikes.

9. Treatment: See comments regarding anticonvulsants in Section IX.

VIII. LATE-ONSET EPILEPSY.

A. Up to the age of 30 years or so, primary generalized epilepsies (previous section) may still present de novo. After that, however, seizures presenting for the *first time* are overwhelmingly due to either acute progressive or acquired static lesions of the brain. Acute lesions include meningitis, encephalitis, cortical contusions from head injury, arterial or venous infarction, or tumors. The acute disturbance may also be a functional, potentially reversible encephalopathy. These include hypoglycemia, hepatic or uremic encephalopathy, hypertensive encephalopathy, or withdrawal syndromes from drugs or alcohol. Seizures starting after the age of 60 years are often due to underlying cerebrovascular disease. Old static lesions are most commonly a result of head injury (posttraumatic epilepsy) or stroke (postinfarction epilepsy) or rarely congenital hamartomas or mesial temporal sclerosis. Slowly progressive tumors may mimic old static lesions.

B. The most common seizure types are partial or focal seizures, which often generalize secondarily, and which usually result from lesions of the temporal lobe (complex partial seizures). Generalized convulsions begin focally and then spread to involve both sides of the body, rather than involving the body bilaterally and symmetrically from the onset. Minimal studies in adults presenting with a first seizure should include EEG (preferably sleep-deprived) and an imaging study such as a CT scan (with and without contrast enhancement) or an MRI. Cerebral angiography and CSF studies may be needed when vascular malformations or an infective cause is suspected.

C. Therapy should be directed toward management of the underlying cause as well as symptomatic treatment of seizures.

IX. ANTICONVULSANTS (ANTIEPILEPTIC DRUGS).
A. General comments.

1. The vast majority of patients should be treated with only *one* drug; once a particular drug *at therapeutic levels* clearly does not completely control the seizures, another

drug should be added; as soon as this drug reaches therapeutic levels, the first drug should be gradually discontinued.

2. For grand mal epilepsy, partial epilepsy, and complex partial epilepsy, the drugs of choice are carbamazepine, phenytoin, primidone, valproic acid, and phenobarbital (Table 11–3). Carbamazepine is sometimes effective when other drugs are not, but it must be taken in at least three daily divided doses, is expensive, has some initial side effects (such as ataxia and confusion), and (rarely) has been associated with bone marrow suppression. Phenytoin is less expensive, can be taken once daily, has fewer initial side effects, but long-term use may result in cerebellar atrophy.

3. Phenobarbital is contraindicated in hyperactive children (administration of this drug may make an uncomfortable situation unbearable). It also causes psychomotor retardation in patients of all ages.

TABLE 11–3.
Drugs of Choice in Treatment of Epilepsy

Seizure Type	Drugs of choice*
Grand mal, focal motor, complex partial	Carbamazepine
	Phenytoin, valproic acid
	Gabapentin
	Felbamate
	Lomotrigine
	Primidone
	Phenobarbital
Petit mal	Ethosuximide
	Valproic acid
Benign centrotemporal epilepsy	Phenytoin
	Phenobarbital
Neonatal seizures	Phenobarbital
Febrile seizures	Phenobarbital
	Valproic acid
Infantile spasms, Lennox-Gastaut syndrome	ACTH
	Felbamate
	Clonazepam

*Drugs are listed in order of preference.

4. Phenytoin produces hirsutism, gum hypertrophy, and coarse facies, and thus should be avoided in young girls.

5. Therapeutic drug levels must be obtained and dose-adjusted based on blood level determinations (see Table 11–2). Trough serum levels should be obtained when there is poor response to dosage regimen, intermittent illness, and when noncompliance is suspected.

6. Knowledge of the elementary clinical pharmacokinetics of the anticonvulsant drugs will make the physician a more skilled therapist. After beginning a maintenance dosage regimen, it takes about five half-lives of the drug before steady state is reached. Therefore, the first blood levels for monitoring purposes should not be taken before that time (see Table 11–2 for half-lives). Trough levels (blood drawn just before a scheduled dose, preferably the first morning dose) should be assessed if seizure control or compliance is in question. If toxicity is the concern, a peak level (blood drawn shortly after a scheduled dose) should be assessed. Drugs with long half-lives (phenobarbital and phenytoin) can be given once a day, making compliance easier. Drugs with shorter half-lives (carbamazepine, valproic acid) need to be given in divided doses daily.

7. Generic carbamazepine and phenytoin, made by different pharmaceutical companies, have different pharmacologic properties. Therefore switching from one brand of generic drug to another may radically alter anticonvulsant (antiepileptic drug) blood levels and precipitate seizures.

B. Phenytoin.

1. The usual dosage is 5 to 7 mg/kg/day (up to about 400 mg/day).

2. Phenytoin should be administered in one to two divided doses daily, since the average serum half-life is 24 hours.

3. The usual therapeutic blood level is 10 to 20 μg/mL, but it is preferable to keep the levels between 15 and 20 μg/mL.

4. Dose-related side effects are:

Blood Level (μg/mL)	Side Effect
1–10	Undertreatment
10–20	Therapeutic dose range (nystagmus in some patients)
20–30	Nystagmus
30–40	Diplopia, dysarthria, ataxia

5. Side effects that are *not* dose-related include gum hypertrophy (which may be prevented by vigorous toothbrushing twice daily), coarsening of features, hirsutism in approximately 40% of patients, and exacerbation of acne. These side effects are especially noticeable in adolescents and may lead to noncompliance in females.

6. Phenytoin rarely may cause a delayed hypersensitivity reaction consisting of fever and pruritic mucocutaneous maculopapular rash with subsequent desquamation, which can be serious or fatal (Stevens-Johnson syndrome).

7. Oral dosage forms are 30- and 100-mg capsules and 50-mg chewable scored tablets.

   Note: Oral suspensions with concentrations of either 25 mg/mL or 6 mg/mL are available, but use of the oral suspension should be avoided since it provides uneven doses owing to the difficulty in achieving uniform mixing of the suspension.

8. Phenytoin is not well absorbed in the neonatal and toddler age group and therefore should be avoided in such patients.

9. The parenteral dosage form is a solution of 50 mg/mL. The solution is highly alkaline and will precipitate if mixed with most other parenteral solutions. The solution should be injected, as much as possible, directly into the vein; saline may be used to flush the IV tubing. IV injection of phenytoin must be at a slow rate (no more than 50 mg/min in adults; no more than 1 mg/kg/min in infants) to prevent cardiac arrhythmias.

   Caveat: Intramuscular (IM) injection should *never* be used since the phenytoin precipitates in muscle, producing necrosis and sterile abscesses, along with unpredictable serum levels of the drug.

C.   Carbamazepine.
1. Effective in partial seizures, particularly complex partial seizures, and generalized seizures.
2. Related structurally to the tricyclic antidepressants, and often effective in ameliorating the behavioral and emotional disturbances that accompany some complex partial seizure disorders.
3. Has been known to produce bone marrow suppression; all patients have a transient fall in white blood cell count on initiation of the drug. Aplastic anemia and agranulocytosis are rare, but serial blood studies are recommended by the manufacturer.
4. Common initial side effects include ataxia, diplopia, and clouding of consciousness.
5. The usual starting dose in adults is 200 mg tid (20–30 mg/kg/day in children).
6. Keep therapeutic level at 4 to 12 μg/mL.
7. Dosage forms available are 200-mg scored tablets and 100-mg scored chewable tablets. A suspension (20 mg/mL) is also available.

D.   Valproate.
1. Valproate is highly effective in absence seizures, both the typical and atypical varieties, and the various forms of myoclonic epilepsies. It is also useful in grand mal and in focal seizures when there is secondary generalization. It is the drug of choice when there is a combination of primary generalized convulsions and absences, myoclonus, or akinetic seizures.
2. Valproate is the only drug, besides phenobarbital, proved to be effective in prophylaxis of simple febrile seizures.
3. Required periodic monitoring with a complete blood count (CBC) and liver function tests for the rare occurrence of bone marrow or hepatic toxicity, especially in children.

Caveat: Fatal hepatotoxicity has been reported in infants receiving multiple anticonvulsants including valproic acid.

4. Relatively few other side effects are seen; gastrointestinal upset is frequent in infants and toddlers, especially at the initiation of therapy. Abnormal platelet count or function may occur and hence platelet count and coagulation values should be checked before planned surgery. Other rare side effects include tremor and hair loss. Although neural tube defects rarely occur, use should be avoided during pregnancy.
5. Usual dose is 250 mg tid in school children (up to 30 mg/kg/day in younger children).
6. Blood levels should ordinarily be between 50 and 100 μg/mL although in some difficult cases, such as Lennox-Gastaut syndrome, blood levels may need to be kept between 100 and 150 μg/mL (as long as there is no toxicity).
7. Available as enteric-coated divalproex sodium tablets (125, 250, and 500 mg) and also as sprinkle capsules (125 mg).

E. Primidone.

1. Primidone is effective for both generalized and complex partial seizures.
2. Since it is partially metabolized to phenobarbital, serum determinations for monitoring drug levels should specify both primidone and phenobarbital levels.
3. Since it is relatively short-acting, should be given in divided doses daily.
4. Children taking this drug may develop irritability and personality changes; therefore it is desirable to avoid its use in children, if possible.
5. The usual starting dose in older adolescents or adults is 250 mg tid, but start at a lower dosage if drowsiness ensues, titrating to toxicity if necessary.
6. Usual therapeutic blood level of primidone is 6 to 12 μg/mL.
7. Dosage forms available include 250-mg scored tablets,

50-mg scored tablets, and as a suspension containing 50 mg/mL.

F. Phenobarbital.

1. The usual dosage is 3 to 5 mg/kg/day (up to about 100–180 mg/day for adult males).

2. May be administered as a single daily dose, since the average serum half-life is about 100 hours.

3. Usual therapeutic blood level is said to be 15 to 30 µg/mL, but the levels aimed for should be 25 ± 5 µg/mL. Most patients will be drowsy when levels are over 40 µg/mL.

4. Because of potential adverse side effects, phenobarbital is not the drug of choice in the initial management of epilepsy.

5. Will produce hyperactivity in many children, particularly if the child has a previous tendency to be hyperactive or is mentally retarded.

6. Can exacerbate depression (affective disorder) in susceptible persons and may be used in overdosage in suicide attempts.

7. Of increasing concern is the issue of whether phenobarbital decreases school performance in children, even at therapeutic dosages.

8. Long-term use may cause mental slowing.

9. Rarely may cause a delayed hypersensitivity reaction consisting of fever and pruritic mucocutaneous maculopapular rash with subsequent desquamation, which can be serious or fatal (Stevens-Johnson syndrome).

10. Oral dosage form is tablets of 15, 30, 60, or 100 mg and syrup of 4 mg/mL; in general, crushed tablets are preferred over the syrup in children, since accurate measurement of dose is difficult with the syrup, and its taste is not pleasing to most children.

G. Ethosuximide.

1. Used when absences of the primary generalized type (petit mal epilepsy) are the sole kind of seizure.

2. Less effective when absences are accompanied by other kinds of phenomena (such as myoclonic seizures or primary generalized seizures). Usually not effective in complex partial absences.

3. Gastrointestinal upset is the most frequent initial side effect.
4. Needs periodic monitoring with CBC and liver function tests for possible bone marrow and hepatic toxicity.
5. Starting dose is usually 250 mg tid.
6. Keep therapeutic level between 50 and 100 μg/mL.
7. Dosage forms available are 250-mg capsules and a syrup containing 50 mg/mL.

H. Clonazepam.

1. A diazepam derivative indicated primarily for myoclonic seizures.
2. Can be used as an adjunct in other primary generalized seizures, such as akinetic seizures.
3. Drowsiness is a frequent initial side effect, so begin with a low dose and build up slowly, using 0.5-mg tablets.
4. Be careful when using in combination with valproic acid: may result in absence status ("electrical status" or "spike-wave stupor").
5. Therapeutic blood levels are usually 0.02 to 0.05 μg/mL, but sedation may be the limiting factor in dosage.
6. Available as scored tablets of 0.5, 1.0, and 2.0 mg.

I. Felbamate.

1. Useful as monotherapy or adjunctive therapy in partial seizures with and without secondary generalization.
2. Effective as adjunctive therapy in controlling the multiple different seizure types seen in patients with Lennox-Gastaut syndrome.
3. Available as 400 and 600 mg tablets and oral suspension 120 mg/mL.
4. Start with 1,200 mg/day in divided doses and gradually increase to 3,600 mg/day.
5. Dose of concomitant medications like phenytoin, valproate, and carbamazepine should be reduced to avoid their toxic side effects.
6. Felbamate causes few side effects, the most common ones being headache, nausea, anorexia, vomiting, and fatigue.

J. Other new antiepileptic drugs: Gabapentin and lamotrigine are two new drugs being introduced in the United States. Both are useful as adjunctive treatment in partial seizures with or without secondary generalization.

K. **Initiating anticonvulsants:** When the diagnosis of epilepsy is established, anticonvulsant (antiepileptic drug) treatment should be instituted promptly. The appropriate drug should be chosen based on the type of seizure (see Table 11–3).

1. Only *one* drug should be started at a time and given to its maximum therapeutic effect.
2. The medication should be initiated at about one-half the suggested therapeutic dosage for 1 week. If no adverse side effects have appeared by that time and the patient has tolerated it well, the full therapeutic dosage may be given. Patients who experience adverse side effects from an excessive initial dose are likely to be poorly compliant in the future. Since it takes four or five half-lives to obtain a steady state, after approximately that elapsed time (see Table 11–2 for half-lives), obtain a serum drug level.
3. The process of instituting anticonvulsant (antiepileptic drug) therapy is essentially a clinical titration. Serum levels are titrated against desired therapeutic effects (lessening or abolition of seizure), keeping in mind that undesirable side effects may limit attainment of the end point. The physician therefore needs accurate observations of the kinds, frequency, and duration of seizures from the patient. The physician can help the patient make these observations by requiring the patient to mail monthly progress reports, in which seizures are charted. The patient should be encouraged to write down a description of the seizure as soon as possible after its occurrence.
4. Monotherapy: Patients should be treated as far as possible with a single anticonvulsant (antiepileptic drug) to avoid drug interactions which may affect efficacy and toxicity. If a single drug is ineffective or only partially effective, a second drug should be added. Then five half-lives later, if the blood level is within the therapeutic range and the seizures are controlled, the first drug should be withdrawn by one dose every five half-lives.

L. **Weaning from anticonvulsants:** Decision regarding drug weaning from anticonvulsants (antiepileptic drugs) depends on the duration of the seizure-free period, seizure type, age of onset, and the presence or absence of EEG abnormalities.

1. Neonates: The best data regarding neonatal seizures indicate that if seizures have stopped, the antiepileptic drugs can be withdrawn at age 3 months. Whether seizures will recur later depends on the degree of cortical damage and underlying cause of neonatal seizures. Severe CNS damage suggests high risk for developing the infantile spasm syndrome later in the first year of life.
2. Childhood and adolescence.
   a. Recent data indicate that in childhood epilepsy (exclusive of neonatal seizures, infantile spasms, or the Lennox-Gastaut syndrome), if a 2-year seizure-free period is obtained, approximately 75% of children will remain seizure-free for at least a 2- to 3-year follow-up period.
   b. The EEG is a good predictor; those with no slowing and no spikes are most likely to remain seizure-free. Those with both slowing and spikes are most likely to recur, while those with either slowing or spikes are intermediate in likelihood of recurrence.
   c. The clinical variety of the seizure is also a factor for prognosis regarding recurrence of seizures following drug withdrawal. The primary partial epilepsies (benign centrotemporal epilepsy and benign occipital epilepsy) probably have the best prognosis and are likely to be "outgrown" (successful weaning of anticonvulsants with no recurrence) in adolescence. The same outcome occurs in approximately half of children with petit mal epilepsy by early adolescence, and most of the other half by the end of adolescence.
3. Late-onset (adult-onset) epilepsy: If epilepsy is defined as at least two or more unprovoked seizures recurring, it is unclear whether the 2-year seizure-free criterion, or any other criterion, is applicable in adult-onset epilepsies. It is likely that in the majority of these patients, lifelong prophylactic anticonvulsant therapy is a necessity. Even though the medical indications for continuing drugs after "good control" are hazy, many social factors conspire to adhere to anticonvulsants, such as the necessity not to have seizures in order to continue having an automobile driver's license, and the fear of losing a job if the patient has seizure recurrences. Finally, many pa-

tients prefer to feel "safe rather than sorry" and do not want to risk the possibility of status epilepticus if seizures recur when off anticonvulsants. When a decision is reached to withdraw anticonvulsants, one drug at a time should be withdrawn. Anticonvulsants should be withdrawn slowly, at a rate of no more than one dose every five half-lives.

M. Compliance.

1. Simple is best. A complex schema of drug administration may be clinicopharmacologically optimal but will be difficult for a patient to follow. A minimal number of daily doses should be used; for phenobarbital, a single daily dose is often effective, and phenytoin can usually be given in no more than two daily doses (once daily may be adequate). Adverse side effects resulting from large initial doses will lead to poor compliance later.

2. The physician must encourage prescription renewal when at least 1 to 2 weeks' supply remains so that the patient will not run out of medications.

3. The patient should be encouraged always to carry on his or her person an extra full day's supply of anticonvulsant in order not to be stranded without medication.

4. When traveling, the patient should carry a letter or card from the physician stating diagnosis and medications in order to obtain an emergency supply of medicines or treatment. This is particularly true when traveling in foreign countries, where strict drug enforcement laws may require confiscation of legitimate anticonvulsant medication if it is not identified and justified.

5. Compliance can be assessed with the aid of serum anticonvulsant (antiepileptic drug) levels.

6. *First impressions count:* The first several months after the diagnosis is made are the most important in establishing a pattern of patient compliance in both medication and follow-up treatment. *Physician availability* is important. When patients first begin taking anticonvulsants, compliance can be fostered by the physician being available for telephone calls, or short, more frequent visits (every 3–6 weeks) to allay the patient's fears about side or toxic effects, what to do if a seizure occurs, and generally to demystify epilepsy.

7. Appropriate patient, parent, and sibling education is necessary to assure compliance. Generally, the more a patient knows about epilepsy, and the more responsibility he or she takes for the management of this disorder, the more likely compliance will occur (see section IX. L. Patient Education).

N. Patient education.
1. When a patient receives the diagnosis of "seizure disorder" or "epilepsy," there is usually initial denial, followed by anger and perhaps depression, before final acceptance. Therefore, the patient and physician should discuss the diagnosis in terms the patient can understand. No information should be released to employers or outside agencies without the patient's consent.
2. Automobile driver's license: The patient should be seizure-free for a period of time determined by law, which varies from state to state. In some states the physician is obligated to report to the state bureau of motor vehicles.
3. School.
   a. If seizures are frequent, a telephone discussion or a personal meeting between the physician and teacher or school nurse is helpful.
   b. The Epilepsy Foundation of America provides information useful for both the patient and family in dealing with the community and school and will sponsor in-service training for teachers and school officials on how to manage persons with seizures.
   c. If seizures are rare, it is not necessary to inform the school.
   d. Learning disabilities and behavior problems can also occur in patients with seizures. These can relate to the seizures, the medications, or may coexist independently.
   e. The physician must encourage vocational planning for patients with frequent seizures *early* in high school or even in junior high school.
4. Employment.
   a. Unfortunately, discrimination against persons with seizures still occurs. State agencies (generally in di-

visions of vocational rehabilitation) may be helpful in assisting persons with seizures in finding employment or minimizing discrimination.

b. Persons with seizures should be encouraged to avoid occupations in which a seizure would be hazardous to self or fellow workers.

5. Alcoholic beverages.

a. Consumption of alcoholic beverages in moderation will rarely increase the incidence of seizures, but alcohol and anticonvulsants have additive effects, usually resulting in lowered alcohol tolerance.

b. An alcoholic with seizures who continues to consume alcoholic beverages should probably not be given anticonvulsants, since compliance is often poor and seizures from medication withdrawal alone may occur. Drinking must stop before anticonvulsant prophylaxis can be effective.

6. Other drugs: Reassure patients that they do not become addicted to anticonvulsants (antiepileptic drugs). Warn about drug interactions (Table 11–4), although most commonly used over-the-counter medications, such as aspirin, have no significant drug interactions. Warn that drug abuse, with "speed," "uppers," or "downers" will result in significant drug interactions and probably exacerbate the epilepsy.

7. Birth control pills: Although it is commonly believed that seizures are exacerbated by oral contraceptives, in reality this is unpredictable in any single patient. Other methods of birth control are available if seizures are exacerbated. Generally, the high-progesterone low-estrogen oral contraceptives are less likely to exacerbate seizures.

8. Pregnancy: The risks of teratogenic effects of anticonvulsants on the fetus must be weighed against the risk of seizures occurring during pregnancy, with attendant effects on the pregnancy. Cleft lip, cleft palate, congenital heart defects, and mental retardation have been reported to result in babies born of mothers taking anticonvulsants during pregnancy. If at all possible, attempts should be made to keep mothers off anticonvulsants at

TABLE 11–4.
Anticonvulsant (Antiepileptic) Drug Interactions

Drug	Serum Level Increased by	Serum Level Decreased by
Phenytoin	Chloramphenicol	Carbamazepine
	Disulfiram	
	Isoniazid	
	Dicumarol	
	Salicylates	
	Felbamate	
	Ethosuximide	
Carbamazepine	Erythromycin	Phenytoin
		Phenobarbital
		Primidone
Valproic acid	Felbamate	Carbamazepine
Phenobarbital	Valproic acid	
	Phenytoin	
Primidone	Valproic acid	Phenytoin
Felbamate		Phenytoin
		Carbamazepine

least in the first trimester of the pregnancy. The usual problem clinically, however, is that the mother has already been pregnant for 6 to 8 weeks when the diagnosis of pregnancy has been made, and if there are teratogenic effects, the damage has already been done. Neural tube defects have been reported with anticonvulsants like valproate and hence ultrasound studies and amniocentesis are recommended if there has been exposure to such drugs in early pregnancy. There is a risk for a bleeding tendency in babies born of mothers taking phenytoin. Giving vitamin K orally to the mother in the last month of pregnancy prevents this.

9. Genetics: The primary generalized epilepsies (petit mal and grand mal) are the most heritable of the epilepsies. The risk of a child having epilepsy when one parent has either petit mal or grand mal is estimated to be as high as 12%. The genetics of the primary partial epilepsies is unclear. Although the secondary partial epilepsies, simple or complex, are due to acquired lesions, whether

these are demonstrable or not, there is some relationship to previous family history of epilepsy. Patients with severe head injury, e.g., are more likely to develop post-traumatic epilepsy if there is a previous family history of epilepsy; however, it is not possible to predict the likelihood of epilepsy developing in offspring of parents, one of whom has an acquired partial epilepsy.

10. Safety: Anticonvulsants should always be stored in locked cabinets to prevent the possibility of theft or accidental ingestion by children.

11. Dentists and dental hygiene: Reassure dentists that there is no great danger of exacerbating seizures in the dentist's chair by giving local anesthetics and that there is no great danger of anesthetics interacting with anticonvulsants. Do instruct patients receiving phenytoin to visit their dentists at least twice a year and to brush their teeth at least twice daily. In addition, they should floss their teeth regularly.

12. Surgical operations: Phenobarbital and phenytoin can be given parenterally at equivalent doses during preoperative and postoperative phases when the patient is taking nothing by mouth (NPO). Phenytoin should *not* be given IM, since it is poorly absorbed through that route. Because the period of NPO following surgery is usually less than 24 hours, parenteral administration of anticonvulsants is usually not necessary.

13. Physical limitations: Patients should be allowed to participate in physical and recreational activities that maintain physical fitness. Perhaps the only activities that require some limitation are swimming (where the caution of never swimming alone should be scrupulously observed) and contact sports, such as American football and ice hockey, in which serious injury could be sustained should a seizure occur on the field or rink (although there is wide room for individual physician judgment here).

14. Resources.
   a. For information regarding services to epileptics, low-cost prescription services, and group life insurance, as well as general programs, the patient should con-

tact the Epilepsy Foundation of America, 4351 Garden City Drive, Suite 406, Landover, MD 20785, telephone: (301) 459-3700 or 800-332-1000.
b. Some reading materials that can be recommended for the patient with seizures include:

Freeman JM, Vining EPG, Pillas DJ: *Seizures and Epilepsy in Childhood: A Guide for Parents.* Baltimore, Johns Hopkins University Press, 1990.

Lagos JC: *Seizures, Epilepsy and Your Child,* New York, Harper & Row, 1974.

Middleton AH, Altwed A, Walsh G: *Epilepsy,* Boston, Little Brown, 1981.

Svoboda WB: *Learning About Epilepsy,* Baltimore, University Park Press, 1979.

Wright GN: *Epilepsy Rehabilitation,* Boston, Little Brown, 1975.

X. **TREATMENT OF CONVULSIVE STATUS EPILEPTICUS (SEE ALSO CHAPTER 20, section II).**
A. **Convulsive status epilepticus** is the state of continual seizures, or more commonly, recurrent convulsive seizures in which the patient does not fully regain consciousness between seizures. Status epilepticus most commonly occurs in known epileptics who stop medication. Rarely, status epilepticus is the first presentation of a seizure disorder, CNS infection (abscess or cerebral meningitis), metabolic disorder (hypoglycemia, hyponatremia, or hypocalcemia), or cerebrovascular disease (acute infantile hemiplegia).
   1. *Do not panic.* The patient should be treated promptly, but carefully.
   2. Establish an adequate airway:
      a. Remove false teeth.
      b. Turn patient or head to one side in order that secretions can drain out of the mouth.
      c. Extend neck (Fig 11–1).
      d. Loosen tight clothing.
      e. Suction mouth as necessary.
      f. Place a padded object between teeth if the mouth is

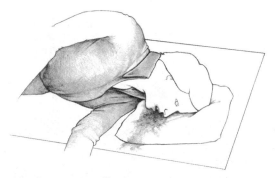

FIG 11-1. Positioning the patient in convulsive status epilepticus.

open (*do not force an object into a tonic, clenched jaw*).
g. Oxygen is not necessary immediately, as long as the airway is adequate.
3. Insert needle into vein and draw blood for glucose, electrolytes, and calcium determinations; through the same needle instill 50% glucose 1 to 2 mL/kg (50 mL in the adult) and then begin continuous IV infusion with 5% dextrose in water (D/W).
4. Initially give diazepam 1 mg every 30 seconds up to a dose of 0.3 mg/kg (maximum dose 10 mg) or lorazepam 0.5 mg every 30 seconds up to a total dose of 0.1 mg/kg (maximum dose 8 mg). *The physician must be prepared to support respiration with an Ambu bag, since brief respiratory arrest may occur after benzodiazepine (diazepam or lorazepam) administration. If unable or unprepared to provide respiratory support, do not give a benzodiazepine.*
5. After diazepam or lorazepam administration, whether or not seizures stop, or if a benzodiazepine is not administered, administer phenytoin 20 mg/kg, up to 1,000 mg. For proper IV injection of phenytoin see section IX. B. 9.

6. If seizures do not stop within 15 to 20 minutes after administration of phenytoin (the drug takes about 10 minutes to reach a sufficient level in the brain to stop seizures), administer phenobarbital IV at a dose of 20 mg/kg. *At this point the patient should be intubated.*

7. Continued seizures despite the previous medications are usually the result of a metabolic disturbance (such as hyponatremia or hypocalcemia) or a serious intracranial lesion (such as abscess or meningoencephalitis), and the seizures will not stop until the underlying disorder is treated. General anesthesia, such as pentobarbital coma, is a last resort and should be administered by an anesthesiologist under EEG monitoring.

8. Maintenance doses of the anticonvulsants should be started immediately and administered *intravenously* until oral doses can be started *(never intramuscularly)*. These are:
   a. Phenytoin 5 to 7 mg/kg/day (300–400 mg/day in adults) IV divided q6h, *or*
   b. Phenobarbital 3 to 5 mg/kg/day (120 mg/day in adults) IV q6h.

XI. TREATMENT OF NONCONVULSIVE STATUS EPILEPTICUS.

A. **Seizures other than generalized convulsions** can occur continuously, and although not life-threatening (because they do not derange respiratory function), they are disabling and must be recognized and treated.

1. *Absence status:* Absence seizures occur either continuously or with only a few seconds break between seizures. The patient appears dazed, blank, or confused, and may intermittently answer questions, usually slowly and irrelevantly. The EEG shows continual 3-Hz spike and wave complexes.

2. *Psychomotor (complex partial) status:* This patient may appear similar to the patient with absence status, except that there may be automatisms continuously. The EEG concomitant is continual 5- to 6-Hz theta waves.

3. These are *not* medical emergencies. However IV diazepam or lorazepam should immediately stop the seizures and confirm the diagnosis. The loading dose of

the appropriate long-term anticonvulsant should then be started.

BIBLIOGRAPHY

Aicardi J: *Epilepsy in Children*. New York, Raven Press, 1986.

Aminoff MJ, Simon RP: Status epilepticus: Causes, clinical features, and consequences in 98 patients. *Am J Med* 1980; 69:657–666.

Browne PR, Feldman RG: *Epilepsy Diagnosis and Management*. Boston, Little, Brown, 1983.

Dalessio DJ: Seizure disorders and pregnancy. *N Engl J Med* 1985; 312:559–563.

Delgado-Escueta AV, Treiman DM, Walsh GO: The treatable epilepsies. *N Engl J Med* 1983; 308:1508–1514, 1576–1584.

Delgado-Escueta AV, Wasterlain C, Treiman DM, et al: Current concepts in neurology: management of status epilepticus. *N Engl J Med* 1982; 306:1337–1340. [*Note:* There is an error in Table 1, procedure 4, line 4 of this article; the correct statement is: "An endotracheal tube should *now* be inserted."]

Engel J Jr: *Seizures and Epilepsy*. Philadelphia, FA Davis, 1989.

Ferry P, Banner W Jr, Wolf R: *Seizure Disorders in Children*. Philadelphia, JB Lippincott, 1985.

Gastaut H, Zifkin BG: Classification of the epilepsies. *J Clin Neurophysiol* 1985; 2:313–326.

Gilman S: Advances in epilepsy. *N Engl J Med* 1992; 326:1609–1615, 1671–1675.

Goa KL, Ross R, Chrisp P: Lamotrigine. *Drugs* 1993; 46:152–173.

Kundt RS, Bickley SK, Shimp LA: Discontinuing antiepileptic therapy. *Am Fam Physician* 1985; 31:177–184.

Lee SK: Nonconvulsive status epilepticus. *Arch Neurol* 1985; 42:778–781.

Mattson RH, et al: A comparison of valproate with carbamazepine for the treatment of complex partial seizures and secondarily generalized tonic-clonic seizures in adults. *N Engl J Med* 1992; 327:765–771.

Nelson K, Ellenberg JH: *Febrile Seizures*. New York, Raven Press, 1981.

Ojemann LM, Ojemann GA: Treatment of epilepsy. *Am Fam Physician* 1984; 30(2):113–128.

Palmer KJ, McTavish D: Felbamate. *Drugs* 1993; 45:1041–1065.

Porter RJ: *Epilepsy: 100 Elementary Principles*. Philadelphia, WB Saunders, 1984.

Resor SR Jr, Kutt H (eds): *The Medical Treatment of Epilepsy*. New York, Marcel Dekker, 1992.

Rothner A.D.: Intractable seizure disorders of childhood. *Cleve Clin Q* 1984; 51:505–510.

Scheuer ML, Pedley TA: The evaluation and treatment of seizures. *N Engl J Med* 1990; 323:1468–1474.

Schomer DL: Partial epilepsy. *N Engl J Med* 1983; 309:536–539.

Shinnar S, Vining EP, Mellits ED, et al: Discontinuing antiepileptic medication in children with epilepsy after two years without seizures: A prospective study. *N Engl J Med* 1985; 313:976–980.

THE STROKE SYNDROME

I. **CLINICAL EVALUATION.**

A. **Stroke, in neurologic terms,** refers to the sudden onset of a focal deficit due to a central nervous system abnormality. Such a clinical presentation does *not* specifically imply cerebrovascular disease, atherosclerosis, hemorrhage, or any other cause. It is true that the most common underlying cause of stroke is a cerebrovascular disorder, but a significant number of stroke patients have curable or remediable causes such as subdural hematoma, tumor, migraine, or postictal (postseizure) paralysis. For this reason, thorough evaluation is mandatory in nearly all patients. The tasks that face the physician are

1. To localize the lesion by neurologic examination (cerebral hemispheres, brainstem, cerebellum, spinal cord).
2. To order the least invasive procedures most likely to reveal the cause of the lesion.
3. To decide, on the basis of available knowledge, the best course of treatment.
4. To provide supportive care while in the hospital.
5. To initiate a program of rehabilitation.
6. Above all, to identify risk factors for stroke (hypertension, hyperlipidemia, smoking, obesity, sedentary life style) and modify or correct these risk factors before a more serious lesion occurs.

B. **By casual inspection,** even before taking a history, the physician can gain a general idea of the location of the lesion.

1. *Cerebral hemispheres:* Paralysis involves the contralateral face, arm, and leg. If the arm is more involved than the leg, suspect a lesion in the distribution of the middle cerebral artery. If arm and leg are equally involved, sus-

pect a deep hemisphere lesion. If the leg is more severely involved than the arm, suspect an anterior cerebral territory lesion. Aphasia or seizures suggest a hemispheric cortical lesion.

2. *Posterior fossa* (midbrain, pons, medulla, cerebellum) abnormalities are *crossed,* e.g., ipsilateral paralysis of face or eye with paralysis of the opposite side of the body. Consciousness is often impaired. Speech is often slurred but not aphasic.

3. *Spinal cord:* Both legs are usually involved, bladder problems are common, and a sensory level exists.

C. **In eliciting the history,** the physician should be guided by the knowledge of the causes of stroke. The following anatomic classification may be helpful.

1. *Intravascular causes:* The physician must consider disease processes that result in hypercoagulable or hyperviscous states which increase the probability of infarction by thrombosis, while hypocoagulable states increase the probability of hemorrhage. Possible diagnostic considerations include leukemia, polycythemia, coagulation disorders, sickle cell anemia, and hemoconcentration from severe dehydration. Increased arterial pressure from hypertension increases the probability of hemorrhage.

2. *Causes related to blood vessel walls:* These include congenital and mycotic aneurysms, infectious causes such as meningovascular syphilis, inflammatory disorders such as collagen-vascular diseases, venous thromboses, and cranial arteritides. Cerebrovascular atherosclerotic disease may result in stroke syndrome either by arterial thromboses or embolism from an ulcerated plaque. Inflammatory diseases may also affect veins and cause venous thrombosis.

Note: Either venous or arterial disease may cause stroke syndrome.

3. *Problems related to the great vessels of the neck:* Disease of the great vessels of the neck (specifically the ca-

rotid arteries) may be surgically correctable. Included are stenosis of the carotid arteries and the subclavian steal syndrome. These are suspected when carotid bruits are heard in the neck but they can only be accurately diagnosed by four-vessel cerebral angiography. Palpation of carotid pulsation is an unreliable index of carotid artery stenosis or occlusion. (A completely occluded carotid artery may have an apparently normal pulse.)

4. *Causes related to the heart:* Patients with cerebral atherosclerosis often also have coronary artery disease. The frequency of heart disease (including myocardial infarction or arrhythmias) in stroke patients is two to three times that of the age-adjusted general population without stroke. In other circumstances, such as bacterial endocarditis or postmyocardial infarction mural thrombus, there is a direct cause-and-effect relationship between the heart disease and stroke. Chronic or recurrent atrial fibrillation has been identified as a major risk factor for stroke. All patients with stroke syndrome need a thorough cardiac evaluation, which minimally would include an electrocardiogram (ECG), but may be extended to include rhythm monitoring procedures and echocardiography. Patients with transient ischemic attacks (TIAs) followed for 5 years die as often of heart disease as of stroke.

5. *Mass lesions:* The neurologic deficits from mass lesions such as chronic subdural hematoma or tumor are usually gradually progressive. Edema around a tumor or hemorrhage into a tumor from erosion of a blood vessel wall can make the clinical picture appear to be of sudden onset. Viral infections such as herpes simplex encephalitis may present as stroke syndrome.

6. *Hypotension:* In orthostatic or postural hypotension, a fall in systemic blood pressure may result in a focal neurologic deficit. Such deficits are usually transient, although in a patient with compromised cerebral circulation the deficit may become permanent. Recognition of hypotension as a contributory cause of cerebral injury is particularly important in the rehabilitation of the patient.

Caveat: Prior to allowing a stroke victim to stand or walk, postural hypotension must be ruled out by carefully measuring blood pressure in the lying, sitting, and standing position.

7. Other causes: Metabolic disorders such as hypoglycemia, hypoxia, and liver or renal disease can cause a preexisting subclinical cerebral deficit to become evident as a focal neurologic abnormality. It is important to emphasize the metabolic causes of stroke syndrome, since prompt intervention may reverse the clinical deficit. It is for this reason that, immediately following the onset of a stroke syndrome, the patient should have studies performed to assess blood sugar, liver and renal function, and arterial blood gases. Following focal seizures, paralysis may persist for 24 or more hours. Rarely, multiple sclerosis may manifest for the first time as an acute hemiparesis resembling stroke syndrome.

II. HISTORY.
A. **The history** may be helpful in determining the cause of the stroke syndrome. It is frequently important to have the patient's story corroborated by a family member or witness. In some cases, such as in comatose patients or patients with aphasia, family members may be the only source of history.
   1. Onset.
      ▶ a. Abrupt onset followed by gradual improvement suggests *embolus* ("While I was washing dishes, my right arm suddenly became paralyzed and I dropped a cup").
      ▶ b. Acute onset with progression to maximal deficit over minutes to hours suggests *thrombosis*.
      ▶ c. Stepwise development or onset during sleep usually suggests *thrombosis*.
      ▶ d. Focal neurologic symptoms usually lasting minutes but no longer than 24 hours suggest a *transient ischemic attack* (TIA).

      Caveat: The diagnosis of TIA is retrospective, made with certainty only after a thorough evaluation.

Some TIAs may represent small areas of damage with rapid functional recovery rather than true transient ischemia. Migraine, postictal (postseizure paralysis), hypoglycemia, and cardiac arrhythmias may also present as TIAs.

▶ e. Onset associated with headache or alterations of consciousness suggests *intracerebral hemorrhage*.

2. Course.

a. Rapid resolution of symptoms and signs in a few minutes is characteristic of TIAs, although by definition symptoms and signs can last up to 24 hours. TIAs are often due to platelet emboli from ulcerated arterial plaques or small emboli from the heart. At least 25% to 40% of patients with TIAs develop a major stroke in 5 years.

Caveat: TIA-like symptoms can occur from other conditions such as hemiplegic migraine, partial seizures, and lacunar infarcts.

b. In progressing stroke, the patient displays increasing deficits during the evaluation period. Differential diagnosis must include mass lesion and metabolic or infectious encephalopathy.

c. In completed stroke, the symptoms have stabilized and may improve.

▶ 1) Rapid improvement suggests cerebral *embolism*.

▶ 2) Gradual improvement over a day to a few weeks suggests *thrombosis*.

▶ 3) Rapid deterioration over a period of several hours suggests *intracerebral hemorrhage*.

3. Questions should be directed to the following symptoms:

a. Alteration of consciousness.

b. Headache (hemorrhage hurts; infarction does not).

c. Visual disturbances (*amaurosis fugax*—monocular blindness of short duration—usually indicates carotid artery disease with embolism to the ophthalmic artery, which is the first branch of the internal carotid artery.

   d. Disturbance of equilibrium (common in posterior fossa disorders).
   e. Motor or sensory disturbances (Fig 12–1).
   f. Precipitating factors and risk factors:
      1) Hypertension.
      2) Atherosclerotic cardiovascular disease in patient or family members.
      3) Elevated serum low density lipoproteins.
      4) Cigarette smoking.
      5) Obesity.
      6) Oral contraceptive use.
      7) Age and sex—middle-aged men and elderly people of both sexes are at higher risk.

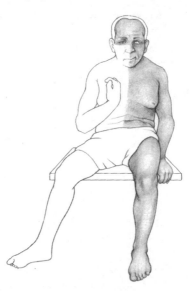

FIG 12–1. Spastic hemiparesis and lower facial weakness suggest contralateral cerebral hemisphere damage—often as a result of medically or surgically treatable carotid artery disease.

4. *Past medical history:* Especially of cardiovascular disease, hypertension, diabetes, head trauma, or recent infection.
5. Family history: Atherosclerotic cardiovascular disease or cerebral aneurysm.

III. EXAMINATION.

A. In addition to the routine examination, the following are especially important:

1. Check for fever or stiff neck (often associated with intracranial hemorrhage or infections).
2. If possible, take the blood pressure in both arms, in lying and standing positions (subclavian steal, postural hypotension).
3. Record level of consciousness using the Glasgow Coma Scale (see Chapter 13, section I.A.4.a).
4. Check heart for arrhythmias, murmurs, and enlargement, and lungs for congestion and friction rubs.
5. Check all peripheral pulses (a cardiac mural thrombus may fragment and occlude arteries of the limbs).
6. Evaluate carotid artery blood flow by listening for carotid bruits. The classic bruit of carotid stenosis is harsh, systolic, emanates from the carotid bifurcation, and radiates to the angle of the jaw. A bruit on the same side as the brain lesion is especially important. Diminished carotid pulse is of no value because an occluded carotid may appear to pulsate normally (the pulsations are transmitted directly from the aorta). A bruit over the supraclavicular fossa suggests stenosis of the vertebral or subclavian arteries. Observe, palpate, and compare the temporal, nasal, and supraorbital artery pulses; these branches of the external carotid artery are significant vessels used for collateral circulation to the brain following internal carotid occlusion (Fig 12–2).
7. Examine optic fundi for
   a. Early signs of papilledema (loss of venous pulsations and wet-appearing retina) indicating subarachnoid hemorrhage or mass lesion.
   b. Retinal infarction or cholesterol embolus (a small, bright-yellow fragment in an artery) suggesting carotid artery ulceration.

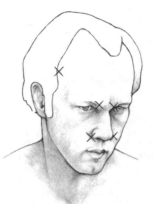

FIG 12–2. Palpation of temporal, nasal, and supraorbital pulses (*X* marks) may provide evidence of collateral circulation following a carotid occlusion.

8. Examine for signs of subacute bacterial endocarditis (SBE) such as petechial conjunctival hemorrhages or hemorrhages beneath the fingernails.

IV. LABORATORY EVALUATION.
A. **The following laboratory studies** are available in all hospitals and should be performed in every patient:
1. An ECG should be done immediately. Over one third of stroke victims will show ECG abnormalities at some time during the first 24 hours.
2. Chest radiograph.
3. Complete blood count (CBC) and platelet count.
4. Erythrocyte sedimentation rate or ESR (an elevated ESR may be related to infection or an autoimmune process such as temporal arteritis or lupus erythematosus).
5. Urinalysis (red blood cells in urine suggest emboli to the kidney as well as to the brain).
6. Blood glucose (before intravenous [IV] infusion is started).

7. Prothrombin time (PT or protime) and partial thromboplastin time (PTT).

8. Liver function and renal function tests such as determination of aspartate aminotransferase (SGOT), alkaline phosphatase, blood urea nitrogen (BUN), and creatinine values.

9. Arterial blood gases if respiratory compromise is suspected.

10. Serologic test for syphilis (the vasculitis associated with syphilis is a treatable cause of the stroke syndrome).

11. If a myocardial infarction is suspected, appropriate serum enzymes should be drawn.

B. **The following studies should be contemplated in every stroke victim.** The decision as to whether they actually will be done or not will depend on availability and economics.

1. *Imaging studies.*

a. A computed tomographic (CT) scan, ideally, should be done on every stroke victim *as soon as possible*. If the deficit is secondary to hemorrhage, this will immediately be apparent (and such patients should NOT be anticoagulated, even with low-dose aspirin or heparin). If the scan is normal or shows an infarct, the physician must immediately consider evaluation of the cerebral vasculature.

Caveat: The CT scan findings must correlate with the patient's neurologic examination; patients may have old or clinically silent infarcts which are irrelevant to the acute situation. Obviously, the CT scan will identify most mass lesions. The physician with no access to a CT scan is indeed handicapped and should treat the patient with supportive measures only.

b. Magnetic resonance imaging (MRI) can identify many abnormalities not evident on a CT scan (such as lacunar infarcts, multiple sclerosis plaques), but may not be available on an emergency basis. Posterior fossa abnormalities are visualized much better with MRI than with CT scans.

2. *Four-vessel cerebral angiography via femoral catheter:* If the CT scan reveals a subarachnoid hemorrhage, angiography is mandatory to identify an aneurysm or arteriovenous malformation. Angiography provides maximal information about the cerebral vasculature. Angiography is also the procedure of choice if carotid endarterectomy is to be performed, since most vascular or neurosurgeons will not operate on the basis of Doppler studies alone. The procedure should be ordered with caution, because it is associated with occasional morbidity and mortality. Ideally, it should be performed by an experienced radiologist trained in neuroradiology. Angiography performed by direct carotid artery puncture is almost never performed in the modern era.

3. *Doppler duplex scanning:* This ultrasound technique is a useful and accurate method of noninvasive assessment of the carotid arteries in the neck. Stenosis and plaques are identified through high-resolution B-mode imaging and the flow velocity is assessed by Doppler signals. The technique is also ideal for serial studies to assess the progression of plaques and degree of stenosis.

4. *Electroencephalography (EEG):* This study is most useful in patients suspected of having a seizure disorder associated with stroke or in identifying an underlying toxic-metabolic disorder. It is also useful in confirming the diagnosis of a superficial hemispheric lesion.

5. *Lumbar puncture:* Immediate lumbar puncture is indicated:
   a. In suspected cases of central nervous system (CNS) infection without evidence of increased intracranial pressure.
   b. When a CT scan is not available and anticoagulant therapy is anticipated; bloody or xanthochromic CSF would be a contraindication to anticoagulation. Normal lumbar puncture (often found with ischemic infarcts) decreases the probability that the deficit is caused by intracranial hemorrhage, tumor, or subdural hematoma.

   Remember: If an infarct is present, cerebral edema will occur in 24 to 48 hours. This edema causes increased intracranial pressure and increases the risk associated with lumbar puncture.

6. *Skull radiographs:* Order only if a skull fracture is suspected and a CT scan or MRI is not available.

V. NOW THAT I'VE MADE A DIAGNOSIS, WHAT DO I DO?. . .
A. What do I do?
1. *Mass lesion:* Aneurysms, subdural hematomas, tumors, and abscesses should be referred to a neurosurgeon.
2. *Lacunar infarct:* The patient has hypertension and a small infarct in the white matter; such patients rarely need four-vessel angiography; treat the hypertension and reduce other risk factors. Aspirin or anticoagulation therapy is not necessary.
3. *Carotid ulceration:* Patient with atherosclerotic ulcerated carotid artery plaques may present with blindness in one eye or contralateral hemiparesis or have a cholesterol embolus visible in the retina; the CT scan or MRI may be normal or show an infarct in the distribution of the middle cerebral artery. The clinical picture may be one of TIAs or a completed stroke. Treat with aspirin 325 mg/day. If attacks continue, consider carotid endarterectomy.
4. *Carotid stenosis:* With stenosis of the internal carotid artery of greater than 80% and symptoms on the opposite side of the body, surgical treatment (endarterectomy) is generally recommended. The outcome depends in part on the experience and skill of the surgeon. The risk of endarterectomy in some practice locations is greater than the risk of conservative therapy, and in such situations medical treatment with aspirin 325 mg/day should be undertaken. If aspirin is not effective, other antiplatelet drugs (such as ticlopidine) or anticoagulants may be necessary.
5. *Cardiac embolus:* Patient may have atrial fibrillation or mural thrombus; if no hemorrhage is evident on the CT scan or MRI, treat immediately with heparin, then later switch to warfarin sodium (Coumadin). The aim is to prevent further embolization. Continue therapy for at

least 6 months. If the infarct is large, it may be preferable to defer anticoagulant therapy for the first few days.

6. *Middle cerebral artery occlusion or arterial occlusion in the posterior fossa:* Extracranial-intracranial bypass operations have been shown to be of no value; if symptoms are progressive, anticoagulant therapy is indicated as long as no hemorrhage is identified on CT scans or MRI.

7. *Seizure or migraine:* Treat specifically (see Chapter 11, section IV, or Chapter 3, section IV).

8. *Venous thromboses* are usually secondary to infection or to an underlying hypercoagulable state. Treat with antibiotics and anticoagulation.

9. *Carotid stenosis and no symptoms:* Endarterectomy is not generally recommended. Treat with aspirin 325 mg/day.

10. *Toxic-metabolic disorders* (e.g., hypoglycemia or blood dyscrasia): Treat specifically.

VI. MANAGEMENT.

A. Supportive therapy for stroke victims.

1. *Nursing orders to monitor neurologic status:* At least during the first 24 hours, the patient should be evaluated hourly. In addition to the Glasgow Coma Scale (see Chapter 13, Section I.A.4.a) and monitoring of blood pressure, pulse, temperature (rectal), and respirations, the nursing staff should be taught to evaluate pupillary size, equality, and reaction to light.

2. *Nursing management:* The following precautions may be beneficial:

   a. Above-knee elastic stockings may minimize the development of phlebothrombosis or thrombophlebitis.

   b. Use dorsiflexion splints or a footboard and sandbags to maintain the foot of the paralyzed leg in dorsiflexion.

   c. Roll towels or other soft objects in the hand to maintain the hand in a position of function.

   d. The physician must be aware of and apprise the nursing staff of hemianopia and hemineglect and position the patient appropriately to accommodate these phenomena.

    e. Frequent turning of the patient prevents bedsores.

    f. If the patient cannot close the eyelids, instillation of artificial tears may prevent corneal ulcers.

    g. In the patient with diplopia, alternate patching of the eyes improves vision and is more comfortable.

    h. In the alert patient with speech difficulty, a communication board containing common requests may be helpful.

    i. Stool softeners should be instituted early to prevent fecal impaction.

    j. In the first few days after paralysis, the patient should be placed in an upright or sitting position intermittently to prevent development of postural hypotension.

    k. A simple explanation of the problem will relieve family anxiety. Especially in the case of the aphasic patient, explain to the family that speech difficulty is not associated with feeblemindedness.

3. *Blood pressure management:* Most stroke victims will have transient hypertension. A diastolic blood pressure of less than 120 mm Hg (torr) is not cause for immediate concern. If the blood pressure is to be lowered, *do so gingerly* over a time period of several days. A moderately elevated blood pressure may be the body's protective mechanism to ensure adequate cerebral perfusion (even in hemorrhage, vasospasm is common).

4. *Nutritional support.*

    a. Intravenous fluids should contain multivitamins, including thiamine to prevent Wernicke's encephalopathy.

    b. Syndrome of inappropriate antidiuretic hormone (SIADH) may occur with stroke; thus the patient should be kept on the "dry" side to treat both this and cerebral edema. Recording of fluid intake and output is important.

    c. Nitrogen and electrolyte balance are best accomplished with nasogastric feedings. The patient should receive nutrition via this route (rather than IV) as soon as possible.

5. *Bladder care:* Urinary retention in the acute phase is common, but an indwelling catheter should be used cau-

tiously. If an indwelling catheter is used, intermittent clamping should be done to avoid loss of bladder tone. Bladder function returns more quickly in patients who have intermittent rather than continuous catheterization. Patients with indwelling catheters tend to have severe urinary tract infections and bladder dysfunction due to chronic scarring.

6. *Pulmonary care:* Frequent suctioning of excess secretions, frequent turning, induced coughing, and deep breathing will help prevent atelectasis. Oxygen should be administered only when arterial oxygen pressure is low.

7. *Cardiac care:* Because there is such a high correlation between cerebral infarction and cardiac abnormalities, continuous cardiac monitoring should (when possible) be instituted.

8. *Physical therapy:* Patients who remain bedridden for any length of time are at risk for developing serious complications such as pulmonary embolism or orthostatic hypotension. With the exception of patients with subarachnoid hemorrhage, those stroke victims who are encouraged to sit or stand as soon as possible, and do so, improve more rapidly and have fewer complications. If the patient is bedridden for any length of time, passive physical therapy may reduce the risk of pulmonary embolism. Physical therapy is also important in preventing contractures, since significant contractures may develop in the shoulder girdle within 24 hours.

9. *Anticoagulation:* Anticoagulation should be instituted only after establishing that the stroke syndrome was not the result of hemorrhage and that there is no gross bleeding into the area of infarction. The main indication for anticoagulation is prevention of subsequent infarction from embolization. The source for emboli should be documented, since heparin and warfarin sodium are most useful for cardiac emboli (antiplatelet agents should be used to prevent platelet emboli from carotid ulceration).

   a. In the acute phase, heparin is given IV by continuous infusion, preferably using an infusion pump. The effects of heparin must be monitored by frequent determinations of the activated partial thromboplastin time (APTT), which should be maintained at 1.5 to 2.5 times the normal value.

b. A coumarin compound such as warfarin sodium may be of value for a period of 6 months or more in those patients who have carotid stenosis or emboli from the heart. This drug reduces the hepatic production of vitamin K–dependent blood clotting factors (factors II, VII, IX, and X). Oral dosage should be individualized to maintain the prothrombin time (PT) at 20 to 25 seconds (1.5 times normal). Initially, one dose of 20 to 60 mg is given followed by maintenance at a dosage of 2 to 10 mg/day. The PT must be determined at least once per week while the patient is receiving warfarin sodium. Once warfarin sodium is started, it probably cannot be stopped without a rebound increased risk of thrombosis. Therapy is complicated by the risk of major hemorrhage.

10. *Antiplatelet drugs*

    a. Aspirin, one tablet (325 mg) per day, inhibits platelet aggregation. It has been found to be useful in decreasing the occurrence of TIAs, stroke following TIAs, and myocardial infarction. Complications include gastric erosion from the aspirin (less likely if buffered) and hemorrhage after surgical procedures.

    b. Ticlopidine, 500 mg/day, is useful in patients who do not respond to or are intolerant of aspirin. Major side effects include diarrhea, skin rashes, and neutropenia.

11. *Treatment of cerebral edema.*

    a. Forty-eight hours after infarction, cerebral edema may develop, causing the patient's condition to deteriorate. Corticosteroids probably have little effect on this edema (as opposed to the dramatic effect of corticosteroids on the edema surrounding a tumor). If steroids are used, dexamethasone in doses of 4 to 20 mg q4h is preferable. The corticosteroid dosage should be rapidly tapered and continued for no longer than 7 to 10 days.

    b. Keeping the patient moderately dehydrated by restricting IV fluids is probably most effective in controlling edema. As an adjunct to this, mannitol (in a 10%–20% solution) at a dose of 1 g/kg in extreme cases will aid in this dehydration. Daily weighing of the patient and monitoring of electrolytes is mandatory with this type of therapy.

12. *Speech and language therapy:* If communication is disturbed by the stroke, speech and language therapy may be helpful. The speech (language) pathologist specifically evaluates auditory processing and retention, reading and writing abilities, and speaking abilities. From this evaluation, a treatment program is designed, utilizing the patient's strengths to improve weakness. The speech therapist identifies the specific problems in communication, consults with the physician and hospital staff, and counsels and advises the family members. The speech therapist can assist the physician in educating the family regarding difficulties, such as those of aphasic patients, and works with the family and patient on a home program. Thorough explanation of the patient's communication difficulties to the family alleviates embarrassment stemming from misunderstanding. The patient should be encouraged to participate in social situations as much as possible. Follow-up treatment is usually arranged for reevaluation and updating of therapy. Speech therapists may note minor changes in speech patterns, which may be subtle signs of recurring disease.

13. *Occupational therapy:* In the rehabilitation of stroke patients, the aims of occupational therapy overlap speech and physical therapy, with strong emphasis on functional skills for the activities of daily living. In cooperation with physical therapy, occupational therapy includes improving or maintaining the range of motion, strength, coordination, and balance, and reduction of spasticity. Therapists provide splints to prevent contracture and slings to prevent subluxation of the shoulder. Evaluation and training is available for patients with perceptual dysfunctions. In conjunction with speech therapy, occupational therapists improve coordination for speech and fine coordination for writing. Special attention is given

to retraining or assistance in the activities of daily living, such as dressing and feeding. Adaptive equipment is provided, and patients are taught how to use it most effectively.

14. *The rehabilitation hospital:* There is increasing pressure on the physician to discharge patients from the acute care hospital as soon as possible. Rehabilitation hospitals offer an environment where physical therapists, speech therapists, occupational therapists, and physicians specializing in neurorehabilitation work as a team to help the patient reach maximal functional capacity. A stroke victim will continue to improve for approximately 6 to 12 months. This alternative should be considered if the patient is moderately to severely disabled and rehabilitation efforts cannot be accomplished on an outpatient basis.

15. Educational materials and other information for patients and families may be obtained from the National Stroke Association, 1420 Ogden St., Denver, CO 80218, (303) 839-1992.

VII. APHASIA.

A. **Aphasia is considered in this chapter because it so commonly occurs in stroke victims,** but it must be remembered that aphasia is a *symptom* (like a hemiparesis) and can occur in any disease process that injures the perisylvian dominant (usually left) hemisphere. It is defined as an acquired disorder of language, and in the absence of other obvious neurologic symptoms, it can easily be confused with dementia and psychiatric disorders.

B. **Aphasia is a disturbance of language** only and must be differentiated from the myriad disorders of *speech*. For example, a patient with cerebellar dysfunction may have a loss of speech melody with an explosive irregular type of vocalization; a patient with vocal cord or tongue paralysis will have a normal speech cadence but a marked change in clarity or tone or both; and a patient with bilateral upper motor neuron lesions will have slow, arduous speech. None of these patients would have any difficulty thinking of words or expressing thoughts appropriately and thus would *not* have a language disturbance (aphasia). Schizophrenic patients on occasion may have a senseless word salad in which there is apparently no connection between one word and the next; speech melody is normal, and when listened to closely, the patient's thought processes will fit into the patient's own private code. Thus, the schizophrenic patient does not have aphasia. Aphasia must also be differentiated from dementia: aphasia is a disturbance of language only, whereas dementia is a disturbance of all cognitive processes, including language.

C. It must be emphasized that the diagnosis of **aphasia should not be a casual diagnosis,** but requires the physician to examine the patient specifically for an aphasic syndrome. In general, the physician should be readily able to differentiate four basic types of aphasic phenomena (Table 12–1):

1) the patient who understands language well but produces little spontaneous speech (*nonfluent* or *Broca's* aphasia);

2) the patient who is unable to understand language, but produces voluminous verbalization with meaningless content (*fluent* or *Wernicke's* aphasia);

3) the patient who has nonfluent speech and poor comprehension (*global* aphasia); and

4) the patient who has good verbal output (fluency), good understanding of language, difficulty with word finding in spontaneous speech, and difficulty naming objects (*anomic* aphasia).

TABLE 12–1.
Simplified Summary of Language Problems in Aphasia

Language Function	Type of Aphasia			
	Broca's	Wernicke's	Global	Anomic
Fluency	−	+	−	+
Comprehension	+	−	−	+
Naming	+	−	−	−

1. Nonfluent patient who understands well (commonly referred to as a motor aphasia, anterior aphasia, nonfluent aphasia, expressive aphasia, or *Broca's aphasia*):

   a. In right-handed persons, this is almost always associated with damage to the left frontal cortex and is usually associated with some degree of paralysis of the right side of the body.

   b. The patient is aware of the speech difficulty and often becomes extremely frustrated and angry; secondary depression may frequently complicate the clinical picture.

   c. Speech is effortful and ungrammatic with short telegraphic phrases poorly articulated. Speech melody and rhythm are abnormal, and perseveration (repeating the same word) is common.

   d. Auditory comprehension is well preserved, and the patient can follow most directions.

   e. In the severe form, the patient may only be able to utter automatic speech such as obscenities and social amenities ("hello"). In the milder form or during recovery, more complicated automatic speech may be observed, such as singing "Happy Birthday" or reciting the Lord's Prayer.

   f. Reading silently for meaning is relatively preserved but slow; reading aloud is impaired, and writing is large, messy, and effortful, paralleling the verbal expression.

   Caveat: The diagnosis of aphasia cannot be made if the patient has absolutely no speech production.

2. Patient does not understand well, but has a voluminous verbal production (commonly called sensory aphasia, *Wernicke's aphasia,* posterior aphasia, receptive aphasia):

   a. In right-handed persons, damage is almost always confined to the left posterosuperior temporal area. This aphasia is usually not associated with a paralysis, although some patients may have a homonymous right visual field defect.

    b. In its pure form, the patient is unaware of the difficulty; usually the patient is pleasant and jovial but may become angry with the examiner's inability to understand his or her speech.

    c. Speech rhythm and melody are normal, but the content is incomprehensible (true in all languages; e.g., the aphasic German appears to be speaking German and the aphasic Frenchman appears to be speaking French, but the language is incomprehensible).

    d. In mild form or during recovery, paraphasias are common; e.g., "Resident pea gun staked on the telegram." for "President Reagan talked on the television." Speech with frequent paraphasias is also called jargon speech.

    e. Patient has very poor auditory comprehension but may respond to whole-body commands such as "stand up," "walk backward," or "open your mouth."

    f. Both reading aloud and reading silently for comprehension are defective; writing is well formed, but contains the same errors and lack of meaning as the verbal expression.

3. Patient who has nonfluent speech and poor comprehension (commonly called *global aphasia*):

    a. As ordinarily used, global aphasia refers to the patient who has both frontal lobe and temporoparietal lobe damage; this is basically a combination of the fluent and nonfluent aphasias involving all aspects of language.

    b. The patient is awake and alert, but for the most part sits silently and is unresponsive.

    c. Global aphasia is almost always associated with right hemiparesis in right-handed patients; there is often a right homonymous hemianopia.

4. Patient with good verbal output and good understanding but with word-finding and naming difficulties *(anomic aphasia)*:

    a. In right-handed persons this is usually due to a lesion of the left angular gyrus (at the junction of the parietal, occipital, and temporal lobes).

b. Speech is fluent, but may be hesitant because of word-finding difficulties (usually nouns).

c. As in fluent or Wernicke's aphasia, paraphasias (sound or word substitutions) are common in spontaneous speech.

d. Because of the word-finding difficulties, this syndrome is often confused with nonfluent or Broca's aphasia, but can be differentiated from it because the anomic aphasic has fluent, nondysarthric, effortless speech, and in the pure form there is no accompanying hemiparesis.

e. Verbal comprehension is intact.

f. When presented with objects, the patient misnames them (often with paraphasic errors) or cannot produce the name, although the patient will select the correct name when given a multiple choice format.

g. Often accompanied by Gerstmann's syndrome (right-left disorientation, finger agnosia, acalculia, agraphia).

5. The aphasic syndromes can be more discretely defined and subcategorized, but familiarity with and identification of these four basic types by the physician will describe most aphasic patients.

D. Treatment.

1. Specific language therapy may accelerate a patient's recovery. Treatment should also be directed at the underlying lesion.

2. Rehabilitation of the patient with aphasia is necessary. For patients with intact understanding, it is important to find mechanisms to assist the patient with communication. The speech and language therapist may be of help in this regard. Simple signboards, letter boards, and other signaling devices are sometimes helpful, but new advances in computer technology in some areas have superseded these devices. The family must be educated to the patient's expressive difficulties and provide a nonstressful environment for the patient's expression. Appropriate reading materials or talking books should be provided for the patient. In the patient with impaired comprehension, supervised care may be necessary.

BIBLIOGRAPHY

Albers GW, Sherman DG, Gress DR, Paulseth JE, Petersen P: Stroke prevention in nonvalvular atrial fibrillation: A review of prospective randomized trials. *Ann Neurol* 1991; 30:511–518.

Brodal A: Self-observations and neuro-anatomical considerations after a stroke. *Brain* 1973; 96:675–694.

Caplan LR: Diagnosis and treatment of ischemic stroke. *JAMA* 1991; 266:2413–2418.

Chesebro JH: Atrial fibrillation—risk marker for stroke. *N Engl J Med* 1990; 323:1556–1559.

Chyatte D, Sundt TM: Cerebral vasospasm after subarachnoid hemorrhage. *Mayo Clin Proc* 1984; 59:498–505.

Damasio AR: Aphasia. *N Engl J Med* 1992; 326:531–539.

DiTullio MD, Sacco RL, Gopal A, et al: Patent foramen ovale as a risk factor for cryptogenic stroke. *Ann Intern Med* 1992; 117:461–465.

EC/IC Bypass Study Group: Failure of extracranial intracranial arterial bypass to reduce the risk of ischemic stroke. *N Engl J Med* 1985; 313:1191–1200.

Easton JD, Sherman DE: Carotid endarterectomy. *Mayo Clin Proc* 1983; 58:205–207.

Grotta JC: Current medical or surgical therapy for cerebrovascular disease. *N Engl J Med* 1987; 317:1505–1515.

Hass WK, Easton JD, Adams HP Jr, et al: A randomized trial comparing ticlopidine hydrochloride with aspirin for the prevention of stroke in high risk patients. *N Engl J Med* 1989; 321:501–507.

Hurwitz BJ, Heyman A, Wilkinson WE, et al: Comparison of amaurosis fugax and transient cerebral ischemia: A prospective clinical and arteriographic study. *Ann Neurol* 1985; 18:698–704.

Kistler JP, Ropper AH, Heros RC: Therapy of ischemic cerebral vascular disease due to atherothrombosis. *N Engl J Med* 1984; 311:27–34.

Levine SR: Acute cerebral ischemia in a critical care unit. *Arch Intern Med* 1989; 149:90–97.

Maggroni AP: The risk of stroke in patients with acute myocardial infarction after thrombolytic and antithrombotic treatment. *N Engl J Med* 1992; 327:1–6.

Meyer FB: Carotid endarterectomy in elderly patients. *Mayo Clin Proc* 1991; 66:464–469.

North American Symptomatic Carotid Endarterectomy Trial Collaborators: Beneficial effect of carotid endarterectomy in symptomatic patients with high grade stenosis. *N Engl J Med* 1991; 325:445–453.

Report of the WHO Task Force on Stroke and Other Cerebrovascular Disorders. *Stroke* 1989; 20:1407–1431.

Ropper AH, Wechsler LR, Wilson LS: Carotid bruit and the risk of stroke in elective surgery. *N Engl J Med* 1982; 307:1388–1390.

Sherokman BJ, Hallenbeck JM: Management of acute stroke. *Am Fam Physician* 1985; 31:190–199.

Till JS, Toole JF, Howard VJ: Management of carotid artery plaques, murmurs, and transient ischemic attacks. *Arch Neurol* 1985; 42:1198–1201.

COMA 13

Coma is a medical emergency. The purposes of this chapter are to: (1) outline immediate measures to care for the comatose patient; (2) establish criteria for deciding whether coma is secondary to a toxic-metabolic disorder (over 80% of cases are) or to a structural central nervous system (CNS) disorder; and (3) provide guidelines for the management of coma secondary to a CNS disorder.

I. THE COMATOSE PATIENT.
A. Immediate measures.
1. Establish and maintain a clear airway. In many cases this requires insertion of an endotracheal tube with ventilatory assistance.
2. Check pulse, blood pressure, and temperature. Apply electrocardiographic (ECG) monitor. If profound hypotension is present, or if there are gross cardiac abnormalities, the cause of coma is evident and should be treated appropriately.
3. Insert an intravenous (IV) line and draw blood for glucose, electrolytes (Na^+, K^+, Cl^-, $^-CO_2$, Ca^{+2}), complete blood count (CBC), blood urea nitrogen (BUN), and creatinine determinations. Arterial blood gases, toxic screening, and thyroid and liver function tests are often also drawn at this time.
4. Administer IV 50 mL of 50% glucose and 500 mg thiamine. Many authorities also suggest administration of naloxone hydrochloride (Narcan) 2 mg, especially if the patient has small pupils; however, if the patient does not respond to a total dose of 10 mg, the diagnosis of narcotic overdose is unlikely.
5. Catheterize the patient's bladder and monitor urinary output.

6. Determine the depth of coma:
   a. The Glasgow Coma Scale (Table 13–1) is commonly used to quantitate the severity of coma; it can be repeated at intervals to monitor the clinical course and effect of therapy.

   Note: This scale is especially useful in determining the prognosis in coma from head injuries and cardiorespiratory arrest. Thus 87% of patients who have a coma score of 4 or less at 24 hours after a head injury die or remain in a vegetative state. Of those with a score greater than 11, 87% show good recovery with mild to moderate disability.

TABLE 13–1.
Glasgow Coma Scale (*Circle the Appropriate Number and Compute the Total*)*

Eyes Open	
Never	1
To pain	2
To verbal stimuli	3
Spontaneously	4
Best Verbal Response	
No response	1
Incomprehensible sounds	2
Inappropriate words	3
Disoriented and converses	4
Oriented and converses	5
Best Motor Response	
No response	1
Extension (decerebrate rigidity)	2
Flexion abnormal (decorticate rigidity)	3
Flexion withdrawal	4
Localizes pain	5
Obeys	6
Total score (range)	3–15

*Sum of highest value in each category is coma score: full mental capacity = 15; highest level of coma = 8; brain death = 3.

b. To evaluate the patient's response to noxious stimuli press the styloid processes of the temporal bone (Fig 13–1). This is an extremely painful stimulus that should be performed with caution; however, it is preferable to rubbing the sternum, twisting the nipples, or squeezing the testicles, which give less information, may leave unsightly marks that the family later questions, and is downright uncivilized. Note the type of response (arousal, decerebrate posturing, decorticate posturing, asymmetric response).

c. *Confused* patients respond to verbal stimuli, but are drowsy, slow, and often disoriented.

d. *Stuporous* patients respond transiently only to vigorous stimuli.

e. *Comatose* patients are unarousable and unresponsive but may exhibit abnormal postures.

B. Examination. Table 13–2 lists the mandatory examinations, which can be completed in a few minutes, and which allow the physician to make a tentative decision as to whether the coma is due to a toxic-metabolic cause or to a CNS lesion.

TABLE 13–2.
Differentiation of Coma Due to CNS Structural Lesion From Metabolic Coma

Examination	Suggestive of Structural CNS Coma	Suggestive of Metabolic Coma
Blood pressure	Increased	Decreased
Respiration	Ataxic	Regular or rhythmic
Temperature	Increased	Normal or decreased
Pupils	Asymmetric	Normal, usually reactive, even when brainstem function is suppressed
Oculocephalic and oculovestibular responses	Asymmetric or absent	Usually intact
Posture	Asymmetric	Symmetric
Fundi	Papilledema	Usually normal
Reflexes	Asymmetric	Symmetric
Neck suppleness	Stiff or normal	Normal
Myoclonus	Rare	Frequent

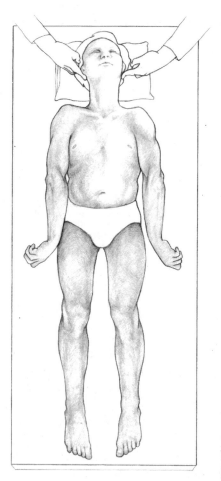

FIG 13–1. The examiner is applying pressure on the styloid processes in the comatose patient and producing decerebrate posturing. This posture is seen in patients with brainstem dysfunction.

1. CNS vs. metabolic coma: This examination may reveal the following types of information:
    a. *Blood pressure and pulse:* If the blood pressure is high and the pulse is low, severe increased intracranial pressure should be suspected. This finding is much more common in children than it is in adults. Most metabolic causes of coma cause hypotension.
    b. *Breathing patterns* that may be seen in coma are:
        1) Normal respiration.
        2) Hyperventilation—metabolic acidosis (e.g., uremia, diabetic ketoacidosis, exogenous toxins such as ethylene glycol) leads to hyperventilation; sustained, regular, rapid, deep hyperpnea is also seen in midbrain lesions (central neurogenic hyperventilation).
        3) Hypoventilation—respiratory depression seen with both medullary lesion and drug overdose.
        4) Cheyne-Stokes respiration—periodic smooth increase and decrease in respirations from apnea to hyperpnea; occurs both in bilateral lesions deep in the cerebral hemispheres and in metabolic coma.
        5) Ataxic respiration—completely irregular pattern due to a low brainstem lesion (as with cerebellar or pontine hemorrhage, medullary infarction, or trauma), but may also occur in severe meningitis.

        Caveat: Use of sedatives in a patient with ataxic breathing may cause respiratory arrest.

    c. *Temperature:* A significantly elevated temperature in the presence of an altered state of consciousness strongly suggests CNS infection; unless signs of imminent cerebral herniation or gross papilledema are present, the cerebrospinal fluid (CSF) must be examined and cultured before antibiotics are started. Subarachnoid hemorrhage may give a mildly elevated temperature, heat stroke a markedly increased temperature.
    d. *Pupils*
        1) Metabolic coma: Symmetric pupils that react to light suggest a metabolic disorder. Bilaterally fixed and dilated pupils are found in anoxia and in glutethim-

ide, scopolamine, and atropine poisoning. The pin-point pupils that occur in narcotic overdose dilate and become reactive with a small dose of a narcotic antagonist.

2) CNS coma is suggested by asymmetric pupils.

   Caveat: Pupillary inequalities of 1 mm or more may be seen in up to 10% of the normal population, and asymmetric pupils may also be the result of previous eye surgery or trauma.

e. *Oculocephalic response (doll's eye movement)* and *oculovestibular (caloric) test:*

   Caution: Do not perform in a patient with trauma.

   1) *Oculocephalic response:* Holding the patient's eye-lids open, passively rotate the head rapidly to both sides. In the comatose patient, the eyes remain as if fixed on an object in the foreground (Fig 13–2).

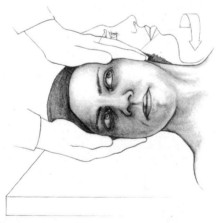

FIG 13–2. Doll's-eye movements. The eyes remain relatively stationary when the head is rapidly turned to one side.

Awake patients have no oculocephalic response. A unilateral response suggests a brainstem lesion. Presence of a normal doll's-eye response in both directions indicates that the brainstem between cranial nerve III (oculomotor nerve) and cranial nerve VIII (vestibuloacoustic nerve) is intact, and this suggests that the cause of coma is not destruction of the brainstem. Absence of the response suggests a metabolic depression of the brainstem or severe brainstem dysfunction.

2) *Caloric test:* If the doll's-eye response is equivocal or if there is some reason the neck should not be rotated (as in head trauma or cervical spine injury), caloric testing (oculovestibular reflex) may provide the same type of information. Check to see that the tympanic membrane is intact and that the external auditory canal is not blocked by wax or blood. Slowly inject at least 10 mL of ice water through a small polyethylene catheter into the external auditory canal. The head should be elevated or flexed to approximately 30 degrees. In patients with suspected cervical spine fracture, instead of bending the neck, the head of the bed should be elevated. Deviation of the eyes toward the ear being stimulated suggests an intact brainstem and a metabolic cause of the coma (Fig 13–3).

f. *Pressure on the styloid process*

1) Decerebrate posture (Fig 13–1): This posture is characterized by extended and internally rotated arms and extended legs with plantar flexion of the feet. Asymmetric posturing (e.g., one side moves, the other does not; or one side is decerebrate, the other decorticate) suggests structural CNS coma. Symmetric posturing is seen in brainstem and metabolic coma.

2) Decorticate posture (Fig 13–4): This posture is characterized by flexion of the upper extremities, extension of the legs, and plantar flexion of the feet. Asymmetric posturing suggests structural CNS coma; symmetric posturing is seen in bilateral hemisphere lesions.

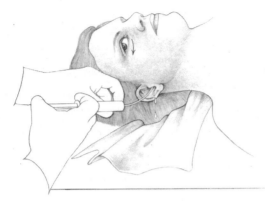

FIG 13–3. Caloric test. In a patient with intact brainstem (cranial nerves III–VIII), cold water in the auditory canal will cause the eyes to deviate toward the cold ear.

    g. *Funduscopy:* Look for early signs of papilledema, including loss of venous pulsations, enlargement of veins, a wet-appearing retina, and blurring of margins of optic discs. Which may be seen in both CNS mass lesions and in metabolic disturbances causing cerebral edema.

    h. *Reflexes:* Asymmetric reflexes suggest structural CNS coma; symmetric reflexes and bilateral Babinski reflexes are seen in both CNS and metabolic disturbances. Suggested techniques for eliciting the patellar and Achilles reflexes are shown in Figs 13–5 and 13–6.

    i. *Neck suppleness:* A stiff neck suggests subarachnoid hemorrhage or infection.

       Caution: The neck should not be manipulated in the case of head trauma in which there is a possibility of cervical spine fracture.

    j. *Myoclonus:* This is manifested as uncoordinated generalized twitches and is more often seen in metabolic

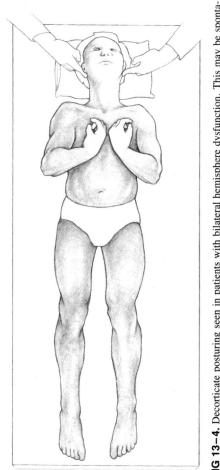

FIG 13–4. Decorticate posturing seen in patients with bilateral hemisphere dysfunction. This may be spontaneous or produced by painful stimulus.

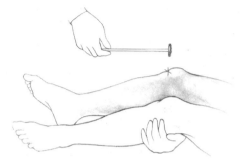

FIG 13–5. Patellar reflex testing in a comatose patient. Place arm under the knees so that they are slightly flexed as illustrated; pay close attention to asymmetries.

coma. Asterixis with flap tremor is another common finding in metabolic encephalopathy.

Note: Rarely, patients with metabolic coma may show focal CNS abnormalities. Asymmetric pupils may be congenital or a result of trauma. Fixed, pinpoint pupils may be secondary to treatment of glaucoma.

C. **History.** The history, when obtainable, often eliminates the need for a number of diagnostic tests and points to a specific cause of the coma. The history may sometimes be obtained from relatives, friends, a family physician, or the police. It should include the following:
   1. Onset: Abrupt onset indicates intracranial hemorrhage or infarction; gradual onset suggests a toxic or metabolic cause.
   2. Preceding neurologic complaints: convulsions, confusion, hallucinations, headache, diplopia, vertigo, numbness, weakness, ataxia.
   3. Recent trauma is suggestive of structural damage.
   4. Past medical history: psychiatric disturbances, diabetes, heart disease, hypertension, renal disease, epilepsy, alcoholism.

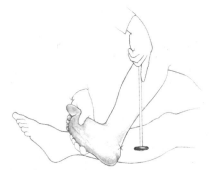

FIG 13–6. Achilles reflex. Cross legs as illustrated and slightly dorsiflex the foot before tapping the Achilles tendon.

5. Drug history: Both prescribed and illicit drugs are important.
6. Social history: Pay particular attention to any traumatic event that might be linked to depression and suicide attempt.

II. STRUCTURAL CNS LESIONS CAUSING COMA (HEMISPHERIC LESIONS).

A. **A unilateral** cerebral hemisphere lesion does not produce coma unless the lesion for some reason (e.g., edema) causes damage to the other hemisphere as well. For coma to occur secondary to a CNS lesion, either both hemispheres must be severely damaged or the reticular activating system in the brainstem must be damaged directly or indirectly because of a shift (usually laterally) in the hemispheres. When both hemispheres are involved, the neurologic examination almost always shows asymmetries; in this situation the computed tomography (CT) scan or magnetic resonance imaging (MRI) should readily lead the physician to the correct diagnosis (massive intracerebral hemorrhage, subdural hematoma large enough to cause herniation, multiple infarcts from emboli, unilateral edema causing shifts in intracerebral contents).

B. Cerebral herniation: The cerebral falx and the tentorium of
the cerebellum are relatively rigid structures, which separate
the cranial contents into three major compartments. Displacement of brain tissue by mass lesions (blood, edema, tumor)
from one compartment to another is termed *herniation* (Fig
13–7). The process is ominous because blood vessels may be
compressed, causing additional damage by ischemia. Secondary hemorrhages (Duret hemorrhages) in the brainstem are
also common.
1. Clinical features.
    a. Uncal herniation of the medial temporal lobe.
        1) Stretching of the third cranial nerve (oculomotor
           nerve) causes ipsilateral pupillary dilation.
        2) Pressure (from edema or mass effect) on the precen-
           tral motor cortex or the internal capsule causes con-
           tralateral hemiplegia.
        3) As the process progresses, the contralateral cerebral
           peduncle is pressed against the sharp edge of the ten-
           torium of the cerebellum, causing ipsilateral paraly-
           sis.
    b. Central herniation—herniation of basal parts of both
       cerebral hemispheres through the incisura of the tento-
       rium of the cerebellum. The clinical picture is not par-
       ticularly distinctive.

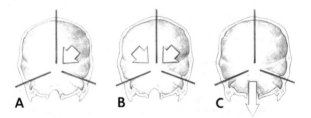

FIG 13–7. Herniation: **A,** beneath the cerebral falx. **B,** through
the incisura of the tentorium of the cerebellum. **C,** through the foramen magnum.

        1) Early: progressive loss of consciousness, small but reactive pupils, Cheyne-Stokes respirations, bilateral motor signs with decorticate posturing

        2) Late: central hyperventilation, hyperthermia, pupils unreactive to light and in midposition, loss of oculovestibular reflexes, decerebrate posturing

  2. Treatment: Herniation may temporarily be halted or reversed by the following agents:

    a. Mannitol 1 g/kg up to 50 g in a 20% solution IV administered over 20 minutes.

    b. Dexamethasone 0.3 mg/kg IV up to 12 mg IV followed by 0.06 mg/kg up to 6 mg q4h.

C. Posterior fossa mass (cerebellar hematoma, posterior fossa subdural hematoma, rapidly expanding posterior fossa tumor).

  1. Diagnostic considerations.

    a. Subacute onset of symptoms.

    b. Usually a past history of hypertension or occipital trauma.

    Note: Cerebellar hematomas are a complication of chronic hypertension; symptoms are rapidly accelerating hypertension, headache, weakness, and confusion.

    c. Rapid progression of symptoms and signs, which may include the following:

      1) Early—occipital headache, repeated vomiting, dizziness, confusion, marked "malignant" hypertension.

      2) Midstage—inability to stand or walk, bilateral extensor plantar responses, urinary incontinence, dysarthria, tonic deviation of eyes away from the side of the lesion, miosis, irregular respirations.

      3) Late—coma, absent doll's-eye responses and caloric responses, respiratory failure, flaccid limbs with diminished deep tendon reflexes.

    Caveat: Lumbar puncture in the presence of a posterior fossa mass carries an especially high risk of cerebellar herniation through the foramen magnum, and death.

2. Treatment: This is a neurosurgical emergency. Immediate surgical decompression can be lifesaving. A definitive diagnosis is best established by CT scan or MRI.

D. Brainstem infarction.

1. Diagnostic considerations.

   a. Acute onset of symptoms with coma and other findings maximal at onset.

   b. Often preceded by transient episodes consisting of diplopia, vertigo, dysarthria, dysphagia, motor weakness, and episodic loss of consciousness.

   c. Respiratory disturbance prominent from onset (periodic breathing, central hyperventilation, or ataxic breathing).

   d. Variable abnormality of pupils, which often are small and react sluggishly to light in a pontine lesion.

   e. Dysconjugate position of the eyes or dysconjugate eye movements (seen in doll's-eye or caloric tests), which suggest lesions of cranial nerves III (oculomotor nerve), IV (trochlear nerve), or VI (abducens nerve); absent or asymmetric doll's-eye or caloric tests; facial paralysis is noted by asymmetric movement of the cheek during respirations.

   f. Quadriparesis with Babinski reflexes (extensor plantar responses) and decerebrate posturing is often present. Cranial nerve abnormalities on one side with paralysis on the opposite side strongly suggest a brainstem lesion.

2. Treatment: Evaluation and treatment are discussed in Chapter 12, section VI.

   Caveat: Certain patients with upper pontine lesions may develop the locked-in syndrome (also referred to as pseudocoma or deafferented state) and have "a mind . . . clogged by a body rendered utterly incapable of obeying its impulses." Such an individual is awake but is unable to communicate except with eye movement ("a corpse with living eyes") like the character M. Noirtier de Villefort in *The Count of Monte Cristo*. These patients may be very much aware of their surroundings, and therefore the physician must be cautious in making comments in the presence of the patient. The locked-in syndrome must be distinguished from the persistent neurovegetative state (imprecisely referred to as coma vigil) in which the patient appears awake (and may even have a waking EEG), but is unable to communicate in any form (thought to be due to a high midbrain lesion).

E. **Summary.**
   1. Assure oxygenation with endotracheal suctioning, a cuffed endotracheal tube, and assisted ventilation with oxygen.
   2. Maintain the circulation by replacing blood volume losses, administering vasoconstrictors, and maintaining cardiac rhythm.
   3. Ensure adequate levels of blood glucose (the major substrate for brain metabolism) by administering 25 g of glucose IV in a 50% solution initially and by frequently monitoring blood glucose levels.
   4. Lower intracranial pressure (optimally the intracranial pressure should be determined by direct measurement with a "bolt" installed by a neurosurgeon, but it is often treated based on clinical judgment alone).
      a. Hyperventilate to lower the carbon dioxide pressure to 25 to 30 mm Hg (torr) thereby decreasing cerebral blood flow.
      b. Mannitol 50 g in a 20% solution is given IV over 20 to 30 minutes.
      c. Dexamethasone 10 mg IV, repeated with 4 to 6 mg q6h.
      d. If cerebral ventricular enlargement is evident on CT scan due to obstruction of CSF pathways, ventricular drainage may be lifesaving.

      Caveat: Hyperventilation should probably not be performed in patients with *ischemia* as a cause of coma. Mannitol is temporarily effective but may have a rebound. Steroids are most effective for edema due to brain tumors, but onset of action requires several hours. Steroids have a minor effect on edema secondary to ischemia. Thus the importance of combining the history, the neurologic examinations, and the CT scan to obtain as accurate a diagnosis as possible.

5. Treat seizures, if present (see Chapter 11, section IV).
6. Treat infection, if present. A patient with fever, stiff neck, and coma should have a lumbar puncture *immediately,* even if a CT scan is not available. The risk from herniation in this situation is much less than the adverse effect of failure to identify the cause of the meningitis, but the physician should be prepared to administer therapy to lower the intracranial pressure (see above).
7. Treat respiratory and metabolic alkalosis and acidosis; abnormalities may further depress respirations or worsen cardiovascular abnormalities.
8. Treat hyperthermia. An elevated body temperature may kill an already damaged brain and, if high enough, kill a normal brain. A cooling blanket is preferred.

III. METABOLIC COMA.
A. Approximately 80% of comas are caused by toxic-metabolic abnormalities; common causes include anoxia (cardiac arrest, pulmonary insufficiency), overdose (barbiturates or other sedatives, alcohol), diabetes (insulin overdose, ketoacidosis), uremia, hepatic failure, heat stroke, and meningitis.

IV. PSYCHOGENIC COMA.
A. Even astute physicians are sometimes fooled by a physiologically awake patient who does not respond to the environment and thus appears comatose. The following tests may be of value in confirming psychogenic coma:
1. The pupils and deep tendon reflexes are normal.
2. Caloric tests: 10 mL of cold water causes *nystagmus with the fast component away* from the irrigated side (in a truly comatose patient, the eyes will deviate to the irrigated side).
3. Doll's-eye movement: This is absent in an awake patient. Patients with absent doll's-eye movement due to a brainstem infarct usually have other, obvious signs.
4. Hold the patient's hand over the face and drop it; the hand will hit the face of the comatose patient, but deviate to the side in an alert patient (see Fig 9–3).
5. Press the styloid processes of the temporal bones; this very painful stimulus will arouse most noncomatose patients.

BIBLIOGRAPHY

Arieff AI, Griggs RC: *Metabolic Brain Dysfunction in Systemic Disorders.* Boston, Little, Brown, 1992.

Brooks DN, Hosie J, Bond MR, et al: Cognitive sequelae of severe head injury in relation to the Glasgow outcome scale. *J Neurol Neurosurg Psychiatry* 1986; 49:549–553.

Fitzgerald FT, Tierney LM, Wall SD: The comatose patient: A systematic diagnostic approach for you to follow. *Postgrad Med* 1983; 74:207–215.

Fraser CL, Arieff AI: Hepatic encephalopathy. *N Engl J Med* 1985; 313:865–873.

Levy DE, Caronna JJ, Singer BH, et al: Predicting the outcome from hypoxic-ischemic coma. *JAMA* 1985; 253:1420–1426.

Maiesek K, Cuvonna JJ: Coma following cardiac arrest: A review of the clinical features, management, and prognosis. *J Intensive Care Med* 1988; 3:153–163.

Plum F, Posner J: *The Diagnosis of Stupor and Coma,* ed 3. Philadelphia, FA Davis, 1980.

Posner JB: The comatose patient. *JAMA* 1975; 233:1313–1314.

Ropper AH: Lateral displacement of the brain and level of consciousness in patients with acute hemispheral mass. *N Engl J Med* 1986; 314:953–958.

Ropper AH, Kennedy SK, Zervas N: *Neurobiological and Neurosurgical Intensive Care.* Baltimore, University Park Press, 1983.

Schewman DA, DeGiogio CM: Early prognosis in anoxic coma: Reliability and rationale. *Neurol Clin* 1989; 7:823–843.

INFECTIONS OF THE CENTRAL NERVOUS SYSTEM

14

Most infections of the central nervous system (CNS) are life-threatening, the exception being the so-called aseptic or viral meningoencephalitis (other than that caused by herpes simplex). Immediate diagnosis and treatment may prevent death or brain damage. Signs and symptoms may mimic other neurologic disorders, so the clinician must have a high index of suspicion. After the initial history and examination, the clinician makes an educated guess as to the likely causative organisms and then selects appropriate antibiotics. Antibiotics and management are subsequently modified, depending on laboratory results.

I. **HISTORY AND EXAMINATION SUGGESTING INFECTION.**

A. **History.** Historical points that direct the physician to consider CNS infection in the patient with developing neurologic signs or symptoms include the following:

1. *Fever* may be 40° C (105° F) or greater in adults, whereas other infections seldom produce fever this high.

   Caution: Fever often may be absent in neonates and elderly patients, and occasionally in all patients.

2. Photophobia is often a historical manifestation in patients with meningitis.

3. Nausea and vomiting are often seen in patients with CNS infection and should not be misinterpreted as being due to gastrointestinal disturbance.

4. Alterations in sensorium or in mentation or behavior.
5. Severe *headache* is worsened by movement of the head or neck, particularly flexion of the neck.
6. Known *bloodborne* infection (such as bacteremia or endocarditis).
7. *Debilitating condition from other disease* (such as chronic renal failure) or from reduced immunity (as in leukemia or lymphoma, administration of immunosuppressant drugs, or in congenital or acquired immunodeficiency syndrome [AIDS]).
8. *Infection of superficial or deep structures adjoining the nervous system* (such as paranasal sinuses, skin of face, vertebral bodies), especially if there has been recent manipulation in the area or if the condition is chronic.
9. *Abnormality of the blood-brain* barrier (as in a recent ischemic infarction or emboli from congenital heart disease).
10. *Exposure of CNS structures secondary to trauma or surgery* (as in compound or basilar skull fractures) or evidence of a fistula connecting with the subarachnoid space (as through the nose, producing cerebrospinal fluid [CSF] rhinorrhea, or through developmental anomalies).

B. **Physical examination.** Following are some aspects of the physical examination that suggest the presence of CNS infection:

1. Fever (especially with decreased level of consciousness, or progressing or fluctuating neurologic signs and symptoms).
2. Nuchal rigidity, a preference for lying in bed with the head extended and the back arched. Kernig's and Brudzinski's signs may be present (Figs 14–1 and 14–2).

Caveat: In infants and some elderly patients, all of these signs may be absent.

3. Neurologic findings suggesting multiple levels of involvement of the nervous system, such as cranial nerve palsies, alterations of sensorium, convulsions, and papilledema.

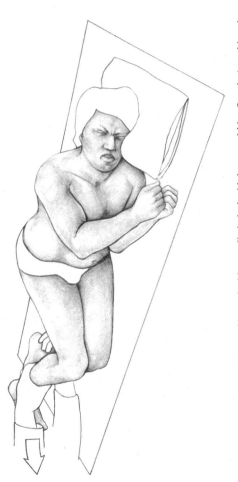

FIG 14–1. Kernig's sign: Patient with meningitis may lie in bed with knees and hips flexed. A positive sign (pain) is elicited when the legs are extended.

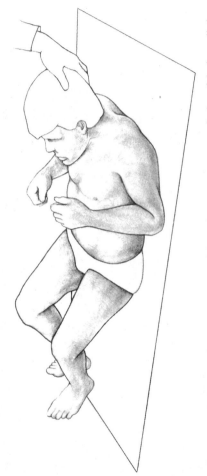

FIG 14–2. Brudzinski's sign: Passive flexion of the neck causes spontaneous flexion of the lower limbs.

    4. Signs of acute or chronic middle ear or mastoid infection, particularly in children

C.   **Cerebrospinal fluid examination** (See Chapter 2, section I).

    1. CSF studies should be done in all patients *without delay* whenever meningitis or encephalitis is suspected. The indication for a lumbar puncture (LP) is *even if you THINK of it*.

       Caveat: If there are focal neurologic abnormalities or papilledema, a CT scan or MRI is strongly recommended before the LP is performed.

    2. Gram stain of CSF sediment will show organisms in 70% of untreated bacterial meningitis cases. India ink preparations for cryptococcus and acid-fast stains for tubercle bacilli are rarely positive but nonetheless should be performed.

    3. Normally, the CSF contains *no* polymorphonuclear leukocytes and no more than five lymphocytes per microliter (cubic millimeter). *More cells* than this suggest CNS inflammation of some type.

    4. A CSF glucose value of less than 40 mg/dL suggests bacterial infection. Simultaneous blood sugars are of little practical value, since blood glucose takes several hours to equilibrate with CSF glucose.

    5. CSF protein and pressure are commonly elevated.

    6. CSF *culture* and sensitivity testing should always include bacteria (aerobic and anaerobic), tuberculosis, brucellosis, and fungi. Although the yield is very low, viral cultures should be obtained when viral meningoencephalitis is suspected and where facilities for viral culture are available.

    7. Antigen-antibody studies:

       a. Cryptococcal antigen (latex particle agglutination test) determinations should be ordered when fungal meningitis is suspected and should be done routinely in all patients who are immunocompromised. Skin test antigen is of no value. Serologic tests for coccidioidomycosis are also warranted in areas in which this disease is endemic.

      b. CSF IgM may be elevated in herpes simplex encephalitis.

      c. Routine countercurrent immunoelectrophoresis (CIE), or more recently, latex agglutination tests may rapidly detect polysaccharide antigens associated with meningococcal, pneumococcal, and *Haemophilus influenzae* type B meningitis.

      d. Routine syphilis serology.

      e. CSF IgG and measles antibody titers must be obtained if subacute sclerosing panencephalitis is suspected.

      f. Dark-field examination and appropriate serologies should be obtained if leptospirosis is suspected.

   8. Whenever possible, a 2- to 3-mL sample of CSF should be stored frozen to enable the physician to perform further studies if clinically indicated during the initial phase of the illness.

   9. Cytologic examinations and cell blocks for pathologic analyses are warranted if lymphomatous or carcinomatous meningitis is possible.

II. ANTIBIOTIC TREATMENT.
A. General principles.

   1. Antibiotics should be started empirically immediately after the LP is done, if there is evidence of bacterial infection. Choose antibiotics that are bactericidal against known or presumed causative organisms.

   2. Antibiotics should be started empirically *before* computed tomography (CT) scan or magnetic resonance imaging (MRI) is done when getting the test will unduly delay performance of the LP.

   3. Combinations of drugs are to be avoided unless a synergistic effect is known to occur. Combinations of drugs may be necessary if:

      a. Sensitivities are initially unavailable.

      b. The organism is believed to be resistant (enteric gram-negative bacilli, fungal infection, tuberculosis, *Brucella*).

      c. The patient is immunosuppressed.

      d. Polymicrobial infection is suspected.

4. The antibiotics must be capable of penetrating into CSF in concentrations well above the mean bactericidal concentration for the infective organism.
5. Intrathecal antibiotic administration is unnecessary in the initial treatment of the patient with acute meningitis and is only useful in certain circumstances (such as resistant fungal meningitis). Select the best antibiotic at the correct daily dosage (Tables 14–1 and 14–2).

TABLE 14–1.
Antibiotic Dosages for Bacterial Meningitis in Children

Age	Antibiotic	Dosage
Birth to 2 months	Ampicillin	150–200 mg/kg/day IV q8h
	Penicillin G	
	<1 wk	150,000 units/kg/day IV q8h
	1 wk–2 mo	150,000–250,000 units/kg/day IV q6h
	Group B *Streptococcus*	250,000–400,000 units/kg/day IV q6h
	Methicillin sodium	100 mg/kg/day IV q8h
	Nafcillin sodium	100 mg/kg/day IV q8h
	Carbenicillin	300 mg/kg/day IV q8h
	Ticarcillin	200–300 mg/kg/day IV q8h
	Piperacillin sodium	200 mg/kg/day IV q8h
	Kanamycin sulfate	
	<1 wk	20 mg/kg/day IM or IV q12h
	1 wk–2 mo	30 mg/kg/day IM or IV q8h
	Gentamicin sulfate	
	<1 wk	5 mg/kg/day IM or IV q12h
	1 wk–2 mo	7.5 mg/kg/day IM or IV q8h
	Tobramycin	
	<1 wk	5 mg/kg/day IM or IV q12h
	1 wk–2 mo	7.5 mg/kg/day IM or IV q8h
	Amikacin	
	<1 wk	15 mg/kg/day IM or IV q12h
	1 wk–2 mo	22.5 mg/kg/day IM or IV q8h
	Moxalactam disodium	100–150 mg/kg/day IV q8h
	Cefotaxime sodium	100–150 mg/kg/day IV q8h
	Vancomycin hydrochloride	
	Birth–1 wk	30 mg/kg/day IV q12h
	1 wk–2 mo	45 mg/kg/day IV q8h

(Continued.)

TABLE 14–1. (cont.).

Age	Antibiotic	Dosage
	Metronidazole	15 mg/kg/day IV q12h
	Chloramphenicol	
	Premature birth–1 mo	25 mg/kg/day IV q12h
	Full-term birth–7 days	25 mg/kg/day IV q12h
	Full-term 7–30 days	50 mg/kg/day IV q8h
	Full-term 1–2 mo	50–100 mg/kg/day IV q6h
Over Age 2 Months	Ampicillin	300–400 mg/kg/day IV q4h
(up to 50-kg	Penicillin G	250,000 units/kg/day IV q4h
Body Weight)	Methicillin sodium	200–300 mg/kg/day IV q4h
	Nafcillin sodium	200 mg/kg/day IV q4h
	Carbenicillin	400–600 mg/kg/day IV q4h
	Ticarcillin	300–400 mg/kg/day IV q4h
	Piperacillin sodium	300–400 mg/kg/day IV q4h
	Chloramphenicol	75–100 mg/kg/day PO or IV q6h
	Gentamicin	4 mg/kg/day IM q8h
	Tobramycin	4 mg/kg/day IM q8h
	Amikacin	15 mg/kg/day IM q8h
	Moxalactam disodium	150 mg/kg/day IV q4h
	Cefotaxime sodium	150 mg/kg/day IV q4h
	Cefoperazone sodium	300 mg/kg/day IV q8h
	Ceftriaxone sodium	100 mg/kg/day IV q12h
	Rifampin	20 mg/kg/day PO q8h up to 600 mg
	Streptomycin sulfate	20–40 mg/kg/day IM q12h (not over 1 g)
	Vancomycin hydrochloride	60 mg/kg/day IV q6h
	Sulfadiazine	150 mg/kg/day IV q8h
	Metronidazole	40 mg/kg/day PO q8h
		30 mg/kg/day IV q6h

6. Be certain the patient is receiving what has been ordered. Serum level determinations can be done for chloramphenicol and the aminoglycosides, and the dosage may be adjusted accordingly.

7. In children, administration of corticosteroids along with the antibiotics may reduce the incidence of complications.

TABLE 14–2.
Antibiotic Therapy for Bacterial Meningitis With a Known Etiologic Agent in Adults

Organism	Preferred Therapy (Antibiotic Dosage/24 hr)	Alternative Therapy (Antibiotic Dosage/24 hr)
Gram-positive		
Pneumococcus	Penicillin G 24 million units IV	Chloramphenicol 4 g IV
Multiply resistant	Vancomycin hydrochloride 2 g IV	Vancomycin 2 mg IV plus 2–5 mg intrathecally
Streptococcus		
Groups A and B	Penicillin G 24 million units IV	Chloramphenicol 4 g IV
Group D (enterococcus)	Penicillin G 24 million units IV + gentamicin sulfate 5 mg/kg IM or IV	Vancomycin 2 g IV + 2–5 mg intrathecally
Staphylococcus aureus	Nafcillin sodium 10–12 g IV	Vancomycin 2 g IV + 2–5 mg intrathecally
Listeria monocytogenes	Ampicillin 12 g IV	Tetracycline 1.5 g IV
Gram-negative		
Haemophilus influenzae	Chloramphenicol 4 g IV	Ampicillin 12–14 g IV
Meningococcus	Penicillin G 24 million units IV	Chloramphenicol 4 g IV
Escherichia coli, *Klebsiella*, *Proteus*, *Pseudomonas*, *Serratia*, and similar organisms	Carbenicillin 30–40 g IV + aminoglycoside IV	Aminoglycoside 2–5 mg intrathecally

III. BACTERIAL MENINGITIS IN NEONATES.

A. Meningitis in the full-term and premature newborn has serious consequences.

 1. Mortality rates are about 20% for *Escherichia coli* and group B streptococcal meningitis, which together account for 60% to 75% of cases.

2. Long-term sequelae range from blindness, deafness, seizures, or hydrocephalus, to cognitive disorders such as mental retardation, attention disorders, and learning disabilities.

3. Brain abscess may complicate meningitis in the neonate.

B. Diagnosis.

1. Early diagnosis is difficult because signs and symptoms may be nonspecific or minor (irritability, poor feeding, jitteriness, respiratory difficulty, lethargy) and the index of suspicion must be high.

2. CSF changes are delayed, especially in the premature infant, and the relatively poor defense mechanisms of newborns allows rapid progression of the disease.

3. Neonates require treatment based on suspicion alone.

4. Pretreatment blood, urine, and CSF cultures are obtained and treatment is discontinued if these do not provide evidence of treatable infection.

5. Normal neonatal CSF protein may be as high as 150 mg/dL, the cell counts up to 25 white blood cells (WBCs) and 650 red blood cells per microliter, and peripheral WBCs as high as 25,000/μL. By 1 month of age these values decrease to adult values.

6. CSF pressure is almost always greater than 180 mm H_2O, but values greater than 400 mm H_2O indicate impending herniation.

C. Treatment.

1. Care of the neonate with meningitis may be complicated by respiratory insufficiency, hypoglycemia, dehydration, shock, or convulsions and is best undertaken in a neonatal intensive care unit. Unless the primary care practitioner has considerable experience with neonates, it is best to refer the patient to a pediatrician or neonatologist.

2. Recommendations for initial therapy are third-generation cephalosporins combined with ampicillin (to ensure coverage for *Listeria monocytogenes*). Cefotaxime sodium 50 mg/kg intravenously (IV) q6h, or moxalactam disodium are preferred in combination with ampicillin until the pathogen is known. See Table 14–1 for other specific drug dosages.

3. Third-generation cephalosporins offer higher levels than the aminoglycosides; however, hard data indicating therapeutic advantage over aminoglycosides are lacking.

4. All medication is given IV and usually continued for 21 days after the CSF has been sterilized.

IV. BACTERIAL MENINGITIS IN INFANTS AND CHILDREN.

A. Bacterial meningitis is primarily a disease of early childhood.

1. Ninety percent of cases occur from age 1 month to 5 years.

2. The most common cause is *H. influenzae* type B, which accounts for 90% of cases from 3 months to 5 years of age, and 50% of all cases in childhood, although this may be altered by recent widespread immunization against *H. influenzae* type B.

3. Pneumococci *(Streptococcus pneumoniae)* and meningococci *(Neisseria meningitidis)* account for most of the rest.

4. All three of these organisms colonize the nasopharynx of healthy children, and most children with meningitis have a preceding or concurrent nasopharyngitis.

B. Diagnosis. Signs and symptoms pointing to CNS invasion are more easily elicited in this group, compared to neonates.

1. Often the main difficulty is distinguishing between acute viral and acute bacterial meningitis, since the early symptoms are similar.

2. Antibiotics frequently have already been administered when the child presents, so that the differential diagnosis often is between partially treated bacterial meningitis and viral meningitis, both of which may show similar CSF profiles.

3. Appropriate smears and cultures should be obtained anyway, and countercurrent immunoelectrophoresis (CIE) or latex precipitation on the CSF performed. Therapy should be continued in all cases of partially treated meningitis, but in other instances, if there is no evidence of bacterial infection, therapy can be discontinued.

C. **Treatment.**
1. *Initial therapy:* Ampicillin 300 to 400 mg/kg/day IV q4h, maximum daily dose 12 g to avoid cerebral irritability, plus chloramphenicol 75 mg/kg/day IV q6h.
2. A single antibiotic should be used whenever possible once sensitivity patterns have been determined. See Table 14–2 for drug dosage and regimens.
3. A second LP should be obtained within 48 hours of starting antibiotic therapy, unless the patient has become completely asymptomatic. By this time no organisms should be detectable on stained CSF smears, or they should be greatly reduced; otherwise therapy must be reevaluated.
4. CSF cells, glucose, and protein return to normal slowly and so may still be abnormal at 48 hours. If the clinical course is satisfactory, it may not be necessary to perform a third lumbar puncture.
5. Duration of treatment is at least 14 days but should be at least 21 days for gram-positive enterococci and 28 days for gram-negative enteric bacilli.

Note: A new vaccine against *H. influenzae* type B is available and should be administered routinely to all infants. Its widespread use will potentially eliminate the majority of cases of this form of meningitis.

V. BACTERIAL MENINGITIS IN ADULTS.
A. With treatment, fatality rates of adult bacterial meningitis are usually less than 10%, but severe neurologic sequelae are possible. The two leading causes in the adult are pneumococci *(S. pneumoniae)* and meningococci *(N. meningitidis)*.
1. Pneumococcal meningitis is usually preceded by pneumonia and often associated with alcoholism, debilitation, and old age, and usually occurs sporadically, except in developing countries. Confused elderly patients should be assumed to have meningitis until a clear and adequate diagnosis can be made.
2. Meningococcal meningitis occurs in epidemics (serogroups A or C) in the pediatric age group, and may be acquired by susceptible adults.

3. Meningitis caused by gram-negative enteric bacteria is almost always a disease of the hospitalized or nursing home patient and often follows bacteremia from other foci such as cellulitis or urinary tract infection or may be seen in patients with head-penetrating head trauma.

B. Treatment.

1. *Initial therapy:* Penicillin G, aqueous, 2 million units IV q2h and chloramphenicol 1 g IV q6h. See Table 14–2 for other drug regimens.

2. Patients are customarily treated through 5 afebrile days, but not less than 1 week for meningococci, 10 days for *H. influenzae,* and 14 days for pneumococci.

VI. COMPLICATIONS OF BACTERIAL MENINGITIS.

A. Seizures: Drug therapy is outlined in Chapter 11. These seizures may be transient and not require prolonged anticonvulsant (antiepileptic drug) therapy or may persist for many years following brain destruction and scar formation. If a patient has a seizure during the acute episode, treat with anticonvulsants for 1 year. At that time, the drug may be discontinued, according to the guidelines in Chapter 11.

B. Increased intracranial pressure: This is usually a transient problem due to cerebral edema; if necessary, treat with fluid restriction, mannitol, or steroids (see Chapter 12, section V). CSF shunting may become necessary if progressive ventricular enlargement occurs.

C. Subdural effusions: These are especially common after *H. influenzae* meningitis in children; suspect with persistent fever and focal seizures. The effusions are usually treated by repeated subdural taps but occasionally require neurosurgical intervention.

D. Subdural empyema: This is similar to a subdural effusion, except that the fluid contains live organisms and is consequently much more dangerous. Immediate surgical drainage and reassessment of antibiotic therapy are indicated.

E. Infarction: Venous infarcts may be caused by cortical thrombophlebitis, venous sinus thrombosis, or both. Cortical thrombophlebitis usually presents early with seizures that are difficult to control. Sagittal sinus thrombosis will manifest as increased intracranial pressure and stroke, predominantly with lower extremity findings. Arterial infarcts secondary to an inflammatory arteritis accompanying bacterial infection may not be evident until the recovery phase from the acute toxic illness, particularly in pneumococcal meningitis.

F. **Prolonged fever** may be due to local infection at the IV site, subdural effusion, inappropriate or inadequate antibiotic therapy, drug fever, or the presence of an unsuspected second organism.

G. **Inappropriate antidiuretic hormone (ADH) secretion:** The syndrome of inappropriate ADH secretion (SIADH) is a frequent occurrence during the early phases of meningitis. Diagnosis is made by finding low serum osmolality and high urine osmolality. This is usually prevented by keeping on the low side of daily fluid maintenance requirements.

H. **Communicating hydrocephalus:** The infection may interfere with proper reabsorption of CSF, but more commonly hydrocephalus is a late complication. The symptoms include deterioration of mental and behavioral function and bilateral corticospinal tract signs, especially increased reflexes in the lower extremities. The diagnosis is suggested by large ventricles on CT scan or MRI. If the condition does not spontaneously resolve, shunting of the CSF by a neurosurgeon may be necessary.

I. **Obstructive hydrocephalus:** This is suggested by an abnormal increase in head circumference and widening of sutures in infants or young children. In older children and adults, there will be progressive mental deterioration and ataxia, and the CT scan or MRI will show ventricular enlargement. Shunting by a neurosurgeon is often required. Acute obstruction results in coma and death if the pressure is not relieved promptly.

VII. PROGNOSIS OF BACTERIAL MENINGITIS.

A. **The prognosis of bacterial meningitis depends on the following:**
   1. The nature of the infectious agent and the severity of the initial process (convulsions and coma).
   2. The age of the patient.
   3. The duration of symptoms before treatment.
   4. Appropriate and early antibiotic therapy.

VIII. BRAIN ABSCESS.

A. Diagnostic considerations.

1. Presentation resembles that of any other mass lesion such as a tumor. Fever and leukocytosis may be minimal or absent and thus do not rule out the diagnosis.

2. Abscesses are very irritating to brain tissue and cause edema, increased intracranial pressure, and seizures.

3. Predisposing factors include acute and chronic sinusitis and otitis, cyanotic congenital heart disease, penetrating head wounds, and chronic pulmonary infection.

4. CSF culture is usually negative; CSF cell count is normal or slightly elevated, and protein is slightly elevated.

5. All types of organisms cause abscesses; if neurosurgical intervention is undertaken, both aerobic and anaerobic cultures must be performed.

6. CT scan or MRI usually shows a "doughnut sign"—an area of low density with a rim of higher density (capsule) and marked surrounding cerebral edema.

7. If CT scan or MRI demonstrates an abscess, LP should be avoided owing to risk of brain herniation.

8. Sinus and mastoid radiographs should be performed to look for a source of infection in all cases.

B. Treatment.

1. Antibiotics against anaerobic *Streptococcus* and *Bacteroides* are given IV. Recommended drugs are metronidazole 500 to 750 mg/day in three or four doses and crystalline penicillin G, 100,000 to 400,000 units in four to six doses daily IV (up to 24 million units daily IV) if the organism is unknown.

2. Treatment of the cerebral edema usually requires dexamethasone 2 to 6 mg every 4 to 6 hours.

3. Neurosurgical excision or drainage of the abscess, with instillation of antibiotics locally, occasionally may be required, unless therapy is instituted very early at a "cerebritis" stage.

4. Duration of therapy remains empirical; however, a minimum of 4 to 6 weeks is generally accepted as sufficient in most patients.

IX. TUBERCULOUS MENINGITIS.

A. **The incidence of tuberculous meningitis** is on the rise in the United States. It should be suspected particularly in recent immigrants, in deprived populations, or in those with human immunodeficiency virus (HIV) infection.

1. The diagnosis is elusive because of the following factors:

   a. Onset is usually gradual without meningeal signs. Symptoms are nonspecific—apathy, anorexia, malaise, low-grade fever. Later there may be drowsiness, seizures, cranial nerve palsies, and other focal (particularly brainstem) signs, and papilledema. The illness develops over weeks, not days.

   b. Tuberculous meningitis is seen in association with disseminated disease in young patients. In adults, the disease (secondary reactivation) usually manifests as CNS disease without dissemination.

   c. Only one third of patients have evidence of active pulmonary disease, while one third have a negative purified protein derivative (PPD) test.

   d. Stains for acid-fast bacilli in CSF sediment are frequently negative, and cultures may take 4 to 6 weeks to become positive.

2. Strongly suspect the diagnosis under the following conditions:

   a. A history of recent exposure to tuberculosis.

   b. In any case where there is evidence of active tuberculosis, especially in young adults and children.

   c. In any patient with meningitis in whom the intermediate PPD is positive (especially if there is a recent conversion). CSF findings usually consist of increased lymphocytes with or without neutrophils, a decreased glucose, and marked increase in protein.

   Note: Tuberculoma does not present as a meningitis, but as a mass lesion.

3. For the above reasons, virtually all CSF with increased cells, even if the glucose is normal, should be cultured for acid-fast bacilli. Cultures and stains have a higher

probability of being positive if the CSF is allowed to stand and the resulting proteinaceous precipitate is examined.

B. Treatment.

1. Once the diagnosis has been made on clinical grounds and adequate cultures have been obtained, treatment must be started immediately; delay of weeks until the culture is positive may lead to irreversible brain damage.

2. Treat routinely with triple therapy:

   a. Isoniazid (INH) 15 mg/kg/day PO to a maximum of 300 mg/day for 12 months.

      Note: Pyridoxine 10 to 20 mg/day should be given with isoniazid to prevent polyneuropathy.

   b. Rifampin 600 mg/day PO, or 10 mg/kg/day, for 12 months.

   c. Ethambutol hydrochloride 25 mg/kg/day PO initially should be decreased to 15 mg/kg/day as soon as possible after treatment course is established, then maintained for 12 months.

3. Second-choice drugs that may be substituted for one or more of the above are:

   a. Pyrazinamide 20 to 40 mg/kg/day for a total of 3 g/day PO.

   b. Streptomycin 1 g/day intramuscularly (IM).

      Caveat: Antibiotic recommendations change from time to time, and consultation with an expert in infectious disease is recommended. Treatment must be monitored with repeated CSF examinations. The antibiotics listed here have a serious potential for toxicity with prolonged use; e.g., ethambutol has been associated with optic neuropathy, and streptomycin may cause vestibular damage. Slow acetylators (American Indians, Eskimos, Middle Easterners) do not tolerate high doses of isoniazid, and the addition of rifampin exacerbates this problem. A maximum dose of isoniazid 300 mg combined with rifampin 600 mg should be used.

X. MENINGITIS DUE TO FUNGAL DISEASE.
A. Diagnostic considerations.

1. The diagnosis is often elusive.
2. Onset is often gradual.
3. Systemic symptoms initially may be mild.
4. CSF may show nonspecific findings of normal or low sugar, increased cells, and increased protein. These findings evoke a large differential diagnosis: herpes simplex encephalitis, tuberculous meningitis, leptospiral meningitis, secondary neurosyphilis, partially treated pyogenic meningitis, sarcoidosis, cerebral abscess, and subdural empyema.
5. India ink preparations of CSF for *Cryptococcus* are not a reliable method of diagnosis but nonetheless should be performed. In suspicious cases obtain cryptococcal antigen and antibody tests in the blood and CSF, as well as cultures of blood and CSF for *Cryptococcus*.
6. The index of suspicion should be especially high in *immunocompromised* or *debilitated* patients. Patients with Hodgkin's disease or acquired immunodeficiency syndrome (AIDS) are particularly susceptible.
7. Common organisms are *Cryptococcus neoformans* (low-grade fever, cough, mental disturbance, eye abnormalities) and *Coccidioides immitis* (prolonged respiratory symptoms, subacute meningitis). However, in autopsy series (especially in medical centers with large numbers of immunocompromised patients) the most frequently identified fungal cause of CNS infection is *Candida*.

B. Treatment.

1. Amphotericin B 0.6 mg/kg/day IV in conjunction with flucytosine 150 mg/kg/day is lifesaving in most fungal infections. Because of their potential toxicity, the drugs should be administered by a clinician experienced in their use.
2. The course of treatment is determined by clinical response and CNS response documented by repeated CSF evaluation.
3. Occasionally intraventricular administration of amphotericin B is necessary to control the meningitis.

XI. **NEUROSYPHILIS.**
A. **Diagnostic considerations.**
  1. The clinical presentations of symptomatic neurosyphilis are protean ("stroke," "dementia," CNS mass lesion, meningitis, hydrocephalus); for this reason the CSF test for syphilis must be done on every patient undergoing a lumbar puncture; the diagnosis is most often made in this serendipitous manner.
  2. The serologic tests for syphilis are:
    a. VDRL, (*V*eneral *D*isease *R*esearch *L*aboratories); rapid plasma reagin test (RPR), automated reagin test (ART)—nontreponemal tests.
      1) Nontreponemal cardiolipin antibody tests (VDRL, RPR) are useful for screening.
      2) A decrease in nontreponemal titers documents adequate therapy.
    b. FTA-ABS—fluorescent treponemal antibody absorption test.
    c. MHA-TP—microhemagglutination–*Treponema pallidum* test.
    d. TPI—*T. pallidum* immobilization test.
      1) Treponemal tests confirm the diagnosis.
  3. Patients with a past history of syphilis or who have a positive serum test for syphilis should have a lumbar puncture to rule out asymptomatic neurosyphilis.
  4. In active neurosyphilis there is a high CSF IgM.
B. **Treatment.**
  1. Neurosyphilis is a treatable disease; progression may be stopped in all cases, and most patients will show improvement.
  2. There are several acceptable choices of antibiotic therapy:
    a. Aqueous penicillin G 2 to 4 million units IV q4h for 10 days, followed by penicillin G benzathine 2.4 million units IM weekly, for three doses.
    b. Amoxicillin 3 g/day PO plus probenecid 1 g/day PO for 10 days or aqueous procaine penicillin G IM 2.4 million units/day plus probenecid 500 mg qid PO for 10 days, followed by penicillin G benzathine 2.4 million units IM weekly for three doses.

c. For penicillin allergy, chloramphenicol 2 g/day IV for 15 to 30 days, or tetracycline 500 mg qid PO for 30 days.
3. Patients with neurosyphilis must be followed with periodic serologic testing and repeat CSF examinations for 3 years.

XII. ASEPTIC MENINGOENCEPHALITIS.
A. Diagnostic considerations.
1. This is the diagnosis given to a patient who shows evidence of inflammation of the meninges and brain tissue, but without evidence of bacteria, fungi, spirochetes, or parasites. The CSF shows a slight increase in cells, usually lymphocytes, with normal glucose and protein.

   Caveat: Although laboratory tests do not find the organism, this is not conclusive evidence that organisms are indeed not present.

2. Aseptic meningitis is most commonly caused by viruses. The differential diagnosis, however, is wide and includes:
   a. Parameningeal infections.
   b. Carcinomatous or lymphomatous meningitis. Careful examination of the CSF by a cytopathologist should identify this.
   c. Rarer conditions include Behçet's disease, Vogt-Koyanagi syndrome, Mollaret's meningitis (some evidence suggests this may be due to repeated reactivation of herpes simplex meningitis), and Lyme disease.
3. In cases where the CSF has an increased cell count, normal sugar, and moderately increased protein, the following laboratory tests should be performed:
   a. An acute serum sample should be drawn and frozen; 3 weeks later a second serum should be drawn and both should be sent to a laboratory where serum responses to specific infectious processes can be detected. The ability to make a diagnosis of a spe-

cific agent is of value for epidemiologic purposes (such as elimination of an arthropod vector) as well as care of the patient. If no rise in antibody titer is found, there should be a higher index of suspicion that the aseptic meningitis was caused by something other than a viral infection. Laboratories require that the physician specify which titers are to be checked; this should be done on the basis of a clinical picture of meningitis or encephalitis, season of year, and assorted other factors (Table 14–3).

    b. CSF tests for syphilis should be performed in all cases.

    c. Serum tests for mononucleosis and cytomegalovirus should be performed.

    d. Viral cultures of CSF, pharynx, and stool are helpful in selected cases.

  4. Presumptive diagnosis may be made during epidemics (arboviruses) or when there is a concurrent recognizable illness (such as mumps, measles, or infectious mononucleosis).

B. Treatment.

  1. Supportive therapy, maintenance of fluid and nutrition (see Chapter 12, section VI.A.4).

  2. Control of cerebral edema (see Chapter 12, section VI.A.11).

  3. Control of seizures (see Chapter 11).

XIII. VIRAL DISEASES OF PARTICULAR IMPORTANCE.
A. Acute encephalitis.

  1. Herpes simplex encephalitis: This is the most common sporadic viral encephalitis. It affects primarily the temporal lobes (a focal encephalitis), although brainstem encephalitides do occur.

    a. The classic presentation is of early personality and behavior changes (often with memory deficits), followed by lateralizing and localizing neurologic signs such as hemiparesis or a visual field defect with increased intracranial pressure. Occasionally the presentation may be aseptic viral meningitis without focal findings.

TABLE 14-3.
Common Viruses

Virus	Associated Factors	Season	Prominent Meningitic Symptoms	Prominent Encephalitic Symptoms
Enteroviruses	Appear in epidemics of gastrointestinal illness	Summer, early Fall	X	
Poliovirus types 1,2,3				
Coxsackievirus A9, B1-5				
Echovirus types 3, 4, 6 9, 11, 18, 30				
Arboviruses				
Eastern equine	Atlantic Gulf Coast (mosquito vector)			
Western equine	Western United States (mosquito vector)			
Venezuelan equine	Florida, Southwest (mosquito vector)			
St. Louis	All United States urban areas (mosquito vector)	Summer, early Fall		X
Powassan	Northern United States, (tick vector)			
California	All United States, primarily children (mosquito vector)			

Virus	Clinical notes	Seasonal occurrence		
Herpesvirus				
Herpes simplex type 1	Adult (mimics temporal lobe tumor)	Sporadic, Winter		
Herpes simplex type 2	Neonatal			X
Varicella-zoster	Shingles, chickenpox	Winter, Spring		
Epstein-Barr	Associated with infectious mononucleosis			
Cytomegalovirus	Infants, immunosuppressed adults			
Myxovirus and paramyxovirus				
Influenza	Rare	Winter		
Parainfluenza	Croup/bronchitis in young children	Winter		
Mumps	Parotitis; common cause of aseptic meningitis	Spring		X
Measles (rubeola)	Encephalomyelitis 1–14 days after rash	Peak in April		
Adenoviruses	Primarily in neonates		X	
Lymphocytic choriomeningitis	Contact with excreta of house mouse	Winter	X	X
Rabies	Animal bites		X	

    b. A CT scan or MRI of the brain may be normal early in the course. After 48 hours, abnormalities are often apparent in the temporal lobe(s).

    c. Early in the course of the illness, the electroencephalogram (EEG) characteristically shows periodic focal spikes from the temporal area with focal slowing or periodic lateralizing epileptiform discharges (PLEDs).

    d. There is a reduction in mortality and neurologic sequelae if the diagnosis is established early and treatment with specific antiviral agents is started, particularly if therapy is initiated before coma ensues.

    e. Treatment

      1) The efficacy of acyclovir (acycloguanosine) is established. The relative paucity of side effects makes it the treatment of choice. Acyclovir 10 mg/kg IV q8h should be administered for a full 10-day course; stabilization or improvement of clinical symptoms should be evident within 48 hours of beginning therapy.

      2) Steroids (dexamethasone 10 mg IV initially followed by 4 mg IV q6h) may be used to reduce cerebral edema.

      3) For herpes simplex encephalitis, cultures of CSF, throat swabs, and stools are of no use in revealing the organism but should be performed to rule out other pathogens.

      4) A brain biopsy can be performed for definitive diagnosis, but in most centers the patient is simply treated empirically. However, if the patient does not respond to treatment, brain biopsy may be necessary to establish the diagnosis.

      5) Since herpes simplex infection is ubiquitous in the population and infections outside the nervous system so common, acute and convalescent titers are usually not helpful unless IgM titers are elevated.

2. Summer encephalitides. These occur in epidemics and are usually secondary to arboviruses:

    a. Equine encephalitis should be suspected anywhere

in the United States when the horse population first becomes affected; with eastern equine encephalitis, 80% of cases will have neurologic sequelae, whereas western equine encephalitis is milder, with 5% to 10% of cases having neurologic sequelae.

b. St. Louis encephalitis occurs primarily in the far western United States.

c. Venezuelan encephalitis occurs primarily in the Southwestern United States.

d. California encephalitis (a tick-borne disease) occurs primarily in the midwestern United States.

e. Acute and convalescent viral titers need to be obtained, but treatment is symptomatic and supportive.

3. Poliomyelitis.

a. Poliomyelitis is now a rare disease in developed countries with compulsory immunization programs. Presentation is with a febrile illness followed by asymmetric weakness often involving only one limb (except for bulbar polio) associated with loss of deep tendon reflexes (see Chapter 15, section II.B.4).

b. There is a postpolio syndrome in which years after a stable deficit the patient apparently becomes progressively weaker, presumably due to the futher loss of overstressed neurons. However, in many cases, reduced muscle function is secondary to arthritic changes in long-stressed joints, improperly fitting prosthetic devices, and disuse atrophy of muscles from lack of exercise.

4. Rabies.

a. The presentation is of a brainstem encephalitis.

b. Transmitted by animal bites, domestic or wild; particularly worrisome are unprovoked attacks by wild animals or bites from bats.

c. Most dangerous are multiple bites or bites around the face.

Note: In the case of an animal bite, the animal should be impounded and observed. Vaccination should be instituted with rabies vaccine produced in cultured human diploid cells. Passive immunization with human antirabies antiserum may be used adjunctively. In all suspected cases consult local or state health authorities and an infectious disease specialist.

B.   Chronic encephalitis.

1. Acquired immunodeficiency syndrome.

   a. The HIV that is responsible for AIDS resides chronically in the CNS long before clinical signs of systemic AIDS appear, but appropriate serologic tests can confirm the diagnosis within 6 weeks of onset of infection. However, it can be years after initial infection before the patient develops AIDS.

   b. The neurologic complications of AIDS present as a wide spectrum of disorders from encephalitis to myelitis to neuritis to myositis. Neurologic signs and symptoms in an AIDS patient may be due to one or more of:

      1) Opportunistic infections in an immunocompromised host; e.g., toxoplasmosis, progressive multifocal leukoencephalopathy, cryptococcal and coccidioidal meningitis, cytomegalovirus encephalitis, disseminated *Mycobacterium avium-intracellulare.*

      2) Unusual primary or metastatic malignancies; e.g., primary CNS lymphoma (reticulum cell sarcoma) or metastatic Kaposi's sarcoma.

      3) The direct effect of the AIDS virus itself which seems to have a propensity for causing damage to the deep cerebral white matter.

   c. Every patient with unusual or unexplained neurologic signs or symptoms should have serologic evaluation for the AIDS virus.

   d. CSF studies, together with MRI, will often identify opportunistic infection of the CNS. Occasionally, brain biopsy may be necessary. Biopsy of peripheral nerve or muscle can be used to diagnose problems in the peripheral nervous system.

   e. Treatment. No specific treatment for infection by the AIDS virus is yet available. Treatment specific for any documented opportunistic infection should be offered.

2. Progressive multifocal leukoencephalopathy (PML).
   a. This is a rare condition, occurring in immunocompromised or debilitated patients, presenting as sequential multifocal neurologic signs.
   b. CT scan or MRI shows multiple decreased white matter densities.
   c. The disease is caused by a papovavirus.
   d. *Treatment:* There is no effective treatment.

3. Creutzfeldt-Jakob disease (Jacob's disease, Jakob-Creutzfeldt disease; subacute spongiform encephalopathy; prion disease) is a presenile dementia associated with either myoclonus or extrapyramidal movement disorder caused by an infectious particle now termed a *prion*. No treatment is available (see Chapter 6, section V.B).

   Caveat: The nervous system tissue of patients is highly infective, even after being fixed in formalin (although a solution of 15% phenol in formalin does appear to inactivate the agent). Fluids and tissues of demented patients should therefore be handled with care, unless the cause of dementia is certain. Tissue from these patients should never be used for transplantation.

4. Subacute sclerosing panencephalitis (SSPE).
   a. Subacute sclerosing parencephalitis is a slowly progressive dementing and degenerative disease occurring primarily in children and caused by reactivation of a latent form of an altered measles virus years after clinical measles; its incidence has decreased since widespread compulsory measles immunization in North America but is still prevalent in underdeveloped countries.
   b. Four clinical stages are identified:
      1) Stage I—personality, behavior, and cognitive changes, often with apraxia and agnosia.
      2) Stage II—onset of characteristic slow myoclonus that is periodic, often involving the trunk and axial structures.

       3) Stage III — progression of focal neurologic signs.

       4) Stage IV — a neurovegetative state followed by death.

    c. Characteristic EEG change of periodic complexes (usually generalized) in a relatively normal background occurs in late stage I or early stage II.

    d. Markedly elevated measles antibody titers are identifiable in the CSF.

    e. Treatment: No curative treatment is available. Reports suggest that isoprinosine (Inosiplex) or intrathecal interferon arrests the disease for a while in some cases.

  5. Progressive rubella encephalitis: Progressive rubella encephalitis occurs in children with congenital rubella (see Chapter 16, section I.A.1.c) after 8 to 19 years and is characterized by progressive dementia, seizures, ataxia, and spasticity. CSF shows increased lymphocytosis, mildly increased protein, and markedly increased gamma-globulin. Serum and CSF show markedly increased rubella antibody titers.

    a. Treatment: There is no effective treatment.

C.   **Postinfectious encephalopathies.** There are a number of uncommon acute toxic encephalopathies and acute and subacute hemorrhagic and nonhemorrhagic leukoencephalopathies which are best managed at a specialized center. However, prompt recognition and initial management of Reye's syndrome is imperative prior to referral.

  1. Reye-Johnson syndrome (Reyes syndrome).

    a. Presents with vomiting, then a rapid decrease in consciousness in children with preceding viral infection (usually influenza B).

    b. Differential clinical staging criteria have been proposed, but generally, if the patient reaches the state of coma, the point of irreversibility may have been passed.

    c. Massive cerebral edema may be evident as papilledema, or on CT scan or MRI of the brain. Lumbar puncture and measurement of CSF pressure should *not* be done without preparation for medical (by mannitol) or surgical decompression. Management usually requires an intensive care unit with ability to do continuous intracranial pressure monitoring.

d. Treatment is aimed primarily at decreasing intracranial pressure, supporting vital functions, and preventing complications of a comatose patient (see Chapter 13).

e. There is a probable role of aspirin or salicylates in causing this disease, with recent data indicating a strong association. Therefore, the present recommendation is that no salicylates be given to children with fever. Some evidence also suggests that the risk may be similar in adults.

D. Herpes zoster (shingles).

1. The varicella (chickenpox) virus resides asymptomatically in dorsal root ganglia, and for unknown reasons may occasionally migrate along sensory roots causing pain and later vesicular skin eruption in root distribution.

2. Pain may precede eruption of skin vesicles by several days, making the diagnosis obscure until eruption occurs.

3. Patients should be evaluated for underlying immunodeficiency, especially lymphomas.

4. Acyclovir is useful treatment, decreasing pain and new vesicle formation. The dosage is acyclovir 15 mg/kg IV in three divided doses daily for 5 to 10 days. In otherwise healthy patients, prednisone 60 to 80 mg daily PO for 2 to 3 weeks may reduce the risk of postherpetic neuralgia.

5. Complications:

a. Postherpetic neuralgia occurs in about 15% of patients with shingles. Treatment is symptomatic: amitriptyline hydrochloride 25 to 50 mg at bedtime in combination with carbamazepine 200 mg three or four times daily after meals. Topical preparations containing capsaicin (the active ingredient in hot peppers) may also alleviate this condition.

b. Ophthalmic zoster carries the danger of corneal scarring. Treatment is with local steroids and antibiot-

ics; patients should be referred to an experienced ophthalmologist.
c. Geniculate zoster will present with a peripheral facial palsy. Management is the same as with Bell's palsy [see Chapter 15, section II.A.1.a.(4)(f)].

BIBLIOGRAPHY

Bell WE, McCormick WF: *Neurologic Infections in Children.* ed 2. Philadelphia, WB Saunders, 1981.

Bell WE, McGuinness GA: Current therapy of acute bacterial meningitis in children, Part II. *Pediatr Neurol* 1985; 1:201–209.

Booss J, Thornton GF (eds): Infectious diseases of the central nervous system. *Neurol Clin* 1986; 4:1–325.

Corey L, Spear PE: Infections with herpes simplex viruses. *N Engl J Med* 1986; 314:749–757.

Hirsh MS, Schooley RT: Treatment of herpesvirus infections. *N Engl J Med* 1986; 309:963–969.

Hook WH, Marra CM: Acquired syphilis in adults. *N Engl J Med* 1992; 326:1060–1067.

Johnson GM, Scurletis D, Carole NB: A study of 16 fatal cases of encephalitis-like disease in North Carolina children. *N C Med J* 1963; 29:464–473.

Johnson RT: *Viral Infections of the Nervous System.* New York, Raven Press, 1982.

McArthur J: Neurologic manifestations of AIDS. *Medicine (Baltimore)* 1987; 66:407–437.

Navia BA, et al: The AIDS dementia complex: Clinical features. *Ann Neurol* 1986; 19:517–524.

Smith AL: Neurologic sequelae of meningitis. *N Engl J Med* 1988; 319:1010–1013.

Steele AC: Lyme disease. *N Engl J Med* 1989; 321:586–596.

Whitley RJ: Viral encephalitis. *N Engl J Med* 1990; 323:242–250.

FOCAL AND DIFFUSE WEAKNESS OF PERIPHERAL ORIGIN

15

I. DIFFERENTIATION OF WEAKNESS.

A. Although generalized weakness may be due to a variety of medical problems (such as anemia or cardiac failure) or to psychiatric disturbances, in this chapter weakness is assumed to be due to disease of the peripheral nervous system (PNS) (muscle or nerve) or the central nervous system (CNS). Sometimes it is difficult to differentiate PNS disease from CNS disease. The following guidelines may be helpful:

1. Increased reflexes and extensor plantar responses (Babinski reflexes) are associated with CNS disorders.
2. Decreased reflexes generally indicate weakness of PNS origin, except in the acute phase of CNS disease or in long-standing, extremely severe CNS disease.
3. Involvement of an arm and a leg on the same side is suggestive of CNS disease.
4. Multiple cranial nerve involvement suggests CNS disease, especially when there is motor weakness or sensory disturbance in the contralateral leg or arm.
5. Changes in muscle bulk (such as atrophy or hypertrophy) suggest PNS disease.
6. Trophic changes in skin and hair, especially if associated with changes in muscle bulk, suggest PNS disease.

B. Once the clinician has determined that the weakness is of PNS origin, Tables 15–1 and 15–2 may be helpful for determining whether the problem primarily involves the muscle or the nerve.

II. DIFFUSE WEAKNESS OF PERIPHERAL ORIGIN
A. Polyneuropathies.

1. Diabetic neuropathy: There are three types of neuropathies associated with diabetes, and a patient may have one or any combination of all three neuropathies:

   a. Diabetic peripheral neuropathy is also called diabetic sensory neuropathy because sensory symptoms tend to be prominent.

   ▶ 1) The usual presentation is paresthesias or hyperesthesias of the feet or painless foot trauma; suspect neuropathy when either exaggerated withdrawal response to plantar stimulation or summation (recurrent pinpricks suddenly become painful) is present (see Chapter 1, section I. C.).

   2) Some degree of peripheral neuropathy is evident in almost all diabetic patients.

   3) Significant peripheral neuropathies are almost always associated with absent ankle reflexes.

   4) Severity of neuropathy often is not directly correlated with control of blood sugar.

   5) Very severe diabetic peripheral neuropathy (pseudotabes) may be characterized by recurrent spontaneous pain (described as "deep in the bones"), loss of pain sensation in joints, sensory ataxia, and development of perforating ulcers.

   Note: It is sometimes necessary to differentiate peripheral polyneuropathy (symmetric involvement of all peripheral nerves, usually the result of a metabolic disturbance and affecting the distal portions of extremities more than the proximal) from mononeuritis multiplex (involvement of multiple individual nerves, often asymmetric and proximal and usually the result of traumatic or vascular injury). Both types of peripheral neuropathy may occur in diabetic patients. The "stocking"

TABLE 15–1.
Differentiation of Muscle and Nerve Disease on Clinical Examination*

Sign	Nerve	Exceptions	Muscle	Exceptions
Reflexes	Absent early	Anterior horn cell disease, reflexes preserved	Usually present	In end-stage muscle disease and in polymyositis, reflexes are diminished or absent
Distribution of weakness	Distal	Occasionally in anterior horn cell disease and lead poisoning; weakness is proximal	Proximal	Myotonic dystrophy has distal weakness
Sensory disturbance	Usually present	Anterior horn cell disease, sensory disturbances are absent; motor symptoms appear first in some neuropathies	Absent	In inflammatory myopathy, nerve terminal branches can be involved; pain may be misinterpreted as sensory disturbances

(Continued.)

TABLE 15–1. (cont.).

Sign	Nerve	Exceptions	Muscle	Exceptions
Autonomic disturbance	Often present	Anterior horn cell disease	Absent	In inflammatory myopathy, nerve terminal branches can be involved
Atrophy	Early	Anterior horn cell disease	Late	Muscular dystrophy, "congenital" myopathies
Hypertrophy	Rare	Plexiform neurofibroma	Common in Duchenne's dystrophy	
Cramps	With initiation of exercise		After exercise	

*Characteristic findings are (1) myotonia—found in myotonic dystrophy, myotonia congenita, and periodic paralysis; (2) fasciculations—indicate anterior horn cell disease but may be benign in situations such as excess caffeine intake.

TABLE 15–2.
Laboratory Features That May Be Helpful in Corroborating Clinical Differentiation of Muscle or Nerve Involvement

Test	Nerve	Exceptions	Muscle	Exceptions
Creatine phospho-kinase (CPK)	Normal	Elevated factitiously after injections and trauma; elevated 2–3 times normal in anterior horn cell disease	Markedly elevated 8–200 times normal	End-stage muscle disease, rare cases of inflammatory muscle disease, and "congenital" myopathies
Needle EMG	Fibrillations and fasciculations (large-amplitude units)	May be normal less than 3 wk from onset; in severe disease electrical activity not detectable	Small motor units	Fibrillations may occur in inflammatory disease
Nerve conduction velocity	Usually a decrease	Usually normal in anterior horn cell disease and selective axonal disorders	Normal	
Muscle biopsy	Small atrophic fibers and grouping of fiber types	Normal less than 3 wk from onset or sampling error	Necrotic muscle fibers and abnormal fiber architecture are common	Sampling error

component of the symmetric peripheral neuropathy is always clinically more evident than the "glove" component. When the upper limbs are equally or more affected than the lower limbs, mononeuritis multiplex is the more likely diagnosis.

b. Diabetic autonomic peripheral neuropathy.
   ▶ 1) Commonly the patient complains of excessive sweating on the upper portion of the body (which is due to decreased sweating on the lower portion of the body) and symptoms due to postural hypotension.
   2) Other symptoms may include impotence, atonic bladder, and abnormalities of gastrointestinal motility.
   3) Patients with diabetic autonomic peripheral neuropathy are very susceptible to heat stroke.

c. Diabetic amyotrophy.
   ▶ 1) Characterized by proximal weakness and atrophy; nocturnal pain in thigh, back, and perineum; and presence of fasciculations.
   2) Sensory loss is minimal; knee reflex may be absent while ankle reflex is present.
   3) Important to diagnose because improvement is often noted with better blood sugar control.

d. Treatment.
   1) Diabetic control is important but may not alter the course except in diabetic amyotrophy.
   2) Pain should NOT be treated with narcotics. Amitriptyline 25 to 125 mg/day, or a combination of fluoxetine (Prozac) 20 mg qam and nortriptyline 25 mg qhs offer the best pain control. Phenytoin 200 mg bid or carbamazepine 200 mg qid may also be used to relieve symptoms.
   3) Thiamine 50 to 100 mg/day may be helpful.

2. <u>Polyneuropathies associated with deficiency states and metabolic disorders:</u> Polyneuropathies associated with deficiency states and metabolic disorders are extremely common and in most instances closely resemble the diabetic polyneuropathies, although there are some individual differences in presentation.

<u>a</u>. Vitamin B$_{12}$ deficiency (pernicious anemia, subacute combined degeneration, combined systems disease).

▶ 1) The clinical presentation is variable because the patient may have only one or more of the following disturbances:

a) Peripheral neuropathy: moderate to severe involvement of sensation and, in later stages, distal muscle atrophy and weakness.

b) Posterior column symptoms: markedly diminished or absent vibratory and position sensation (particularly in the lower extremities); sensory ataxia; on examination, patient will fall from a standing position with eye closure (positive Romberg test).

c) Spasticity: corticospinal tract involvement with paraparesis or quadriparesis (tetraparesis); on clinical examination, bilateral extensor plantar responses (Babinski reflexes) are usually present.

d) Dementia: may be clinically indistinguishable from other forms of dementia (see Chapter 6, section III. F).

e) Neuropsychiatric disorder: prominent behavioral and personality changes, particularly depression.

Remember: It may be difficult to demonstrate spasticity or posterior column disturbance in the presence of severe peripheral neuropathy, and demonstrating sensory disturbance may be difficult in the presence of significant dementia.

2) The diagnosis is best established by finding low levels of serum methylmalonic acid. Low serum vitamin B$_{12}$ levels are helpful in establishing the diagnosis but may not be abnormal even in the presence of tissue deficiency. A Schilling test is rarely necessary in modern practice.

3) Anemia or disturbances of blood cell morphology may be absent and should not be used as criteria for excluding this diagnosis.

4) Treatment: Only *after* the diagnosis is *definitely established* should treatment be started. Vitamin B_{12} 1,000 µg *parenterally* every week for ten doses and then monthly for life.

Caveat: Administration of folic acid may mask the hematologic abnormalities of vitamin B_{12} deficiency and can worsen the neurologic symptoms.

b. Folic acid deficiency.
▶ 1) The *clinical presentation* is often indistinguishable from vitamin B_{12} deficiency, except that dementia is usually the most prominent neurologic symptom.
2) The diagnosis is established by low serum folate levels.
3) Treatment: *Before* folic acid is administered, vitamin B_{12} deficiency must be definitely excluded. Folic acid 5.0 mg should be administered daily.
c. Thiamine deficiency–alcoholic polyneuropathy: Thiamine deficiency most commonly presents in alcoholic patients (see Chapter 8, section II) with absent ankle reflexes, paresthesias, and minimal motor weakness. It often occurs in hospitalized patients who have a history of high carbohydrate diet but are now NPO and receiving intravenous fluids into which the physician has neglected to place a vitamin supplementation.
d. Other metabolic causes of peripheral polyneuropathy:
1) Chronic renal disease.
2) Chronic liver failure.
3) Remote effect of carcinoma, particularly bronchogenic carcinoma (serum antibody assays are available to document this cause of peripheral polyneuropathy).
4) Drug-induced peripheral polyneuropathy can occur with many agents, including vincristine, cisplatin, nitrofurantoin, dapsone, isoniazid (INH), disulfiram.
3. Polyneuropathies associated with heavy metal poisoning: Arsenic, lead, mercury, and thallium are the most common metal poisonings associated with peripheral neuropathy. Specific features of these polyneuropathies are summarized in Table 15–3. Bismuth, manganese, gold, anti-

mony, barium, zinc, and copper in large doses have also been associated with neuropathy, but other systemic symptoms usually dominate the clinical picture.

a. Guillain-Barré syndrome (Landry-Guillain-Barré-Strohl syndrome, inflammatory polyradiculoneuropathy, "French polio," ascending polyradiculoneuropathy).

▶ 1) Characterized by symmetric progressive weakness greater distally than proximally, worse in the legs than the arms; usually presents as an ascending paralysis that affects motor nerves more than sensory nerves.

2) Reflexes in the lower extremities are absent early in the disease.

3) The facial nerve may be involved.

Caveat: Bilateral facial weakness of rapid onset accompanied by a motor polyneuropathy is most often due to Guillain-Barré syndrome.

4) Sensory loss is variable, but usually mild; when present, position and vibration sense are more affected than pain.

5) Onset subacute (usually over 1 – 2 days). Over half of the patients have a history of an antecedent "flu-like" illness, which has resolved by the time of onset of polyradiculoneuropathy; 10% of patients have had surgery 1 to 4 weeks previously; postimmunization occurrence has been reported.

6) Autonomic function is usually abnormal, but manifestations are variable and include bladder disturbance, fluctuating blood pressure with postural hypotension, anal sphincter weakness, gastrointestinal motility disturbances (including dysphagia), and sluggishly reactive pupils; abnormalities of cardiac rhythm may occur; loss of sweating in lower extremities may result in increased sweating in upper extremities.

7) After the first 2 or 3 days of paralysis, the cerebrospinal fluid (CSF) protein is elevated, and only a few lymphocytes are present, usually less than

TABLE 15-3.
Principal Metal Toxins

	Arsenic	Lead	Mercury	Thallium
Clinical tip-off	Red hands and burning feet with hyperhidrosis	Peripheral neuropathy which may appear to be single nerve involvement (such as wristdrop or footdrop)	Severe spontaneous arm and leg pain	Alopecia
Exposure	Homicide attempt, insecticides, medicinal arsenic, Paris green, accidental contamination, Fowler's solution (potassium arsenite)	Industrial ingestion; tetraethyl gasoline; lead paint; burning lead batteries; eating from pewter or dishware with glaze containing lead; melting for purposes of molding.	Ingestion of methyl mercury (Minamata disease), especially fish in polluted areas; industrial exposure; antifungal treatment of grain	Homicide, insecticide, rodent poison
Clinical syndrome	"Stocking-glove," mainly sensory neuropathy;	Primarily a motor neuropathy, which	Dementia with primarily motor neuropathy;	Distal sensorimotor neuropathy of

severe pain and paresthesias, especially of feet and hands; "burning feet and hands," red hands with hyperhidrosis and subsequent motor neuropathy involving distal muscles of hands and feet	frequently may appear as though single nerves are involved, such as radial nerve (wristdrop), median nerve (thenar atrophy), peroneal nerve (footdrop); painful joints; in children causes cerebral edema	occasional sensory stocking-glove neuropathy; acrodynia (pink disease) in infants and young children	stocking-glove type with alopecia
Diagnosis 24-hour urine analysis, hair analysis, blood arsenic level	Blood lead level, 24-hr urine analysis	24-hr urine analysis	24-hr urine analysis
Treatment Penicillamine 250 mg qid (may also use BAL or EDTA)*	Penicillamine 250 mg qid (may also use BAL or EDTA)*	Penicillamine 250 mg qid (may also use BAL or EDTA)*	Diphenylthio-carbazone or sodium dicarbamate

*BAL = dimercaprol; EDTA = ethylenediaminetetraacetic acid.

10/μL (so-called albuminocytologic dissociation). Peak levels of CSF protein (may be greater than 2,000 mg/dL) occur 4 to 6 weeks after onset of illness and may continue to rise as clinical improvement occurs.

8) Maximum deficit occurs over 3 days to 6 weeks; spontaneous recovery occurs in a "descending fashion," over 6 weeks to 6 months, and is usually complete.

9) Routine nerve conduction velocities are normal in up to 10% of patients; tests of F-wave latency and the H-reflex are usually abnormal.

10) Neurologic complications of arsenic poisoning or of acquired immunodeficiency syndrome (AIDS) may closely mimic Guillain-Barré syndrome and should be excluded by appropriate tests.

Note: Sometimes the first presentation of chronic relapsing polyneuropathy may mimic Guillain-Barré syndrome. However, such patients have multiple relapsing episodes at varying intervals and of varying duration, often without complete recovery between exacerbations.

11) Treatment.
  a) The availability of an intensive care nursing unit is vital for managing the acute life-threatening complications of Guillain-Barré syndrome (see also Chapter 20, section IX).
  b) Respiratory function initially must be closely monitored with frequent (at least hourly) bedside measurements of forced vital capacity (FVC) and inspiratory force (a direct pulmonary reflection of muscular strength). Respiratory function must be closely monitored, even in patients with no apparent respiratory involvement, since rapid progression of weakness over several hours may produce respiratory failure. If FVC falls below 1,400 mL in the 70-kg individual, endotracheal intubation or tracheostomy

must be very seriously considered. An inspiratory force of less than 25 cm H_2O also indicates probable need for endotracheal intubation. The frequency of monitoring of respiratory function may be reduced as the patient shows signs of clinical improvement.

Caveat: The use of paralyzing agents (such as succinylcholine) to facilitate endotracheal intubation may lead to dangerous hyperkalemia.

c) Ventilatory assistance must be provided at the first sign of dyspnea or decreased blood oxygen saturation. Dysphagia can result in aspiration of food, and nasogastric feeding may be necessary. Paroxysmal hypertension, cardiac arrhythmias, and abnormal thermoregulation can occur and must be individually treated. Intercurrent infections must be treated vigorously. Pulmonary embolism can occur secondary to venous stasis in paralyzed limbs; thigh-length elastic stockings are recommended.

d) Treatment of the precipitating illness may be necessary; about 5% of cases have a preceding mycoplasma infection requiring antibiotic therapy. Also, the syndrome of inappropriate antidiuretic hormone (SIADH) may occur in some patients and should be treated with careful fluid restriction.

e) Nursing care and physical therapy are necessary adjuncts. Frequent turning is important to avoid pressure sores. Pressure on peripheral nerves (especially the ulnar nerve at the elbow and peroneal nerve at the fibular head) can destroy the still intact nerve axons as well as the delicate regenerating myelin, resulting in permanent nerve palsies; this should be avoided by appropriate patient positioning and cushioning. Passive range of motion is important to prevent contractures. Early mobilization of the extremities is necessary to avoid the development of thrombophlebitis with subsequent pulmonary embolization; low-dose heparin therapy may also be useful in preventing this complication.

f) Corticosteroids have not definitely been shown to benefit Guillain-Barré syndrome, although in chronic relapsing polyneuropathy, there is definite benefit with corticosteroid therapy.

g) If available, plasmapheresis *early* in the course of the disease (during the first week) is highly recommended and will hasten recovery.

B. Diseases of the anterior horn cell.

1. Amyotrophic lateral sclerosis (ALS).

▶ a. Characterized by gradually progressive muscle weakness associated with fasciculations of arms, legs, and tongue. The initial weakness may be proximal and resemble a muscle disease. The weakness is not necessarily symmetric, and bulbar musculature may be affected first. Signs of upper motor neuron disease (hyperactive reflexes and extensor plantar responses) may be present initially but are later masked by severe loss of anterior horn cells.

Caveat: Simultaneous occurrence of upper and lower motor neuron paralysis in the same muscle (spastic hyperreflexia along with fasciculations and atrophy) is almost diagnostic of ALS.

b. There are no significant sensory abnormalities.

c. Occasionally minor elevations of serum creatine phosphokinase (CPK) up to three times normal and elevation of CSF protein to 70 to 80 mg/dL may be noted.

d. Since the disease is fatal within several years in 80% of patients, ALS must be very carefully differentiated from the following potentially treatable conditions:

1) Diseases of the cervical spinal cord (see Chapter 18), such as syringomyelia, spondylitic myelopathy, tumors (fasciculations only in the upper extremities and upper motor neuron signs in the lower extremities).

2) Parathyroid disease (elevated serum calcium).

3) Diabetic amyotrophy (improvement with blood sugar control).

4) Benign fasciculations (often seen in patients with excessive caffeine intake).

e. Treatment.

1) The intellect in ALS is preserved; careful counseling of the patient and family concerning the poor prognosis and early death are mandatory.

2) If severe dysphagia is present, a feeding gastrostomy or pyriform sinus feeding tube may make the patient more comfortable.

3) Most physicians will not use ventilatory assistance, since this results in a totally paralyzed patient (eventually even eye movements become paralyzed) who suffers a prolonged and agonizing death.

4) Further information on services available to patients with ALS can be obtained from the Muscular Dystrophy Association, 810 Seventh Ave., New York, NY 10019, telephone (212) 586-0808; or from the ALS Association, 21021 Ventura Blvd., Suite 321, Woodland Hills, CA 91364, telephone (818) 340-7500.

2. Inherited anterior horn cell disease (spinal muscular atrophies).

a. Infancy *(Werdnig-Hoffmann disease)*.

▶ 1) Presents as a floppy baby (Fig 15–1) with progressive weakness and feeding difficulties.

2) Fasciculations are easiest to see in the tongue but are difficult to see in the extremities because of baby fat.

3) Death usually occurs in the first few years of life due to respiratory insufficiency.

4) This disorder results from an autosomal recessive gene.

b. Childhood or adolescence *(Kugelberg-Welander disease)*.

▶ 1) Presents as progressive, proximal weakness sometimes associated with large calves.

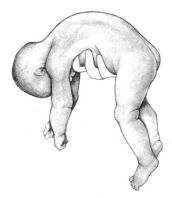

FIG 15–1. A 1-year-old "floppy baby" with infantile spinal muscular atrophy (Werdnig-Hoffmann disease). Note that there is a marked lack of muscle tone.

   2) Fasciculations may be visible in the extremities and tongue. Upper motor neuron signs are absent.
   3) This disorder may result from an autosomal recessive or autosomal dominant gene.
 c. The diagnosis is made on the basis of the clinical presentation, evidence of denervation on electromyographic (EMG) studies, and characteristic pathologic findings in histochemically stained muscle biopsies.
 d. Treatment.
   1) There is no specific treatment, but physical and occupational therapy should be directed toward maintaining limb function and preventing deformity.
   2) Genetic counseling is necessary.
   3) Emotional support for the family should be provided.
   4) Further information on services available to patients can be obtained from the Muscular Dystrophy Association, 810 Seventh Ave., New York, NY 10019, telephone (212) 586-0808.

3. Peroneal muscular atrophy syndrome (Charcot-Marie-Tooth disease; idiopathic dominantly inherited hypertrophic polyneuropathy; hereditary motor and sensory neuropathy).

▶ a. This autosomal dominant disorder is associated with slowly progressive foot deformity (pes cavus and hammer toes) and atrophy of lower legs resulting in "stork legs" or "inverted champagne bottle legs" (Fig 15–2). The most common early presentation is bilateral footdrop.

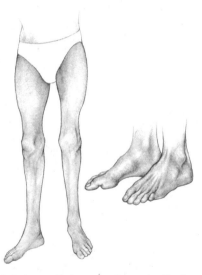

FIG 15–2. Patients with the peroneal muscular atrophy syndrome (Charcot-Marie-Tooth disease) have a "stork-legs" appearance due to atrophy of the lower leg and distal one third of the thigh musculature. Hammer toes and pes cavus may also be an early sign of this disorder.

b. Diagnosis is suggested by appropriate clinical findings, family history, and abnormal nerve conduction studies and EMG.

c. Clinical presentation of this disorder varies from family to family, but within a single family the symptomatology of affected family members tends to be similar.

d. In some families other neurologic signs may be present, such as sensory loss, enlarged nerves, or cerebellar ataxia.

e. Treatment: There is no specific treatment for this disorder, although disability is usually mild and compatible with long life. Genetic counseling is necessary. Prevention of injuries to limbs that have reduced sensibility is imperative. Supportive physical and occupational therapy can often be provided through the Muscular Dystrophy Association, 810 Seventh Ave., New York, NY 10019, telephone (212) 586-0808.

4. Poliomyelitis.

▶ a. Poliomyelitis is an acute viral infection of the anterior horn cells. The weakness is often preceded by gastroenteritis.

b. The disease is usually asymmetric, with flaccid weakness.

c. There may be paralysis of the bulbar muscles.

d. Poliomyelitis is associated with aseptic meningitis.

e. The diagnosis is confirmed by acute and convalescent serologic titers.

f. Many years after the acute paralysis with varying degrees of subsequent recovery, occasional patients may experience apparent progressive weakness, sometimes accompanied by pain. Most often this weakness is due to

1) Normal age-related loss of muscle power (which compromises already marginal muscle function).

2) Degenerative arthritis (developing in joints subjected to abnormal stresses from the longstanding muscle pareses) limiting joint and muscle function and resulting in pressure neuropathies or radiculopathies.

3) Bracing and prostheses, which are currently inappropriate (often not having been reevaluated since the time of the initial polio episode).

4) The "postpolio syndrome" of premature loss of anterior horn cells, which presumably have been overtaxed in having to maintain a massive motor unit because of the reinnervation of the huge number of muscle fibers denervated during the acute phase of polio.

g. Treatment.

1) There is no specific treatment for the infection.

2) Respiratory function may need to be supported.

3) The disease is now rare in North America owing to prevention with appropriate vaccination. Contacts should be vaccinated if not previously done.

C. Diseases of the neuromuscular junction.

1. Myasthenia Gravis.

▶ a. This is a disease of the neuromuscular junction in which weakness develops after repetitive muscle contraction ("fatigable weakness"); it usually presents with some degree of ophthalmoplegia. Myasthenia gravis should be strongly suspected in any patient who reports excessive weakness at the end of the day. The complaints of weakness are frequently bizarre and are often interpreted as a psychiatric disturbance, especially since the routine neurologic examination is normal in most patients.

b. When the physician entertains the diagnosis of myasthenia, the following examinations should be performed:

1) Since the eyes are most frequently involved, have the patient maintain a sustained upward gaze for at least 3 minutes without interruption. In the myasthenic patient, one or both eyelids will often begin to droop or the gaze will cease to be conjugate (Fig 15–3).

2) Have the patient perform repetitive muscle contractions related to the complaint, and observe for evidence of developing weakness. For example, if the

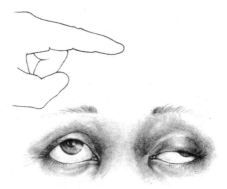

FIG 15–3. In myasthenia gravis fatigable weakness is evident on examination of eye movements. There is usually ptosis which becomes more evident as the patient attempts to sustain upward gaze.

patient complains of weakness in climbing stairs, repetitive deep knee bends will become progressively more difficult to perform. If the patient complains of weakness in the hands, repetitive squeezing of a manometer cuff will show a progressive decrease in power. If the patient complains of difficulty in swallowing, repeated sips from a large glass of water will be normal at first but will subsequently result in choking.

c. Involvement of respiratory or pharyngeal muscles may occur with variable severity in the disease, and can lead to fatal respiratory failure or aspiration.

d. Definitive diagnosis.

1) Tensilon (edrophonium chloride) test.

a) Establish criteria for success or failure of this test, e.g., the disappearance of ptosis or restoration of strength after weakness had been produced by repetitive action.

b) Be sure that there is adequate preparation to deal with complications, which may include respiratory arrest and cardiac arrhythmias.

c) Establish an intravenous (IV) line in the patient and prepare the following solutions:

   i) An IV bottle of either normal saline or 5% D/W.

   ii) Normal saline is drawn up into a 1-mL syringe and labeled *A*.

   iii) Tensilon (as a 10-mg/mL ampule) is drawn up into a 1-mL syringe and labeled *B*.

d) The physician should be positive in statements about the effectiveness of each injection. First, inject contents of syringe *A* (saline placebo) in 0.5-mL increments and appear very disappointed when there is no effect.

e) Then contents of syringe *B* (Tensilon) should be injected in 0.5-mL increments; often an effect will be evident with as little as 5 mg.

f) A dramatic improvement in the selected criterion should occur within 30 seconds after the injection of the Tensilon and revert to its original state after 2 minutes. Effects occurring with saline placebo or before 30 seconds and after 2 minutes with Tensilon injection should be suspect.

Caveat: Atropine sulfate 0.4 mg should be readily available in a syringe for IV administration to reverse muscarinic side effects such as increased weakness or fasciculations.

2) Repetitive motor nerve stimulation (Jolly test) results in a characteristic decrementing pattern in myasthenia gravis; single-fiber EMG is also abnormal.

3) Provocative tests for myasthenia (such as curare tests) are rarely essential for diagnosis and may be extremely dangerous if not carried out under carefully controlled in-hospital conditions.

4) Anti-acetylcholine receptor antibody (AChR-Ab) titers are elevated in up to 90% of myasthenic patients.

e. In certain circumstances myasthenic crisis (acute or subacute onset of respiratory failure) may be induced by drugs or infection, and treatment of this constitutes a neurologic emergency (see Chapter 20, section X). Some of the drugs that can produce a myasthenic crisis are curare, succinylcholine, streptomycin, dihydro-streptomycin, kanamycin, polymyxin, lincomycin, tetracycline, oxytetracycline, gentamicin, and quinine (tonic water).

Note: Agents which are safe in myasthenia gravis include penicillin, cephalothin, rifampin, vancomycin, amphotericin, and nystatin.

f. Thymic abnormalities (hyperplasia or thymoma) occur in about 80% of myasthenic patients, and thymectomy can sometimes result in long-term remission.

g. During the neonatal period, 20% of infants born to myasthenic mothers have transient feeding difficulties, weak cry, breathing difficulties, floppiness, and other myasthenic symptoms (neonatal myasthenia), and require only supportive treatment.

h. D-Penicillamine can occasionally induce myasthenia gravis, which usually resolves within 1 year of discontinuing the drug.

i. Treatment.

   a) Initial treatment is usually with anticholinesterases (such as pyridostigmine bromide) for a trial period, although nearly all myasthenic patients require treatment in a tertiary hospital setting where therapy includes thymectomy (sternal splitting approach), plasmapheresis, alternate-day corticosteroids, and immunosuppressive therapy.

   b) Respiratory failure may occur during a crisis and is a neurologic emergency requiring ventilatory support (see Chapter 20, section X).

2. Lambert-Eaton (myasthenic) syndrome.

   a. The Lambert-Eaton syndrome resembles myasthenia gravis with complaints of tiredness and weakness, but unlike myasthenia gravis, ocular involvement is rare.

b. Strength may improve temporarily after voluntary contraction, but prolonged effort results in fatigue.

c. Muscle tendon reflexes are depressed but may improve after exercise.

d. Response to Tensilon is usually equivocal, and the diagnosis is established by characteristic findings with repetitive motor nerve stimulation.

e. Often associated with an occult malignancy (particularly lung carcinoma) or with autoimmune disease.

f. An antibody directed against the nerve terminal has been identified in affected patients; rare patients also have anti-acetylcholine receptor antibodies and may have signs and symptoms of both myasthenia gravis and the Lambert-Eaton syndrome.

g. Treatment.

1) For the non-neoplasm–related syndrome, treatment includes plasmapheresis, prednisone 30 to 60 mg qid, or azathioprine 1.5 to 2.0 mg/kg/day, singly or combined. For neoplasm-associated disease, antitumor therapy is required; plasmapheresis or prednisone, or both, may be used in addition, but immunosuppressive therapy should be avoided.

2) Symptomatic improvement of strength and exercise tolerance may be achieved with guanidine 10 to 35 mg/kg/day or 4-aminopyridine 40 to 200 mg/day; potential side effects of guanidine include ataxia, gastrointestinal distress, bone marrow depression, and renal failure; side effects of 4-aminopyridine include seizures and a confusional state.

3. Botulism.

a. Botulism presents as subacute paralysis of extraocular muscles with subsequent involvement of pharyngeal muscles.

b. Respiratory compromise secondary to skeletal muscle weakness occurs 24 to 48 hours after onset.

c. Botulism is caused by ingestion of toxin produced by *Clostridium botulinum,* which may be found in improperly canned non-acidic foods such as green beans.

d. Diagnosis can be confirmed by characteristic findings on repetitive nerve stimulation.

    e. Treatment.
        1) Polyvalent botulinum antitoxin should be adminis-
           tered, and stomach and intestinal contents re-
           moved.
        2) Respiratory failure is a major concern and should
           be monitored and treated in a manner similar to the
           respiratory problems of Guillian-Barré syndrome.

D. Diseases of Muscle.
  1. Myotonic dystrophy (Steinert's disease)
  ▶ a. Characterized by complaints of muscular stiffness (due
      to myotonia), which is relieved after repetitive activity,
      associated with slowly progressive distal weakness, es-
      pecially in the upper extremities; footdrop may develop
      later.
    b. Myotonia is a delayed relaxation of muscles, clinically
      recognized by:
        1) Having the patient make a tightly clenched fist for
           30 seconds and observing the difficulty in opening
           the hand.
        2) Percussion of the thenar eminence with a reflex
           hammer will cause the thumb to oppose the little
           finger and remain in that position for several sec-
           onds.
        3) Percussion of the gastrocnemius produces a tran-
           sient hard lump in the gastrocnemius.
        4) EMG shows a characteristic pattern with "dive-
           bomber" sounds.
    c. Facial features are often distinctive (Fig 15–4); other
      characteristics include pronounced frontal balding, pto-
      sis, cataracts, cardiac conduction defects, glucose intol-
      erance, disturbed gastrointestinal motility, sleep prob-
      lems (daytime somnolence), and psychological distur-
      bances (depression).
    d. The disorder is transmitted by an autosomal dominant
      gene on chromosome 19.
    e. Myotonic dystrophy may present in infancy as a floppy
      baby with respiratory distress and difficulty in feeding,
      usually in myotonic infants born to myotonic mothers.
    f. Other diseases with myotonia include myotonia con-
      genita and hyperkalemic periodic paralysis.

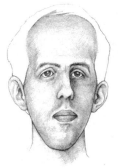

FIG 15–4. Patients with myotonic dystrophy have characteristic facial features of frontal baldness, depression of the temporal region (due to atrophy and loss of bulk of the temporalis muscle), and a long thin face with a pointed chin.

g. Treatment.
1) Most patients do not require treatment of the myotonia, but for occasional patients with incapacitating myotonia, phenytoin 100 to 400 mg/day is the preferred drug for relief of symptoms, although alternative drugs are available on an experimental basis.
2) Genetic counseling should be provided.
3) Cardiac evaluations are mandatory and a pacemaker insertion may be necessary to prevent fatal cardiac arrhythmias.
4) Depressive psychological (and other personality) disturbances may be improved by imipramine hydrochloride 50 to 150 mg qhs.
5) Pregnant women with myotonic dystrophy should be warned that there may be difficulty with the delivery and that the infant may have respiratory and feeding difficulties (neonatal presentation of myotonic dystrophy).

2. Duchenne's dystrophy (X-linked pseudohypertrophic muscular dystrophy; "common muscular dystrophy").

▶ a. Hereditary disorder that affects only boys and is first manifested around the age of 3 years by difficulty in climbing stairs.

b. On clinical examination, the following are seen:
   1) Calves that are larger than normal and have a rubbery feel on palpation.
   2) When the boy attempts to rise from a lying to a standing position, he will attempt to climb up on his legs (Gowers' maneuver) (Fig. 15–5).

c. The diagnosis is confirmed by an extremely high serum creatine phosphokinase (CPK) (8–200 times greater than normal), by characteristic pathologic findings in histochemically stained muscle biopsies, and by biochemical analysis of muscle specimens revealing absence of the membrane protein *dystrophin* manufactured by a gene on the short arm of the X chromosome. DNA studies can be used to reveal the exact gene mutation (most often a deletion) in the patient or in female carrier relatives.

d. Associated intellectual impairment is common.

e. A slowly progressive variant form of the disease with onset in late childhood or adolescence has been termed *Becker's muscular dystrophy*.

f. Treatment: Patients should be referred to the local clinics directed by the Muscular Dystrophy Association, 810 Seventh Ave., New York, NY 10019, telephone (212) 586-0808. These clinics provide diagnostic facilities, genetic counseling, physical therapy, appliances such as braces and wheelchairs, and social services.

3. Polymyositis and Dermatomyositis.

a. The patient (child or adult) presents with subacute onset of proximal weakness and muscle pain (a common complaint is difficulty in climbing stairs).

b. Neurologic examination is usually normal except for the presence of proximal weakness demonstrated by difficulty performing deep knee bends or arising from a chair (Fig 15–6)

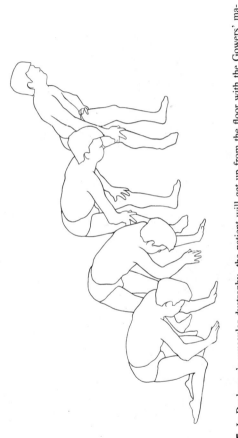

FIG 15–5. In Duchenne's muscular dystrophy, the patient will get up from the floor with the Gowers' maneuver. The boy will "walk up" his body with his hands as he arises.

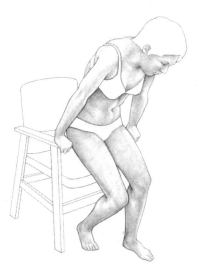

FIG 15–6. The proximal muscle weakness found in polymyositis results in difficulty arising from a chair. Note that the patient must use her arms to push off the chair to come to a standing position.

    c. Skin lesions may be present and include malar flush, reddening at the base of the fingernails, a scaly rash over the extensor surface of the joints, and subcutaneous calcifications.

    d. Diagnosis is established by elevated serum CPK, elevated erythrocyte sedimentation rate (ESR), and characteristic pathologic findings in histochemically stained muscle biopsies.

    e. Occasionally associated with occult malignancy, autoimmune disorders, or AIDS.

    f. Treatment. Prednisone in a dose of 60 mg/m^2 (children) or 100 mg (adults) every other day will often result in a remission, but treatment with other additional immunosuppressive drugs may be necessary.

4. Muscle weakness associated with systemic disease (type II muscle fiber atrophy).
   a. Patient presents with proximal weakness of subacute or chronic onset.
   b. This is the most common cause of proximal muscle weakness.
   c. Associated with disuse (disuse atrophy) or with various chronic disorders such as cachexia, hypercorticism ("steroid myopathy"), hyperparathyroidism, cancer ("carcinomatous myopathy"), or hyperthyroidism ("thyroid myopathy").
   d. EMG, nerve conduction studies, and serum CPK are usually normal.
   e. Definitive diagnosis is by characteristic pathologic findings in histochemically stained muscle biopsies.
   f. Treatment.
      1) Weakness is generally reversible if the underlying cause can be corrected.
      2) This potentially treatable cause of muscle weakness must be carefully differentiated from the untreatable causes of proximal muscle weakness.
5. Malignant Hyperthermia (Hyperpyrexia).
   a. Malignant hyperthermia is characterized by sudden onset of marked hyperthermia (body temperature of 42° C [107° F] and higher) during general anesthesia with halogenated anesthetics (halothane, enflurane) or succinylcholine. Additional symptoms are extreme muscular rigidity, hyperkalemia, tachycardia, tachypnea, severe metabolic and respiratory acidosis, and myoglobinuria.
   b. Frequently familial; occasionally associated with neuromuscular diseases, including central core disease and myotonia congenita.
   c. Susceptible patients often have elevated serum CPK in preoperative blood studies.
   d. Treatment.
      1) Death occurs in over 60% of patients in whom treatment is delayed. Immediate IV administration of dantrolene in a dose of 1 to 10 mg/kg will usually abort an episode, followed by oral dantrolene 1 to 2 mg/kg qid for 1 to 3 days to prevent recurrence.

2) Prevention is most important. If there is a family history of anesthetic-associated deaths, the known precipitating anesthetic agents should be avoided. If surgery in a known susceptible person is indicated, preoperative treatment with dantrolene 1 to 2 mg/kg q6h for 1 or 2 days before surgery with a last dose of 2 mg/kg 3 hours preoperatively may prevent development of the syndrome.

III. FOCAL WEAKNESS OF PERIPHERAL ORIGIN.

A. **Nerve lesions.** Localized weakness is frequently due to injury of the peripheral nerve, plexus, nerve root, or nerve cell body (Fig 15–7). In most cases, there is both motor and sensory disturbance. The specific site of the nerve injury is recognized by the pattern of muscle weakness and by the distribution of the cutaneous sensory disturbance. Sometimes it is difficult to determine the exact muscle involvement by clinical examination, and in such circumstances, EMG may determine the specific muscles involved. Since most clinicians do not often evaluate patients with peripheral nerve lesions, help is available from a thin inexpensive paperback book from the Medical Research Council that can be readily carried in a physician's bag: *Aids to the Examination of the Peripheral Nervous System* (Her Majesty's Stationery Office, 51 Nine Elms Lane, London SW8 5DR, England). Although specific causes of focal peripheral nerve weakness are not discussed in this chapter, root lesions are most commonly caused by a herniated intervertebral disc, plexus lesions by trauma or infection, and peripheral nerve lesions by trauma, pressure, or vascular occlusion. Multiple individual nerve lesions may occur in a single extremity (as in trauma, vascular injury, or infection) or in multiple extremities (mononeuritis multiplex). The following is a description of common peripheral weakness patterns that should be recognized by the clinician:

1. Root lesions: Common cervical root syndromes involve the C6 and C7 roots and are discussed in Chapter 18. The relationship of the cervical roots, brachial plexus, and peripheral nerves are shown in Figure 15–7. Common lumbar root syndromes involve the L4, L5, and S1 roots and are discussed in Chapter 17, section II. B. 8.

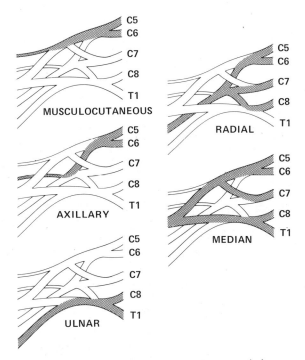

FIG 15-7. Diagram of the relationship between cervical nerve roots, brachial plexus, and peripheral nerves.

    a. Peripheral nerve lesions.
        1) Radial nerve (Fig 15-8).
        ▶ a) Characterized by weakness of extension of wrist and fingers (wristdrop) and only a small area of sensory loss along the dorsum of the base of the thumb (anatomic snuff-box).
           b) Known as "Saturday night palsy" because paralysis commonly occurs from prolonged pres-

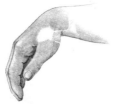

FIG 15–8. With a radial nerve palsy, there will be a wristdrop (due to weakness of the radial-innervated wrist extensor muscles) and a small patch of sensory disturbance in the area of the "anatomic snuff-box."

sure on the nerve in the upper arm, as might occur in an intoxicated person in a semistuporous state resting with an arm hanging over a park bench.

  c) Treatment.

    i) If the injury is due to pressure, spontaneous recovery will usually occur over a 2- to 6-month period.

    ii) Until recovery occurs, a cock-up splint for the wrist may make the hand more functional.

2) Median nerve.

  a) Carpal tunnel syndrome (median nerve lesion at wrist).

    ▶ i) The patient will complain of pain and paresthesias in the hand, especially the thumb and index finger. The patient may also complain of pain more proximally in the forearm, upper arm, or shoulder. The pain is frequently worse at night, often awakening the patient; pain relief may be obtained by rubbing or shaking the hand and arm or letting the hand hang over the side of the bed.

ii) Although the patient may complain of reduced sensibility in the thumb and index finger, actual sensory loss may be difficult to demonstrate on formal testing.

iii) Weakness and atrophy of the thenar muscles are usually late signs.

iv) Tinel's sign (Fig 15–9) may be helpful. This is obtained by lightly tapping the median nerve at the wrist, with such a tap reproducing the symptoms. Hyperextension or hyperflexion of the wrist may produce the same effect.

v) May be bilateral, but is usually worse in the dominant hand. Finding prolongation of the distal latency on nerve conduction velocity studies of the median nerve at the wrist and EMG abnormalities in the thenar muscles establishes the diagnosis.

vi) Associated with rheumatoid arthritis (collagen-vascular disease), hypothyroidism, obesity, acromegaly, gout, and multiple myeloma; carpal tunnel syndrome ini-

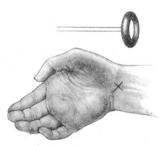

FIG 15–9. Tinel's sign is a burning-tingling sensation in the fingers, produced by tapping over the median nerve at the site of entrapment under the carpal ligament in the carpal tunnel syndrome.

tially presenting during a pregnancy usually resolves after delivery.

vii) Treatment: Treatment of any underlying disease is necessary. Symptomatic relief is usually obtained with a wrist splint, which keeps the wrist in a neutral position and prevents repetitive motion. Most patients with the carpal tunnel syndrome do not necessarily require surgery, although sectioning of the carpal ligament will relieve pressure on the nerve in severe cases.

b) "Bridegroom's palsy" (median nerve lesion in upper arm).

▶ i) Characterized by weakness of the prehensile abilities of the thumb, including difficulty opposing the thumb to the little and index fingers; after many months atrophy of the thenar eminence may occur with recession of the thumb to form a "simian hand."

ii) Results from injury to the median nerve along its course beside the brachial artery in the medial portion of the upper arm following unsuccessful attempts to catheterize the brachial artery or from an abnormal sleeping position (the name is derived from the sleeping position of the bridegroom's outstretched arm under the bride's head).

iii) Sensory loss over the entire thumb, index, and middle fingers, and the lateral half of the ring finger may be demonstrated.

3) Ulnar nerve.

a) Characteristic clinical features are:

i) In slight or early injury: weakness of finger extension (especially the ring and little fingers); weakness of little finger abduction; slight weakness of wrist flexion.

ii) In severe or longstanding injury: atrophy of the hypothenar eminence; atrophy of the intrinsic hand muscles with hollowing between the metacarpal bones (especially evident in the space between the thumb and index finger; see Fig 15–10); clawhand or "beer stein holder's hand" deformity.

iii) Sensory loss of little finger and medial half of ring finger may be found.

b) The commonest location of injury is at the condylar (ulnar) groove at the elbow; the commonest modes of injury are pressure and arthritis; previous fracture or a shallow condylar groove predisposes to injury; "tardy ulnar palsy" refers to recurrent injuries to the ulnar nerve at the elbow, resulting in a slowly progressive loss of ulnar nerve function (frequently involving the dominant hand).

c) Treatment.

i) Padding the elbow and educating the patient to avoid ulnar nerve injury at the elbow may result in return of ulnar nerve function.

ii) Anterior surgical transplantation of the nerve may be necessary to avoid repeated injury.

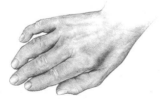

FIG 15–10. Lesions of the ulnar nerve produce atrophy of the interossei of the hand, which is evident as a "guttering" between the carpal bones.

Caveat: The radial, ulnar, and median nerves all supply the muscles of the thumb. Extension is served by the radial nerve, adduction by the ulnar nerve, and opposition by the median nerve (Fig 15–11).

4) Facial nerve (Bell's palsy).
   ▶ a) Characterized by acute or subacute onset of complete or partial unilateral paralysis of the facial muscles including the forehead (Fig 15–12). This paralysis may be associated with a previous nonspecific viral illness and is not associated with any other neurologic abnormalities.
   b) Patient may complain of hypersensitivity to noise on the same side, owing to paralysis of the stapedius muscle.
   c) If the injury to the facial nerve is proximal to the chorda tympani, loss of taste on the anterior two thirds of the tongue on the same side as the paralysis can be demonstrated by careful exami-

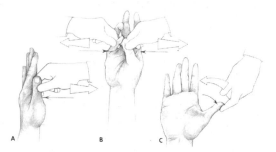

FIG 15–11. Functional integrity of the radial, median, and ulnar nerves can be tested by examining the strength of the thumb: **A,** adduction: ulnar-innervated muscles. **B,** opposition: median-innervated muscles. **C,** extension: radial-innervated muscles.

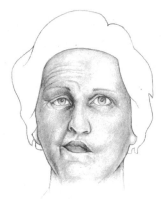

FIG 15–12. The patient with Bell's palsy (facial nerve palsy) will demonstrate an unwrinkled forehead, widely opened eye (with weakness of eyelid closure), flattening of the nasolabial fold, and a droop of the corner of the mouth.

nation; however, patients rarely complain of any change in taste.

d) Patient may complain of difficulty chewing because of accumulation of food in the paralyzed cheek (due to buccinator muscle paralysis); there is no true dysphagia.

e) Bell's palsy is an idiopathic disorder with a good prognosis for spontaneous recovery. However, it must be differentiated from other causes of facial paralysis, including the following:

  i) If there is decreased hearing or a decreased corneal reflex, suspect a cerebellopontine angle tumor such as an acoustic neuroma (schwannoma) or meningioma.

  ii) If there are vesicles in the external auditory canal, suspect the Ramsey-Hunt syndrome (infection of the geniculate ganglion with herpes zoster); there may be an underlying lymphoma.

iii) Chronic otitis media or mastoiditis may damage the facial nerve.

iv) Since the facial nerve passes through the parotid gland, infection or inflammation (including sarcoidosis) of the parotid can cause facial nerve paralysis.

f) Treatment.

i) Spontaneous recovery usually occurs.

ii) Corticosteroids have not been shown to be of definite benefit, although it is common practice to administer prednisone 80 mg/ day for 5 days if the patient is seen within 3 days of the onset or if pain in or behind the ear is prominent.

iii) The eye is vulnerable because lid closure is impaired, and the cornea must be protected with ophthalmic ointments, patches, or goggles.

5) Femoral nerve.

▶ a) The patient presents with difficulty in climbing stairs owing to weakness of one or both quadriceps muscles (sometimes incorrectly called "quadriceps myopathy"). The patient may compensate for this weakness by walking with the knee rigid. With a longstanding or severe lesion there is wasting of the quadriceps and, in children, development of genu recurvatum.

b) The patellar (knee) reflex is reduced or absent.

c) Sensory loss may be detected over the anteromedial thigh.

d) Femoral neuropathy is often associated with diabetes mellitus or trauma. Femoral neuropathy must be differentiated from disuse atrophy (in which the knee reflex is preserved) and polymyositis (in which the serum CPK is elevated or the muscle biopsy is abnormal).

6) Peroneal nerve.

▶ a) The patient presents with footdrop ("slapping foot"). A peroneal nerve lesion causes weakness of extension of the foot and toes and weakness of eversion (turning out) of the foot. In longstanding or severe lesions, there is wasting of the anterolateral compartment of the lower leg (Fig 15–13).

   b) Sensory loss may sometimes be demonstrated

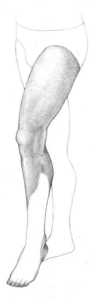

FIG 15–13. In longstanding or severe lesions of the peroneal nerve there is wasting of the anterolateral compartment of the lower leg.

over the lateral and anterior portions of the lower leg and dorsum of the foot.

c) Injury to the common peroneal nerve in the lateral knee (where the nerve courses around the head of the fibula) often results from:

   i) Sitting with legs crossed.

   ii) Pressure during sleep, coma, or anesthesia.

   iii) Pressure by casts, garters, boots, or braces.

   iv) Trauma or laceration to the area of the fibular head (as in climbing over a barbed wire fence).

> *Caveat:* A peroneal nerve injury resembles an L5 root lesion; however, the internal hamstring reflex is diminished in an L5 root lesion but not in a peroneal nerve lesion (see Chapter 17), and the posterior tibial muscle (which inverts a plantar-flexed foot) is weak in an L5 root lesion but not in a peroneal nerve lesion.

7) Lateral femoral cutaneous nerve (meralgia paresthetica).

▶ a) Patient presents with a sensory disturbance on the lateral aspect of the thigh (Fig 15–14). The abnormal sensation may be reduced sensibility, a pins-and-needles feeling, or burning discomfort, and may be exacerbated by touching the skin (as from clothing or stockings) or by prolonged standing or walking.

   b) Since the lateral femoral cutaneous nerve is a sensory nerve to the skin, weakness is never present.

   c) Symptoms are due to compression of the lateral femoral cutaneous nerve in its passage under the inguinal ligament.

   d) This condition is common in obesity, pregnancy, diabetes, trauma to the inguinal area, or after wearing tight-fitting corsets.

2. Brachial plexus lesions: Lesions of the brachial plexus are difficult to diagnose but should be suspected when there is

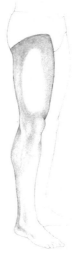

FIG 15–14. Meralgia paresthetica is an uncomfortable (burning) sensation in the distribution of the lateral femoral cutaneous nerve. Both the hypersensitivity to sensory stimulation and loss of normal sensibility can usually be demonstrated in this distribution.

more extensive involvement than would be produced by a lesion of a single nerve or root.

a. Upper trunk of the brachial plexus lesion (Erb-Duchenne palsy).
   ▶ 1) The patient presents with weakness about the shoulder and the elbow. The arm may dangle at the side with the fingers slightly flexed and the palm facing backward (the so-called porter's tip position; see Fig 15–15). This is due to inability to abduct and externally rotate the shoulder and to supinate and flex the forearm.
   2) Biceps and brachioradialis reflexes are absent.

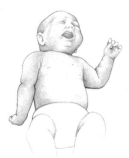

FIG 15–15. Erb-Duchenne palsy (lesion of the upper trunk of the brachial plexus) results in inability to abduct and externally rotate the arm with weakness of wrist extension leading to the characteristic "porter's tip" posture. Such an injury is not uncommon in infants owing to traction on the head and neck during delivery.

3) Sensory loss is minimal but, if present, may be found over the lateral shoulder, thumb, and index finger.
4) The patient usually complains of a diffuse discomfort or pain in the shoulder.
5) Lesions are produced by sudden traction that pulls the shoulder downward or pulls the neck away in the direction opposite to the shoulder; may occur during anesthesia, motorcycle accidents, in "rucksack paralysis," or as a birth injury.

Note: An upper trunk plexus injury resembles a C6 root lesion; external rotation and abduction of the shoulder are severely affected in the upper trunk plexus lesion but not in the C6 root lesion. Also, sensation is often intact in the upper trunk plexus lesion but a sensory disturbance is usually present in the C6 root lesion (see Chapter 18).

b. Lower trunk of the brachial plexus lesion (Klumpke-Déjérine palsy).

▶ 1) The patient presents with weakness of forearm flexors and all intrinsic muscles of the hand; in longstanding or severe lesions, there will be atrophy of the intrinsic muscles of the hand, recession of the thumb into the plane of the hand, and extension of the wrist.

2) Triceps reflex is absent.

3) Often there is no sensory disturbance but, if present, may be found along the posteromedial aspect of the forearm and the ulnar side of the hand.

4) Patient will frequently complain of a diffuse pain in the shoulder and axilla.

5) May be associated with Horner's syndrome (ptosis, miosis, and facial anhidrosis on same side as the injury) due to damage to preganglionic sympathetic nerve fibers in the T1 root.

6) Results from sudden upward pull on the shoulder, e.g., parent jerking upward on the arm of a falling child.

c. Brachial plexus neuritis (brachial plexitis).

▶ 1) Patient will present with the sudden onset (usually at night) of severe pain in the shoulder or arm, which is exacerbated by arm movement and elbow flexion. This is followed (within 2 weeks of the onset of the pain) by progressive weakness usually involving the shoulder girdle musculature innervated by the upper trunk of the brachial plexus, with lesser diffuse involvement of the musculature innervated by the rest of the plexus.

2) Reflexes will be variably reduced depending on the extent and degree of involvement.

3) Sensory loss is minimal or not detectable.

4) May involve both arms but is usually asymmetric with greater involvement in the dominant arm.

5) CSF is normal.

6) Treatment: Spontaneous recovery usually occurs but may take up to 2 years. Contractures may develop unless physical therapy range-of-motion exercises are undertaken until strength returns.

B. Other Lesions Causing Focal Weakness.

1. Cervical bony anomalies: The most common problem is the *thoracic outlet syndrome* (also see Chapter 18, section II. B. 9):

    ▶ a. Often patients complain of arm pain with no objective signs, but a severe thoracic outlet syndrome is characterized by weakness and atrophy of the thenar musculature with lesser weakness and atrophy of other intrinsic hand muscles and flexor muscles of the forearm.

    b. The finger and wrist extensors and the proximal arm musculature are preserved.

    c. Biceps and triceps reflexes are preserved.

    d. Intermittent aching pain in the arm is often present for many years, particularly in the ulnar side of the forearm and hand (frequently exacerbated at night), with numbness and tingling in the forearm.

    e. Can be differentiated from carpal tunnel syndrome by the presence of weakness in nearly all intrinsic hand muscles (only the thenar muscles are weak in the carpal tunnel syndrome) which may be associated with denervation demonstrable on EMG. Nerve conduction velocities may be slightly, but uniformly, slow without localized delay at the wrist (as in carpal tunnel syndrome) or at the elbow (as in tardy ulnar palsy)

    f. The diagnosis is based on correlating the clinical and electrophysiologic findings with radiographic evidence of a long down-curving transverse process of C7 or a rudimentary cervical rib.

    g. Treatment: If symptoms are not relieved by physical therapy, surgical release of the dense fibrous band connecting the first rib to the transverse process of C7 or to a rudimentary cervical rib may be necessary to free the C8 and T1 roots stretched and angulated over this band. Before surgery, angiography should be performed to confirm the exact location of the compression.

2. Focal myositis.

    a. Muscle inflammation may occur secondary to bacterial infection (*Staphylococcus* or *Streptococcus* abscess), parasitic infestation (toxoplasmosis, trichinosis, *Toxocara*), or granulomatous disease (tuberculosis, histoplasmosis, actinomycosis, sarcoidosis).

    b. The patient presents with swelling, weakness, pain, and tenderness in the affected muscles. This may be confused clinically with peripheral nerve, plexus, or root lesions, but may be differentiated by finding elevation of serum CPK.

    c. Definitive diagnosis may be made by muscle biopsy with histochemical staining, bacterial and fungal stains, and culture.

    d. Treatment: Treatment is of the basic disease process. Fasciotomy may be necessary to prevent ischemic necrosis if associated swelling is marked.

3. Dupuytren's contracture.

    a. There is progressive flexion contracture of the proximal joints of the ring finger, little finger, and middle finger, frequently bilateral. Thickened bands of palmar fascia may be seen and palpated (Fig 15–16).

    b. May be confused with a carpal tunnel syndrome because of associated mild dull ache or tingling sensation in the palm.

    c. Muscles and nerves are not involved, although secondary disuse atrophy of muscles may develop.

    d. Treatment: Orthopedic surgical fasciotomy or fasciectomy.

4. Volkmann's ischemic contracture.

    a. After acute trauma or embolism to the forearm (usually within 6–48 hours of the injury) swelling of injured tissue may occlude blood vessels, causing acute ischemia and infarction of muscles and nerves.

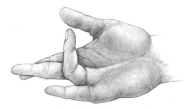

FIG 15–16. A bandlike thickening of the palmar fascia is evident in Dupuytren's contracture.

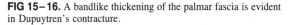

b. Subsequent contracture may be confused with brachial plexus injury because of pronation of the forearm, flexion of the wrist, flattening of the hand (paralysis and atrophy of intrinsic hand muscles with loss of the thenar and hypothenar eminences), hyperextension of the fingers at the proximal joints, flexion of the fingers at the middle joints (clawhand), and glove sensory loss (Fig 15–17).

c. Treatment.

1) Acutely, surgical intervention (fasciotomy) often is necessary to relieve the forearm congestion and prevent ischemia and infarction.

2) Once the contracture develops, orthopedic procedures may be performed to provide some hand function.

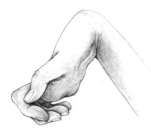

FIG 15–17. In Volkmann's ischemic contracture there is atrophy and fibrosis of the forearm and hand resulting in a fixed posture.

BIBLIOGRAPHY

Anderson NE, Cunningham JM, Poser JB: Autoimmune pathogenesis of paraneoplastic neurological syndromes. *CRC Crit Rev Neurobiol* 1987; 3:245–299.

Asbury AK, Johnson PC: *Pathology of Peripheral Nerve*. Philadelphia, WB Saunders, 1978.

Barohn RJ, Schenk Z, Warmolts JR, et al: The Bruns-Garland syndrome (diabetic amyotrophy) revisited 100 years later. *Arch Neurol* 1991; 48:1130–1135.

Brooke MH: *A Clinician's View of Neuromuscular Diseases,* ed 2. Baltimore, Williams & Wilkins, 1986.

Brumback RA, Gerst J (eds): *The Neuromuscular Junction.* Mount Kisco, NY, Futura, 1984.

Brumback RA, Leech RW: *Color Atlas of Muscle Histochemistry.* Littleton, Mass, PSG, 1984.

Brunch TW: Polymyositis: A case history approach to the differential diagnosis and treatment. *Mayo Clin Proc* 1990; 65:1480–1497.

Carpenter S, Karpati G: *Pathology of Skeletal Muscle.* New York, Churchill Livingstone, 1984.

Drachman DB: Present and future treatment of myasthenia gravis. *N Engl J Med* 1987; 316:743–747.

Dubowitz V: *Muscle Disorders in Childhood.* London, WB Saunders, 1978.

Dyck PJ, Thomas PK, Lambert EH, et al (eds): *Peripheral Neuropathy,* ed 3. Philadelphia, WB Saunders, 1992.

Engel AG, Banker BQ (eds): *Myology.* New York, McGraw-Hill, 1986.

Gamstorp I, Sarnat HB (eds): *Progressive Spinal Muscular Atrophies.* New York, Raven Press, 1984.

Horati Y: Diabetic peripheral neuropathies. *Ann Intern Med* 1987; 107:546–559.

Kelly JJ Jr: Peripheral neuropathies associated with monoclonal proteins: A clinical review. *Muscle Nerve* 1985; 8:138–150.

Lund H, Nilsson O, Rosen I: Treatment of Lambert-Eaton syndrome. *Neurology* 1984; 34:1324–1330.

Mitchell BM, et al: Effects of desipramine, amitriptyline, and fluoxetine on pain in diabetic neuropathy. *N Engl J Med* 1992; 326:1250–1255.

Mulder DW (ed): *The Diagnosis and Treatment of Amyotrophic Lateral Sclerosis.* Boston, Houghton Mifflin, 1980.

Nakano KK: *Neurology of Musculoskeletal and Rheumatic Disorders*. Boston, Houghton Mifflin, 1979.

Ropper AH: The Guillain-Barré syndrome. *N Engl J Med* 1992; 326:1130–1136.

Vinken PJ, Bruyn GW, Ringel SP (eds): *Handbook of Clinical Neurology*. Vol 40. Part I—*Diseases of Muscle*. Amsterdam, North Holland, 1979.

Vinken PJ, Bruyn GW, Ringel SP (eds): *Handbook of Clinical Neurology*. Vol 41. Part II—*Diseases of Muscle*. Amsterdam, North Holland, 1979.

Walton J: *Disorders of Voluntary Muscle,* ed 4. New York, Churchill Livingstone, 1981.

THE CHILD WHO IS NOT DEVELOPING OR LEARNING NORMALLY

16

Children are frequently brought to the physician for evaluation of neurologic problems. Apart from the focal neurologic symptoms described elsewhere in this book, children may be referred for evaluation of deviation from the expected normal pattern of development. In this chapter, the problems are categorized according to the age at which the child is most likely to present to the physician for evaluation and treatment. For many of the disorders, a multidisciplinary approach to evaluation and treatment is required. For the child under 3 years of age, the physician usually needs to coordinate the services of these various disciplines, but for the child over 3 years of age school systems (as required by Public Law 94-142, Education for All Handicapped Act of 1975) may coordinate services, with the physician acting as a member of the multidisciplinary team. Table 16–1 lists some of the kinds of problems.

Every child under age 3 years who visits a primary care physician should be screened for developmental delays, as part of the general physical examination or well-baby visit. This task can be simplified by providing a growth and developmental questionnaire for parents to fill out in the waiting room, by routinely plotting heights, weights, and head circumference measurements (see Appendix A), and by training an office assistant or nurse to administer the Denver Developmental Screening Test (see Appendix A). Observations of the child's behavior in the waiting room by a per

TABLE 16-1.
Developmental, Learning, and Behavior Problems of Children

Age	Assessable Responses	Types of Abnormalities
Infants and toddlers (birth–3yr)	Developmental screening Gross motor Speech Dysmorphic features Neurometabolic urine screening Denver Developmental Screening Test	"Cerebral palsies" Dysgenetic ("Funny Looking Kid") syndromes Inborn errors of metabolism Chromosomal disorder
Preschool years (3–6 yr)	Language Fine motor Adaptive and social development	Hearing loss Mental retardation syndromes Developmental language disorders
School age (6–12 yr)	Cognitive development Emotional/social development Moral development Behavioral development Minor neurologic signs ("soft signs") through special neurologic examination	Hyperactivity-attentional disorders Learning disability syndromes Childhood depression Behavior disorder Petit mal epilepsy
Adolescence (12–18 yr)	Emotional health Neuropsychological assessments	Attentional disorders Written language disabilities Adolescent adjustment reactions Psychiatric disorders Alcohol and drug abuse

ceptive receptionist or secretary are also helpful. Remember that during the first 2 years of life, the child's responses are limited and consist mainly of motor responses. After that period, language develops and makes assessment of intellectual functioning easier. Once the child enters school, abnormalities of attention and learning and various types of behavior disorders may also become evident.

One of the most important roles of the physician is to determine whether the child's deviation from normal is the result of slow development, developmental arrest, or developmental deterioration, since this will determine the types of disease processes considered and hence the evaluation undertaken (Fig 16–1). The rate of acquisition of new milestones provides dynamic clues to developmental disabilities. By schematically graphing time against courses of abnormal development for any given series of developmental milestones, it is possible to show three different schematic graphs. Children with slow development (Fig 16–1,A) require evaluation by psychosocial and educational services and referral to appropriate community resources. The presence of developmental arrest (Fig 16–1,B) or deterioration of functioning (Fig 16–1,C) will almost always require referral to a specialized diagnostic center.

I. INFANTS AND TODDLERS.

A. How to identify an infant who is not developing normally. Obtain the history to determine whether the child has any of the risk factors such as those listed below. The infant at risk for later developmental, learning, or behavioral problems is one:

1. Whose prenatal and perinatal history reveals certain risk factors. For example:
   a. Maternal diabetes.
   b. Maternal toxemia.
   c. Maternal viral infection (rubella, human immunodeficiency virus [HIV]).
   d. Maternal alcoholism or drug addiction (cocaine).
   e. Teenage mother.
   f. Mothers over 35 years, especially if first pregnancy.
   g. Fetal distress during delivery.
   h. Breech presentation.
   i. Prematurity.
   j. Infant small for gestational age (assessed by Dubowitz scale of newborn age and Lubchenko charts).
   k. Neonatal respiratory distress.
   l. Neonatal seizures.
   m. Neonatal infection (especially meningitis).
   n. Prolonged neonatal jaundice.

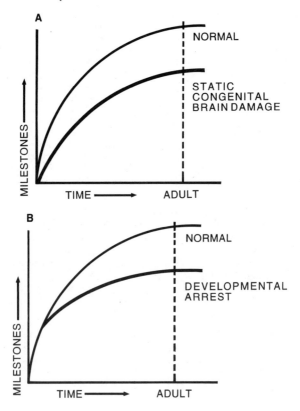

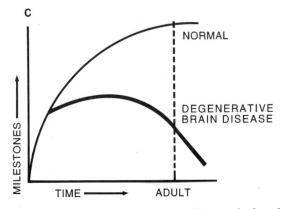

FIG 16–1. A, in slow development the child starts slowly and gradually falls further behind his or her normal peers, because the rate of development is also slow. This type of developmental curve is seen in the child with a static congenital encephalopathy or with Down syndrome. **B,** developmental arrest occurs in the child who has shown normal development from birth, but stops acquiring new skills. This type of developmental curve may be found in the child who has been successfully treated for bacterial meningitis or who has sustained significant head trauma. This type of curve may also be seen in the early phases of a degenerative process when the natural acquisition of developmental milestones may balance the deterioration. **C,** deterioration of functioning (the actual loss of previously acquired milestones) implies an ongoing destructive process in the brain. This type of curve may be found in hydrocephalus, untreated galactosemia or phenylketonuria, or rare CNS neurometabolic diseases.

2. Who acquires illnesses that may injure the brain, such as head trauma, meningitis or encephalitis, stroke, brain tumor, or malnutrition.
3. Whose rate of acquisition of developmental milestones deviates from normal expectancy.

   Note: Risk factors are not only biological, but more important are often psychosocial, such as poor maternal-child interaction, inappropriate parenting by primary caregivers, and child abuse or neglect. Other risk factors are poverty, with its attendant cultural deprivation and accompanying emotional and nutritional deprivation, although wealth, with its tendency for overindulgence, can also inhibit emotional and behavioral development. The physician cannot alter the nonbiological risk factors but can exert great indirect influence by compassionate parent education and sensitive referral to psychological and social services. Any infant in the high-risk category should receive special attention.

4. The majority of causes of mental retardation tend to fall into a few broad categories:
   a. Perinatal hypoxia and ischemia.
   b. Infection—prenatal, perinatal, or neonatal.
   c. Down syndrome.
   d. Fragile X syndrome.
   e. Other cerebral dysgenesis (including neuronal migration disorders).

B. History: Obtain a history of developmental milestones in infancy. In particular look for evidence of:
1. Absence of social smile after 8 weeks.
2. Poor head control while sitting on mother's lap after 4 months.
3. Inability to sit unsupported after 8 months.
4. Inability to play games such as peekaboo, bye-bye, and pat-a-cake after 12 months.
5. Inability to walk independently by 15 months.
6. Persistent hand preference before 12 months.
7. Delay in speech milestones (Tables 16–2 and 16–3).
8. Peculiar postures or modes of crawling (lying frog-legged, crawling on one side, kicking of legs symmetrically after 4 months).

TABLE 16–2.
Important Speech and Language Milestones (Ages 6–30 Months)

Receptive Language	Age (mo)	Expressive Language
Turns to sound of bell	6	Cries, laughs, babbles
Waves bye-bye	9	Imitates sounds and makes dental sounds during play ("da-da")
Knows meaning of "no" and "don't touch"		
	12	1–2 words ("dada," "mama," "bye")
Responds to "come here"	15	Jargon (speechlike babbling during play)
Points to nose, eyes, hair	18	8–10 words (1/3 are nouns); puts 2 words together ("more cookies"); repeats requests
Points to a few named objects and obeys simple commands	24	Asks 1- to 2-word questions ("Where kitty?")
Repeats 2 numbers and can identify by name "What barks" and "What blows?"	30	Uses "I," "you," "me"; names objects; uses 3-word simple sentences

TABLE 16–3.
Important Speech Milestones (Ages 3–6½ years)

Receptive Language	Age (yr)	Expressive Language
Responds to prepositions *on* and *under*	3	Masters consonants b, p, m
Responds to prepositions *in, out, behind, in front of*	4	Speaks in 4- to 5-word sentences, uses future and past tenses, and masters consonants d, t, g, k
Can repeat a sentence of 7 words	5	Masters consonants f, s, v, and names red, yellow, blue, green
	6½	Masters the consonantal digraph *th,* uses sentences of 6–7 words, and says numbers up to 30s

C. **Physical examination of the infant:** The essential parts of
the pediatric neurologic examination include the following:
   1. Head circumference: Measure frontal-to-occipital head
      circumference (Fig 16–2) and plot on an appropriate
      growth chart (see Appendix A). Values less than the fifth
      or greater than the ninety-fifth percentiles are abnormal.
      Serial measurements are more reliable than single mea-
      surements. Growth should be along a percentile line, and
      deviation is abnormal. Head circumference growth should
      be correlated with growth in height and weight.
   2. Transillumination of the head (Fig 16–3) is performed
      in the newborn period and before age 1 year. A flash-
      light with an appropriate rubber adaptor should be used
      to perform this in a light-tight, darkened room after ap-
      propriate dark adaptation. A small rim of light on the
      scalp should surround the rubber adaptor symmetrically

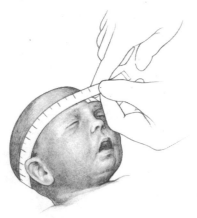

FIG 16–2. The occipital-frontal circumference (OFC) is measured
by using a steel or paper centimeter tape measure, which is placed
over the forehead and the occipital protuberance (see also Appendix A).

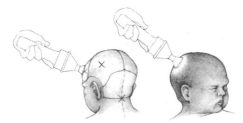

FIG 16–3. Transillumination of the head. The flashlight with rubber adaptor is placed over symmetric frontal and parietal skull areas. The rim of light around the edge of the rubber adaptor is usually no more than a few millimeters and should be symmetric (the illustrated rim is abnormal). The flashlight is placed in the midline below the occipital protuberance to inspect posterior fossa transillumination.

in similar positions on each side of the head and in the midline posteriorly at the base of the skull. Excessive transillumination suggests absence of brain tissue, necessitating further evaluation. This procedure has generally been neglected with the advent of neurosonography, computed tomography (CT) scans, and magnetic resonance imaging (MRI).

3. The skin is examined for café au lait spots, vitiliginous spots, hairy patches over the midline, ichthyosis, nevi, port-wine stains (or other neurocutaneous stigmata). A Wood's lamp (ultraviolet lamp) may be helpful in detecting vitiliginous patches.

4. Observe for abnormal facial features in the eyes, ears, nose, and chin. Does the child look significantly different from the parents?

5. Observe for leg postures, particularly:
   a. Frog legs (suggests hypotonia; see Fig 16–4).
   b. Kicking legs symmetrically beyond 4 months of age (suggests spastic diplegia).
   c. Kicking only on one side (suggests spastic hemiplegia involving the less mobile side).

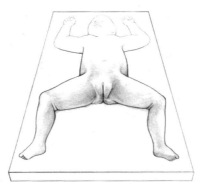

FIG 16–4. Frog-legged posture, suggesting hypotonia. Extremities are abducted proximally and flexed at elbows and knees.

6. An asymmetric tonic neck response present from 2 to 6 months of age is normal; it is abnormal if the child is unable to move out of the posture (too obligatory) or if the response persists beyond age 6 months (Fig 16–5).
7. The Moro (or startle) reflex (Fig 16–6) in the waking

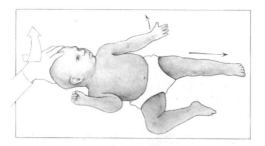

FIG 16–5. Tonic neck response: with the infant supine the arm (and leg) extend on the side toward which the head is turned, while the other arm (and leg) flex ("fencing posture").

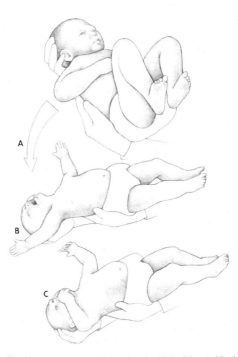

FIG 16-6. The Moro (startle) reflex is elicited by suddenly extending the baby's head (**A**). The normal response has two phases: first, sudden extension and abduction of the arms and extension of the legs (**B**); and second, slower adduction of the arms (**C**).

state is normally present from birth to age 3 months. Persistence beyond this time is abnormal. Asymmetry in this reflex at any time is abnormal and may suggest hemiparesis, brachial plexus injury, or spinal cord defect.

8. Observe for excessive opisthotonic posturing, either spontaneously or upon being handled. This is an early

sign of "cerebral palsy," which may be present before obvious diplegia or other major motor deficits.

9. In testing the child on the pull-to-sit (traction) test, the child's arm resistance, as well as head control, must be observed. By 5 months of age the head should come up with the body and not lag. The child should pull symmetrically against the examiner with both arms (Fig 16–7). Persistent head lag is associated with hypotonic disorders. Asymmetric arm pull suggests a hemiparesis.

10. Test for joint hyperextensibility—extending the knee beyond 180 degrees, extending the wrist back on the arm, and dorsiflexing the foot on the shin. Abnormalities are found in hypotonic children with a variety of neurologic defects.

11. Observe postural responses at 6 months in a sitting position (Fig 16–8):
    a. When pushed to the side, the child should extend the arms to catch self.

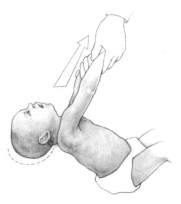

FIG 16–7. Pull-to-sit (traction) maneuver. This is tested from the newborn period to 6 months. The pull of the child's arms as well as the degree of head lag is observed.

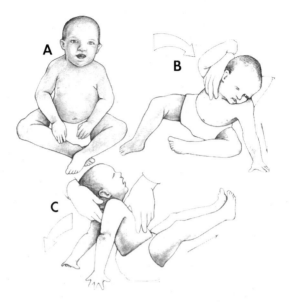

FIG 16–8. Responses to thrust in an infant in the sitting position (**A**). When pushed to the side, the baby extends the arm on that side outward, as if to catch the fall (**B**). At 6 months, when the infant is suddenly pushed backward, the legs should kick out symmetrically (**C**).

      b. When pushed backward, the child should extend the legs. Asymmetry suggests hemiparesis, and nonextension of the legs suggests a diparesis.
12. Test for the parachute response (Fig 16–9).
13. A Denver Developmental Screening Test should be done on initial contact and on the first few subsequent visits, if developmental delay is suspected. Serial developmental assessments are more predictive of later outcome than single assessments (see Appendix A).

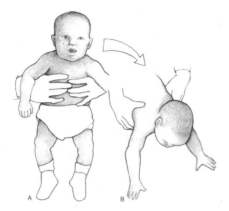

FIG 16–9. The parachute response appears at 8 months. It is elicited by suspending the baby in the upright position (**A**) and then rapidly propelling the head toward the examining table (but stopping short of hitting the table). The arms should thrust out symmetrically, as if to break the fall (**B**).

D. Laboratory studies.

1. If there is *developmental delay,* the following screening procedures may be done:

a. Urine neurometabolic screening.

b. Neurosonography: This simple portable procedure (necessitating no radiation exposure or sedation) should be performed in all neonates with abnormal head circumference, dysmorphic features, or in whom intraventricular hemorrhage or hydrocephalus is suspected.

c. Thyroid testing: Serum thyroid-stimulating hormone (TSH), triiodothyronine (T_3), thyroxine (T_4).

d. If congenital intrauterine infection is suspected, TORCHES (*t*oxoplasmosis, *r*ubella, *c*ytomegalovirus, *he*rpes simplex, *s*yphilis) titers, hepatitis B titers, and HIV titers for acquired immunodeficiency syndrome (AIDS) need to be done.

e. If dysmorphic features are prominent, chromosome karyotyping and banding studies are warranted. Chromosome breakage syndromes and the fragile X syndrome require special media and methods, and the cytogenetics laboratory must be so alerted.

f. Skull radiographs (specifically for abnormal calcification, suture synostosis or splitting, and beaten copper appearance).

g. If developmental anomalies of the brain are suspected, such as lissencephaly or polymicrogyria or other neuronal migration disorders, CT scan or MRI of the brain is warranted.

2. If there is *developmental regression,* referral to a center with a pediatric neurologist is indicated (see 3.d–f below).

3. Diseases in which there is *developmental arrest and then regression* tend to fall into only a few categories:

a. Previously diagnosed cerebral palsy, which turns out to be a misdiagnosis and is really a slowly progressive, rather than static, encephalopathy.

b. Complications of developmental brain anomalies, such as the development of hydrocephalus.

c. Resistant seizure syndromes—infantile spasms, Lennox-Gastaut syndrome, and infantile myoclonic epilepsy.

d. Infectious disease, such as AIDS, SSPE (subacute sclerosing panencephalitis), or rare slow virus infections, such as progressive rubella encephalopathy or progressive multifocal leukoencephalopathy.

e. Neurometabolic disease, such as certain aminoacidurias, organic acidurias, lysosomal storage diseases, peroxisomal diseases, or mitochondrial diseases involving primarily gray matter, or white matter, or both.

f. Rare syndromes of episodic neurologic disturbance, associated with lactic acidosis, hyperammonemia, hypoglycemia (organic acidurias, mitochondrial diseases), or degenerative disorders of unknown cause such as neuronal ceroid lipofuscinosis. Neuroimaging studies of the brain, particularly MRI and MR spectroscopy, can be very helpful diagnostically in suggesting a neurometabolic disease.

E. Identifiable causes of developmental delay.

1. Neonatal hypothyroidism.

   a. Profound mental retardation will develop if treatment is delayed beyond the neonatal period. If treatment is instituted under age 3 months, 80% of infants may be normal; if treatment is delayed beyond 3 months, less than 30% will be normal.

   b. Lethargic floppy infant with poor sucking.

   c. Prolonged neonatal jaundice.

   d. The presence of a triad of large tongue, abdominal distention, and constipation is rare and is usually found only in severe cretinism.

   e. Diagnosis by heel-stick blood sample analysis for T_4; this is done as a routine neonatal screening in most states.

   f. Treatment: Immediate oral T_4 supplementation, desiccated thyroid 15 mg/day. Patient should be followed closely with thyroid studies.

2. Phenylketonuria (PKU).

   a. Usually a normal-appearing neonate who fails to gain weight and has feeding difficulties in the first weeks of life.

   b. Seizures, poor growth, and profound mental retardation develop if untreated.

   c. Autosomal recessive pattern of inheritance.

   d. Diagnosis by heel-stick blood sample (drawn after milk feeding) analyzed for phenylalanine level (this screening procedure is done by law in all states) or by positive urine ferric chloride test.

   e. Treatment: A diet low in phenylalanine (formula such as Lofenalac) is necessary. Genetic counseling should be provided to the family.

3. Galactosemia.

   a. Normal-appearing infant who develops vomiting, diarrhea, or seizures of variable severity after several days or weeks of milk feeding, including breast-feeding.

   b. Prolonged neonatal jaundice is often present.

    c. Blood glucose levels are in the hypoglycemic range only if assayed immediately after a milk feeding.

    d. Autosomal recessive mode of inheritance.

    e. Cataracts, hepatosplenomegaly, seizures, and profound mental retardation will develop if untreated.

    f. Diagnosis after a feeding by finding low blood glucose, positive urine sugar (Clinitest tablets), but negative urine glucose (glucose oxidase urine dipsticks); quantitative galactose levels also can be obtained.

    g. Treatment: A galactose-free diet is necessary. Genetic counseling should be provided to the family.

4. Down syndrome.

    a. The clinical diagnosis of Down syndrome is made by the following criteria:

       1) Oblique palpebral fissures.

       2) Epicanthal folds.

       3) Brushfield's spots (light speckling) of the iris.

       4) Flat nasal bridge.

       5) Clinodactyly of the fifth fingers and bilateral transverse palmar creases.

       6) Wide spacing of the first and second toes.

       7) Hypotonia.

    b. Down syndrome is more frequent in pregnancies of women aged over 40 years.

    c. There is a high incidence of associated problems such as congenital heart disease, tracheoesophageal fistula, duodenal atresia, megacolon, and lymphoreticular malignancies.

    d. The diagnosis is confirmed by chromosomal studies—95% of cases have trisomy 21, the remainder have translocations or mosaicism.

    e. Hip radiographs that show a characteristic change in the acetabulum may be helpful.

    f. Progressive upper cervical spine abnormalities may result in spinal cord symptoms in late childhood or early adolescence.

    g. Progressive personality changes and intellectual deterioration begin in the late twenties or early thirties, and by age 40 years all patients have histopathologic Alzheimer's disease.

  h. Treatment.
   1) Although no specific medical treatment is available, there is evidence now that early intensive developmental stimulation programs and early special education programs, as well as psychosocial support, result in achievement of higher functioning than what might have been predicted in the past. The degree of psychomotor retardation varies from mild to moderate and allows placement into trainable or educable special education classes. Employment as adults in sheltered situations is possible, and independence in self-care the rule.
   2) The recurrence risk after trisomy 21 is 1% to 2%. Referral to a pediatric geneticist is advisable.
   3) Support groups for families are available.
   4) Patient and physician information materials can be obtained from the National Down Syndrome Society, 666 Broadway, New York, NY 10012, telephone 800-221-4602; or the National Down Syndrome Congress, 1800 Dempster St., Park Ridge, IL 60068-1146, telephone 800-232-NDSC.
5. Fragile X syndrome.
  a. Associated with moderate to severe mental retardation.
  b. Dysmorphic features include large ears, prominent jaw and forehead, broad nose, high-pitched voice, macro-orchidism.
  c. Often associated with seizures.
  d. An X-linked disorder affecting only males, but females are carriers.
  e. Chromosome studies show excessive breaks when cultured in special media.

   Note: Because special culture media are required to demonstrate the chromosomal abnormality, it is imperative to alert the laboratory if this diagnosis is considered.

    f. Treatment.
        1) No specific treatment is available; seizures should be treated symptomatically (see Chapter 11, section IV.); genetic counseling of the family is necessary.
        2) Patient and physician information materials can be obtained from the Fragile X Foundation, 1441 York St., Denver, CO 80206, telephone: (303) 861-6630.
6. Congenital intrauterine infection.
    a. Depending on the type and duration of the prenatal infection, the presentation of the child may vary from a small-for-dates, premature, severely microcephalic infant with hepatosplenomegaly, purpura, and severe jaundice to a normal-appearing child, who does well in infancy but who develops poorly in late childhood.
    b. Most common agents are in the TORCHES groups, but other agents include the hepatitis B virus, enterovirus, and, increasingly, HIV.
    c. Diagnosis is by determination during the neonatal period of elevated (preferably from cord blood) serum IgM (and disease-specific IgM). The agents can sometimes be cultured from the stool, urine, or throat. Serologic tests are available through state health laboratories.
    d. Skull radiographs or CT scans of the brain reveal punctate periventricular calcifications in cytomegalovirus infection, and larger, scattered calcifications of toxoplasmosis.
    e. The degree of neurologic impairment varies with the severity of infection:
        1) Seizures and severe retardation are more common with herpes simplex, toxoplasmosis, and cytomegalovirus.
        2) Visual disturbances are more common with toxoplasmosis and rubella (cataracts), and hearing loss alone with cytomegalovirus.
        3) Hearing impairment together with autism is more common with rubella. A progressive rubella en-

cephalitis continuing after the neonatal period and
through the first year is now recognized.

4) Cytomegalovirus is the most common infectious
cause of mental retardation and also the most un-
derdiagnosed.

5) Developmental delay, "failure to thrive," and recurrent infections can be associated with HIV-
related central nervous system (CNS) involvement, as either progressive or static encephalopathy. Neonatal HIV infection is transmitted by less
than 40% of infected mothers either in utero or at
delivery. Confirmation of the infection is difficult
because of the presence of maternal antibodies in
the infant up to 6 months. Prevention of maternal-
infant transmission is imperative. An infectious
disease specialist needs to be consulted if there is
suspicion of HIV infection, AIDS-related complex
(ARC), or AIDS.

f. Treatment:

1) In congenital syphilis procaine penicillin G 50,000
units/kg intramuscularly (IM) in single daily dose
for 14 days must be administered.

2) Toxoplasmosis is treated in the child less than 1
year of age with pyrimethamine 1 mg/kg/day PO
(with leucovorin calcium 5 mg twice weekly) and
sulfadiazine 50 mg/kg/day PO in divided doses for
21 days. If there is evidence of active disease, additional corticosteroid (prednisone 1–2 mg/kg/
day) may be necessary. Complicated cases requiring additional or other courses of treatment should
be referred to an infectious disease center. Chori-
oretinitis should be managed by an ophthalmologist.

3) Since the child with any congenital infection is potentially contagious, contact with other infants and
with pregnant women should be avoided (excre-
tion of high titers of virus may continue for several months in congenital cytomegalovirus and rubella infections).

4) General supportive care only is available for rubella and cytomegalovirus, while acyclovir is available for herpes simplex encephalitis (usually secondary to type 1, or genital herpes).

5) Currently zidovudine (azidothymidine [AZT] or Retrovir) is available for AIDS, and other drugs are being investigated, but the mother should be counseled about the risk of having further infected children.

7. Static congenital encephalopathy with predominant motor involvement (cerebral palsies).

a. The *static encephalopathies* are defined as a group of disorders in which there is a major motor deficit secondary to a brain lesion acquired at or around the time of birth. Hypoxia and ischemia, infection, hemorrhage, and brain anomalies account for the majority of static encephalopathies.

b. Infant has delay in achieving motor milestones, while social and behavior development may be normal. The infant often has normal or above-normal intelligence, but 40% have varying degrees of mental retardation.

c. The development of neonatal intensive care units has been a major reason for survival of very low-birth-weight (<1,500 g) and extremely low-birth-weight (<1,000 g) babies, but with probably increasing risk of long-term neurologic and developmental disability, including cerebral palsies.

d. Some specific patterns of motor involvement can be recognized. Children may display combinations of these patterns (mixed forms) and may show variation over time (note that the mixed forms have a worse prognosis):

1) Hemiplegia or hemiparesis (involvement of arm and leg on same side; undergrowth and abnormal posturing of that side).

2) Diplegia or diparesis (both legs involved, with minimal to absent involvement of the upper extremities) is the most common form. Usually there is delayed standing, early walking on tiptoes, and

walking with scissoring or knees crossing, and in the first years of life hypotonia and decreased reflexes, but later with increased tone and hyperreflexia.

Note: The term *paraplegia* refers to acquired leg paralysis secondary to spinal cord injury, usually at the thoracolumbar level.

3) Tetraplegia or tetraparesis (involvement of both legs and arms; very poor head control and trunk control on sitting) is better described as a bilateral hemiplegia, since the lesions responsible are usually bilateral hemispheric.

Note: The term *quadriplegia* usually refers to paralysis of arms and legs secondary to cervical spinal cord injury.

4) Ataxic or atonic (presentation of hypotonia in infancy, then marked unsteadiness and incoordination when the upright posture is attempted).

5) Choreoathetosis (abnormal choreoathetoid posturing of arms and legs) is the least common pattern of motor involvement. Presentation in infancy is usually with hypotonia, which then evolves into rigidity and choreoathetoid movements.

e. Speech may be abnormal in tone, rate, rhythm, and pronunciation owing to impairment of the motor aspects of articulation, while basic language expression and reception are normal. The most severe motor speech disorders, sometimes to the point of anarthria, are seen in the choreoathetoid syndromes. Occasionally the speech disorder is disproportionately severe relative to the involvement of the extremities, and compared to preservation of intellect.

f. Epilepsy occurs in one third or fewer of cases, primarily in those with spastic cerebral palsies (hemiplegic, diplegic, tetraplegic). When some combination of major motor defect, mental retardation, and epilepsy occurs, with or without deafness or blindness, the term *multiply handicapped* is often applied. Such distinctions are important because they determine the kind of intervention programs that are appropriate.

g. Of importance in the neurologic examination is the observation of postures—early excessive opisthotonos, obligatory spontaneous asymmetric tonic neck postures, and the persistence of developmental reflexes that should have been inhibited. The persistence of the asymmetric tonic neck reflex after age 6 months and the absence of a parachute response after 1 year augurs for a poor prognosis for walking.

h. Many diagnoses of "cerebral palsy" attributed to birth asphyxia are now known to be due to prenatal causes:

1) Preexisting brain malformations, which may predispose the newborn to neonatal problems, including asphyxia.

2) Placental abnormalities with consequent fetal ischemia or embolization resulting in brain injury.

Note: Pathologic study of the placenta should be performed in any infant with neonatal difficulties in order to identify causative placental abnormalities.

Caveat: "Minimal cerebral palsy" occurs in a number of children, and presents as a clumsy child, or one with "visual-perceptual" difficulties, or sometimes as an attentional-hyperactivity disorder. The diagnosis is made upon finding minimal, but definite neurologic signs, such as shortened Achilles tendons, with hyperactive lower extremity reflexes and Babinski reflexes, or mild but definite signs of congenital hemiparesis. Usually the children have no real functional handicap from the motor deficits.

i. Treatment.

1) Physical therapy, occupational therapy, and developmental stimulation programs must be estab-

lished *early,* preferably in the first year of life, to permit maximum socialization and education of the child and to minimize the development of fixed skeletal deformities.

2) The infant that does best is the child with "pure" spastic diplegia or hemiplegia.

3) Many forms of neurodevelopmental therapies are available, which are usually administered along with routine physical-occupational therapy.

4) Follow-up care needs to be monitored and coordinated, particularly since multiple disciplines, especially orthopedics and physical-occupational therapy, are involved. Regional crippled children's service clinics are available. If the family can identify with one central primary physician, or agency, as the care coordinator, compliance of therapeutic regimens by the family is better assured.

5) Information for physicians and patients may be obtained from United Cerebral Palsy Associations, 330 West 34th St., New York, NY 10001, telephone (212) 947-5770.

Caveat: In patients with cerebral palsies in whom there is a change in motor or mental functioning for the worse, or where there is a "family history" of cerebral palsy or early death from neurologic conditions, suspect hereditary neurometabolic disease or familial brain dysgeneses, and refer to a pediatric neurologist.

II. THE PRESCHOOL YEARS (AGES 3–6).

A. Identifying the child who is not developing normally.
During the preschool period, the child develops language and behavior patterns that indicate temperament or personality. Delay in speech and language is the most important disorder to assess during this period. Speech or language delay is the single most consistent predictor of later learning disabilities, particularly in reading and writing. Motor disabilities are less commonly noted for the first time during this period. Parents may bring a child to the physician with a primary complaint

of delayed speech or language. However, the astute physician must be able to recognize delayed or aberrant speech and language:

1. During routine physical examinations.
2. During follow-up of children who have been identified earlier as high risk.
3. During examination for another complaint, such as a cold.

B. **Risk factors.** In the preschool years physicians should become aware of risk factors that warn of academic or behavior difficulties when first grade begins:

1. The presence of attention-deficit hyperactivity disorder (ADHD): This can be suspected by reports from nursery school or kindergarten teachers that a child is more "immature" than expected for his or her age. Teachers will report discipline problems and problems in playing with peers.
2. Delayed speech and language: If a language disorder (developmental dysphasia or acquired aphasia) is present, there is a high risk for specific learning disability involving delayed acquisition of reading and writing skills (dyslexia and dysgraphia). Speech disturbances alone (developmental articulation disorders, stuttering) do not presage learning disabilities.
3. The Landau-Kleffner syndrome is an acquired language disorder associated with seizures and electroencephalographic (EEG) epileptiform abnormalities that has a subacute onset, but a chronic course.
4. Lack of achievement of academic readiness skills at the end of kindergarten (counting, reading and writing the alphabet, naming colors, etc.), which are predictive of readiness for the first grade.
5. Poor drawing abilities for age, clumsiness, or incoordination does not necessarily presage academic learning disabilities, although it may lead to difficulties in handwriting and in art classes.

C. **Therapeutic services.** The physician has many therapeutic services open to patients at this age. Private or public community agencies, Headstart programs, preschool handicapped programs, and formal speech therapy are available in most communities even before the formal kindergarten period.

Various nursery schools that provide more than baby-sitting by incorporating child development approaches are becoming more widely available. The special services of special education departments of the public school systems are mandated to provide educational services for preschool children, beginning at age 3 years, under the Education for All Handicapped Act (PL 94-142), depending on state law.

D. Identifiable disorders.
  1. Hearing loss.
     a. Deviation from the normal rate of development of sound reception and expression (Tables 16–2 and 16–3) suggests possible hearing impairment.
     b. There may be a delay in the development of speech or abnormal tone or quality of speech sounds. For example, with mild hearing loss, words with high-frequency sounds will be misunderstood by the child, and the high-frequency sounds in words will be omitted from the child's speech ("stop" will be heard and spoken as "top").
     c. The most common and frequently neglected cause of hearing loss is middle ear disease.
     d. The child may display autistic features.
     e. The child will be fascinated by loud sounds (especially vibrating bass sounds), and the parents may complain of the child's turning the radio or television on very loudly.
     f. The child may develop lip reading, gestures, and pantomime to communicate.
     g. Diagnosis necessitates detailed audiometry by an audiologist experienced with young children. Recording of brainstem auditory evoked potentials may be necessary in younger children.

     Caveat: An apparent normal response to a bell in office testing is an inadequate assessment of the child with possible hearing loss. Screening audiograms in the school usually will not detect the child with anything less than profound hearing loss.

     h. Treatment. Thorough otologic and audiologic assessment is usually necessary. Amplification devices or cochlear transplants may be helpful in some children. Modification of the classroom environment or special schooling for the deaf may be necessary.

2. Mental subnormality (mental retardation).

   a. In the child with normal hearing (after thorough audiologic testing) who has delay in speech or language, the most common cause is a global deficit in intellectual-cognitive skills, i.e., mental retardation.

   b. The most important gross language milestone is a *two- to three-word sentence (must be a subject-verb sentence) by 24 to 30 months.*

   c. Testing by a psychologist experienced in assessing children must be done in order to discriminate appropriately the presence of the intellectual-cognitive deficit. Such tests as the Bayley Scales of Infant Development, the Stanford-Binet Form L-M, the Wechsler Preschool and Primary Scale of Intelligence (WPPSI), and the Kaufmann Assessment Battery for Children (K-ABC) are useful. Extreme caution must be exercised in predicting future performance potential based on test numbers alone.

   d. Mental retardation is documented not only by intellectual-cognitive testing but by social-behavioral testing as well. Significant deficits in both areas must be present for the diagnosis to be accurately applied.

   e. Mental retardation is actually only a description of a symptom complex (intellectual-cognitive and social-behavioral deficit that occurs before the age of 18 years) and may be the end result of multiple possible causes.

   f. There are a number of conditions that may mimic mental retardation (pseudo–mental retardation):

      1) The most common are developmental language disorders (developmental dysphasias). These will give test results showing a low Wechsler Full Scale IQ (intelligence quotient) score, with the Verbal Scale IQ score usually 15 to 20 points below the Performance Scale IQ score.

      2) Multiple specific disabilities but normal intellectual potential, as indicated by normal adaptive be-

havior, age-appropriate play, and social functioning, and average or better IQ subtest scores on
subtests indicative of cognitive ability (Wechsler
Similarities and Information subtests).

3) Borderline intellectual potential, but complicated
by specific developmental disabilities, attention
disorder, emotional disorders, or sensory impair-
ments.

4) Other conditions include deafness or severe hearing impairment (presenting as speech and language delay), behavior disorders (including childhood depression), ADHD, bilingualism (and
ethnic-cultural differences), and pharmacologi-
cally induced cognitive dysfunction.

g. Etiologic screening: Look for treatable causes (see
section I.D). More and more genetic diseases are able
to be treated by dietary restriction, cofactor supplementation, detoxification, bone marrow transplantation (storage diseases), enzyme transfusions, and possibly (in the near future) gene transplantation. Known
genetic causes require genetic counseling of parents
and siblings of childbearing age; referral to a pediatric geneticist is helpful. If any screening tests are
positive, refer to an appropriate specialist in neurology, genetics, or metabolism for further in-depth diagnostic assessment.

3. Infantile autism.
  a. Onset before age 18 months.
  b. Abnormal interpersonal relationship ("doesn't relate
  to people as people but to people as objects"): the
  child avoids eye contact and tactile contact; the child
  may, for example, use the mother's hand "as a tool"
  to grasp a doorknob; does not cuddle as an infant.
  c. Bizarre mannerisms (motor stereotypies): repetitive
  movements resembling tics, such as flapping arms at
  sides, rocking, or other self-stimulating maneuvers;
  whirling and spinning.
  d. Abnormal play: Child uses toys inappropriately in a
  stereotyped manner e.g., trucks are lined up (never
  rolled) while buildings are rolled.

   e. Aberrant language.
     1) Variable acquisition rates; e.g., markedly delayed verbal comprehension and production, but in later childhood, "cocktail party chatter."
     2) Reading acquired before spoken language.
     3) Pronoun inversion ("I" for "you").
     4) Echolalia and perseveration.
   f. On formal intellectual testing, child's scores are in the "retarded" range, but the child appears to be functioning at a much higher level.
   g. Splinter skills may be present. These are precociously developed but isolated abilities such as calendar skills (e.g., being able to tell what day of the week it was on September 25, 1896).
   h. Compulsive need for sameness in environment and in routine.
   i. This is a rare disorder. However, in autistic children who are aggressive, hyperactive, and nonverbal, it is often misdiagnosed as severe or profound mental retardation.
   j. Similar disorders, with milder features (e.g., less severe language disability), begin in children after age 18 months. These autistic-like disorders have been termed pervasive developmental disorders or autistic spectrum disorders.
   k. Treatment.
     1) Neuropsychopharmacologic management is at present entirely symptomatic and empirical:
       a) Haloperidol may be used if there is much hyperactive aggression, self-mutilation, or marked motor stereotypes (the bizarre mannerisms). Starting dose: 1 mg bid to tid.
       b) Amitriptyline hydrochloride may be used, starting with 10 mg at bedtime, if there is much hyperactivity, trouble sleeping at night, or reversal of the diurnal cycle.
       c) Carbamazepine, beginning at 200 mg bid to tid, may be used if there is much aggressive behavior, and the child also has seizures.
       d) Lithium carbonate, beginning with 300 mg qd

to tid, may be used for sustained hyperactive behavior akin to mania.

   e) The CNS stimulants methylphenidate (Ritalin), dextroamphetamine, and pemoline hydrochloride may also be used for prominent attentional disturbances or hyperactivity.

2) Psychoeducational management: Refer patients less than age 3 years of age to community infant stimulation programs; after age 3 years they should be referred to the public school department of special education for preschool handicapped programs and development of an Individual Education Plan (IEP) under the Education for All Handicapped Act. Physician and parent information may be obtained from the Autism Services Center, P.O. Box 507, Huntington, WV 25710, telephone (304) 525-8014.

4. Developmental hyperactivity (attention-deficit hyperactivity disorder, ADHD).

   a. Parents describe the child as "always on the go" from birth (may even have been more active in utero).

   b. The child may never crawl but walks early enough and runs rather than walks.

   c. The child characteristically is impulsive, distractible, immature, and clumsy, with a short attention span, and difficulty in following directions, often racing from task to task without completing any one task.

   d. Frequently parents and other caretakers have difficulty tolerating the child. Many behavior problems may develop. Peers have difficulty tolerating the child.

   e. There is a "paradoxical reaction" to certain drugs—the barbiturates (sedative in normal persons) markedly increase the hyperactivity, whereas stimulants such as amphetamines, methylphenidate, and pemoline reduce the hyperactivity and increase the attention to tasks.

   f. Boys are more frequently affected than girls.

   g. Subtle neurologic signs on special extended neurologic examinations may be demonstrated.

   h. The initial presentation of Gilles de la Tourette's syndrome to the primary care physician can be with hyperactivity and attentional problems.

   i. Treatment.

      1) The physician's immediate task is parental education about both the nature of the condition and the appropriate management of the attention, behavior, and academic problems. Parents should be referred to the appropriate literature on dealing with the hyperactive child.

      2) Pharmacologic management is effective, if given in conjunction with a comprehensive program of behavior modification and environmental adjustment in the school and home, along with appropriate pedagogical intervention, cognitive-attentional training, and training in organizational skills. Modification of the school and home environment is necessary—more structure, less distraction, short circumscribed tasks, a checklist for developing self-monitoring abilities, and home chores to develop time-management ability and responsibility.

      3) Pharmacologic management utilizes primarily the CNS stimulant drugs methylphenidate, dextroamphetamine, or pemoline. Dosage is clinically titrated to achieve a therapeutic effect. Hyperactivity may abate with a lower dose than is necessary to improve attentional or behavior disturbance. Failure with one drug does not necessarily mean that the other drugs will also fail.

      4) Before initiating treatment with the selected medication, the physician must establish a baseline assessment of motor, attentional, and behavioral parameters; a variety of standardized questionnaires and continuous performance tests, now often computer-administered and scored, are available. The use of central auditory processing tests by an audiologist experienced with children is also a good method to establish a baseline for attentional tasks, and for follow-up monitoring. These mea-

sures will ensure that data from a number of sources, other than the physician's own observation of the child in the examining room (which is often misleading), are available for an accurate view of the child's functioning.

a) Methylphenidate (Ritalin) is the recommended first drug of choice. If treatment is unsuccessful, discontinue and treat with dextroamphetamine. Medication should be given in a twice-daily regimen, just before breakfast and lunch, to avoid anorexia and maximize absorption. Medication after 4 P.M. should be avoided to prevent insomnia. Suggested beginning doses are:

   i) Methylphenidate 5 mg bid.

   ii) Dextroamphetamine 5 mg bid.

   iii) Pemoline may be used as a single morning dose after breakfast starting with a dose of 18.75 mg every morning for young children or 37.5 mg for older children.

b) Medication should be given daily, although some children who display symptoms only during school need not be given the drug on weekends, school holidays, or during summer vacation.

c) The child should be carefully followed on a weekly basis with upward adjustment of dosage if necessary to achieve the desired therapeutic effect. After a maintenance regimen has been established, height and weight should be monitored and charted at least monthly to detect growth failure. A drug-free holiday is necessary if growth failure is documented. The child on a maintenance regimen must be followed regularly to monitor for undesirable side effects.

III. THE SCHOOL-AGE YEARS (AGES 6–19).

A. **Entry into school** can be a traumatic period in which intellectual, motor, and emotional disorders may become more prominent. Disorders as previously described, such as hyperactivity-attentional syndromes, may become more obvious during this period. However, difficulty in school performance may be the first indication of a developmental or learning disability. Some specific behavior and educational disorders may first become evident at this time. This is a particularly trying time not only for the child but for the family as well. It is imperative that all professionals provide the family with accurate, comprehensive, and noncontradictory information. Because of the presence of a disabled child, family interactions may be tumultuous, affecting the psychosocial adjustment of siblings and parents, as well as family unity. A well-coordinated support system for the family may be as beneficial as any intervention prescribed for the child individually.

B. Childhood depression.

1. Endogenous major depression in a child may first present during school age (also see Chapter 9, section I.B.2).

2. The family history is often strongly positive for depression, mania, nervous breakdown, mental illness, suicide, or alcoholism.

3. There is a history of recurrent episodes of change in behavior, including:

   a. Changed activity level, either hyperactivity (especially fluctuating) or reduced activity.

   b. School problems secondary to distractibility or decreased attention span or a new learning disability.

   c. Excessive moodiness or irritability.

   d. Appetite disturbance, sleep disturbance.

   e. Medically unexplained headaches, recurrent abdominal pain, or recurrent vomiting.

   f. Secondary enuresis (see Chapter 5, section VI.A) without demonstrable urologic or neurologic abnormality.

   g. Phobias or excessive fears.

   h. Preoccupation with death, suicide attempts, setting fires, running away.

4. Sadness and low self-esteem are encountered in long-standing learning disabilities, underachievement, or school failure, but in these situations are not associated

with the variety of other symptoms characteristic of depression.

5. Treatment. Antidepressant pharmacotherapy is usually necessary along with supportive psychotherapy and family therapy and is generally best accomplished by referral to appropriate specialists.

C. **Educational dysfunction.** There are many non-CNS factors that can account for below-expected academic performance. Some of these are:

1. Sensory deprivation (blindness or deafness).
2. Schools with deficient teaching programs.
3. Belonging to a minority group with different values from those of the predominant culture.
4. Bilingualism.
5. Primary emotional or psychiatric disturbance.

D. **If non-CNS factors cannot be identified** as the cause of poor achievement, then one or more of several kinds of educational dysfunction may account for poor academic performance.

1. *Mild to moderate mental retardation.* The child has global intellectual, cognitive, adaptive, and social-behavioral deficits. Formal psychological testing as well as serial developmental and neurologic assessments over time are required to make this diagnosis.

   Caveat: Skepticism must be used in evaluating intelligence test scores that report "characteristic of mental retardation." Psychological tests produce numerous false-negative and false-positive results. Careful, detailed neuropsychological testing is necessary for precise characterization of mental retardation.

   a. Treatment. Usually public schools have resources rooms or special classes for the educable or trainable retarded. An IEP is required for each child according to the Education for All Handicapped Act.

2. Borderline intelligence: The child with borderline intelligence shows on formal psychological testing cognitive potential below normal but above that of mental retardation. Although not mentally retarded the child will perform more slowly than normal because his or her potential is lower than normal.

    a. Treatment. The child will require an IEP, usually incorporating more tutoring at a slower pace than that of the comparable regular classroom. This is the group correctly referred to as "slow learners." More information for parents may be obtained from the Center for Slower Learners, 1700 Preston Rd., #400, Dallas, TX 75248, telephone (214) 407-9277.

3. Attention-deficit disorder with or without hyperactivity: These are children with developmental hyperactivity in which the short attention span and distractibility, and not necessarily the motor hyperactivity, are the presenting features and the reason for academic underachievement. Girls, more than boys, are apt to have attention disorders without hyperactivity. This group of disorders is one of the most common problems for which schools refer children to physicians. The referral information usually has terms such as "immaturity," "underachievement," "learning disability," or "behavior problem." Motor hyperactivity tends to abate with age, but the attention disorder may persist through high school and even into adulthood. The older the child, the more the physician must look for complicating secondary emotional problems, such as conduct disorder.

    a. Treatment. All management previously discussed in section II.D.4 applies. In addition, continual and clear communication with school teachers and administrators is necessary for effective monitoring of the child's responses to pharmacologic intervention.

4. Specific learning disabilities. Children with specific learning disabilities have normal intellectual potential but greater than expected difficulty in acquiring one or more of the basic academic skills of reading, writing, arithmetic, or spelling. The incidence is about 3% of the school population. Specific reading disabilities (sometimes termed *developmental dyslexia*), with later spelling and written language disabilities, are the most common specific learning disabilities.

    a. The classic neurologic examination is almost always normal, but subtle neurologic signs can sometimes be demonstrated. A neurodevelopmental evaluation may reveal aberrant or delayed functioning.

b. Speech articulation can be tested by repetition of test phrases—*la-la, mi-mi, go-go.*

c. Spoken language can be rapidly screened by repetition of sentences of varying length and syntax.

d. Arithmetic ability can be screened in the early school-age child by addition and subtraction of single digits, and in the older school-age child by multiplication of two-digit numbers by two-digit numbers (written).

e. Note whether errors in reading, writing, or arithmetic may be due to attention problems (e.g., skipping lines, wrong lining up of columns) or are impulsive errors (e.g., writing down the first things to come to mind, frequent erasing). These are clues to the presence of an attention disorder that may be presenting as a learning disability.

f. Ascertain if there is a family history of reading or other learning disabilities or of attention-activity disorders.

g. Screen for visual-motor problems by Draw-a-Person test, drawing a clock, or copying geometric figures.

h. The specific learning disability syndromes such as the developmental Gerstmann's syndrome, developmental dyslexia, developmental dyscalculia, developmental clumsiness or apraxia, developmental dysgraphia, and developmental dysphasia are described in numerous texts.

i. Although psychometric testing may be helpful in elucidating these disorders, many psychological tests produce false-positive and false-negative results. Therefore detailed neuropsychologic testing is often necessary to characterize more precisely a clinically diagnosed learning disability.

j. Learning disability syndromes may occur alone or in combination, and also may coexist independently with ADHD.

k. Many neurobiological correlates of learning disabilities are now known and may suggest techniques in the future for supplementary diagnosis.

1. Physician and parent information is available from the Association for Children with Learning Disabilities, 4900 Girard Rd., Pittsburgh, PA 15227, telephone (412) 881-2253; and The Orton Dyslexia Society, Chester Building #382, 8600 LaSalle Rd., Baltimore, MD 21286, telephone (410) 296-0232 or 800-ABCD123.

BIBLIOGRAPHY

Aicardi J: *Diseases of the Nervous System in Childhood.* Oxford, Mackeith Press/Blackwell, 1992.

American Psychiatric Association: *Diagnostic and Statistical Manual of Mental Disorder,* ed 3, revised [DSM–III–R]. Washington, DC, American Psychiatric Association, 1987.

Amir N, Rapin I, Branski D (eds): *Pediatric Neurology: Behavior and Cognition of the Child with Brain Dysfunction.* Basel, Karger, 1991.

Barlow CF: *Mental Retardation and Related Disorders.* Philadelphia, FA Davis, 1978.

Bodensteiner J (ed): Pediatric neurology. *Neurol Clin* 1990; 8:483–779.

Bodensteiner J (ed): Pediatric neurology. *Pediatric Clin North Am* 1992; 39:591–953.

Brumback RA, Bodensteiner JB, Roach ES: Support groups for pediatric neurologic disorders. *J Child Neurol* 1990; 5:344–349.

Capute AJ, Accardo PJ: Linguistic and auditory milestones during the first two years of life. *Clin Pediatr* 1978; 17:847–853.

Denckla MB: Neurological examination for subtle signs (PANESS). *Psychopharmacol Bull* 1985; 21:273–800.

Denckla MB, James LS (eds): An update on autism: A developmental disorder. *Pediatrics* 1991;87 (suppl 5).

Desnick RJ (ed): *Treatment of Genetic Diseases.* New York, Churchill-Livingstone 1991.

Dmitriev V, Oelwein PL (eds): *Advances in Down Syndrome,* Seattle, Special Child Publications, 1988.

Gascon G, Johnson R, Burd L: Central auditory processing and attention deficit disorder. *J Child Neurol* 1986; 1:27–33.

Gascon GG, Ozand PT, Brismar J (eds): Neurogenetic/neurometabolic diseases. *J Child Neurol* 1992; 7(suppl):51–140.

Golden G: Neurobiological correlates of learning disabilities. *Ann Neurol* 1982; 12:409–418.

Haas R, Rapin I, Moser H (eds): Rett syndrome and autism. *J Child Neurol* 1988; 3(suppl):51–593.

Levy HB, Harper CR, Weinberg WA: A practical approach to children failing in school. *Pediatr Clin North Am* 1992; 39:895–928.

Lott IT, McCoy EE: *Down Syndrome. Advances in Medical Care.* New York, Wiley-Liss, 1992.

Morgan SB: Helping parents understand the diagnosis of autism. *J Dev Behav Pediatr* 1984; 5:68–85.

Ozand PT, Gascon GG: Organic acidurias: A review—part 1. *J Child Neurol* 1991; 6:196–219.

Ozand PT, Gascon GG: Organic acidurias: A review—part 2. *J Child Neurol* 1991; 6:288–303.

Paine R, Oppe T: *Neurological Examination of Children. Clinics in Developmental Medicine,* vol 20/21. Philadelphia, JB Lippincott, 1966.

Palfrey JS, Mervis RC, Butler JA: New directions in the evaluation and education of handicapped children. *N Engl J Med* 1979; 298:819–824.

Pennington BF: *Diagnosing Learning Disorders.* New York, Guilford Press, 1991.

Rourke BP, Bakker DJ, Fisk JL, et al: *Child Neuropsychology.* New York, Guilford Press, 1983.

Touwen BC: *The Examination of the Child With Minor Nervous Dysfunction,* ed 2. Philadelphia, JB Lippincott, 1981.

Voeller K (ed): Attentional deficit hyperactivity disorder. *J Child Neurol* 1991; 6(suppl):51–5131.

Volpe J: *Neurology of the Newborn,* ed 2. Philadelphia, WB Saunders, 1987.

LOW BACK PAIN *17*

Low back pain with or without leg pain, is one of the most common complaints seen in medical practice. It is estimated that up to 80% of the American population may suffer at least temporary disability from low back pain. Low back pain is only a *symptom* which can result from several conditions and hence the term should not automatically be equated with herniated lumbar disc. Each patient must be evaluated with a detailed history, an adequate physical examination, and relevant investigations so that a correct diagnosis is reached and appropriate treatment initiated.

I. **DIAGNOSIS.**
A. **Etiologic factors.**
    1. Trauma:
        a. Acute lumbosacral sprain.
        b. Fracture of lumbar vertebrae.
    2. Tumors:
        a. Metastases to the spine: Common sources are prostate, breast, and kidneys.
        b. Tumors compressing the cauda equina.
    3. Metabolic: Osteoporosis (particularly in postmenopausal females), myeloma, and hyperparathyroidism.
    4. Degenerative processes involving the intervertebral disc or the joints between the articular processes of adjacent vertebrae; a posterolateral herniation of the nucleus pulposus usually compresses a nerve root.
    5. Other structural lesions of the spine:
        a. Spinal stenosis.
        b. Spondylolisthesis.
    6. Infections of the disc space or vertebrae.
    7. Inflammatory disorders involving:
        a. Vertebrae, e.g., ankylosing spondylitis.
        b. Meninges, e.g., arachnoiditis.

8. Vascular:
   a. Abdominal aortic aneurysm eroding the vertebrae.
   b. Occlusive vascular disease causing radicular or plexus ischemia.
9. Direct involvement of lumbosacral plexus or sciatic nerve, e.g., trauma, tumors, injections into or close to the sciatic nerve.
10. Psychogenic, especially when litigation is involved.

B. **History.** It is of utmost importance that the history be derived *without using leading questions*. Patients with pain problems are often overly susceptible to suggestion. Leading questions may only provide misinformation to the initial examiner and allow the patient to develop a symptom complex that will mislead subsequent examiners. For example, do not ask whether specific activities aggravate the pain; ask whether there are any known factors that aggravate the pain. Do not ask whether the pain goes into the leg; ask whether the pain extends into any other part of the body from the lower back. The answers to such questions may help to differentiate organic from functional problems. With experience, the examiner should (in approximately 15 minutes) be able to take a history regarding the back pain problem that will provide the following information:

1. The chronological sequence of the events involved in the pain problem leading up to the time of examination: "Tell me the whole story of your problem from the very beginning."
2. An exact description of the type of pain, its location, extent, and radiation, if any: "Tell me exactly what this pain is like."
3. Factors that precipitate the pain and activities that exacerbate or relieve the pain: "Does anything affect this pain?"
4. A description of any back injury (and whether there is litigation related to that injury): "Have you ever injured your back?"
5. Associated motor or sensory complaints—nature and extent: "Have you noticed any weakness or loss of feeling?"
6. Interference with bowel, bladder, or sexual function:

"Do your bowels and bladder work all right?" "Have
you had any problems with your sexual function?"

7. A detailed description of previous therapy for the pain
and what effect it may have had: "Have you ever had
any treatment for your back? If so, describe." (Be alert
to drug-seeking behavior.)

C. **Hypothesis formation.** From the history a hypothesis as to
the possible source of pain should be formulated:

1. If the pain is localized to the low back, without radiation to the leg, it is unlikely that there is nerve root involvement. Osteoporosis, spinal metastasis, degenerative disc disease, disc space infections, all can present
with low back pain alone.

2. If the pain radiates to the lower extremity, take into consideration the following:

   a. Root pain:
   1) Worse with factors that increase intraspinal pressure (coughing, sneezing).
   2) Distribution is usually in the L4, L5, or S1 dermatome.

   b. Claudication:
   1) Related to exertion—especially with iliofemoral
   occlusive vascular disease.
   2) Lumbar spinal canal stenosis: Pain is worse with
   exertion.

   Caveat: Stenosis commonly produces numbness and weakness; vascular disease does not.

   c. Posterior longitudinal ligament involvement (most
   often a bulging disc which does not stretch a nerve
   root):
   1) Seldom radiates below knee.
   2) Pain is vague, not associated with paresthesia.

   d. Hip joint disease and pelvic abnormalities may also
   cause lower extremity pain.

3. Back pain in the elderly population (over age 60 years)
often presents differently from that in the younger adult
(under age 60 years) population:

   a. Back pain is often present at rest.

b. Spinal claudication is more common and can occur without severe spinal stenosis.
c. Reflex changes are often evident, but reflexes may be normal if the spinal cord is primarily involved.
d. Bladder dysfunction is often occult and may only be evident with a cystometrogram.
e. Reduced mobility can obscure significant vascular disease.

D. Physical examination.

1. Examination of *gait* is a very important part of the physical examination of patients with back pain. The physician must pay particular attention to the following:

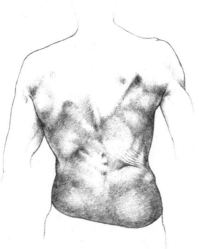

FIG 17–1. A patient with an organic back pain problem frequently walks with forward flexion of the trunk and with one iliac crest higher than the other. A lateral curve of the spine is often present.

    a. Whether the patient is walking with a list of the spine; this is highly indicative of an organic back problem (Fig 17–1).

    b. Whether the patient can support weight on the toes and heels (motor weakness in muscles below the knee).

    c. Whether the patient can hop on one foot or the other (weakness of quadriceps or gluteus muscles).

2. Examination of the *back* should be carried out with the patient in the upright standing position. Conditions to be noted include the following:

    a. Muscle spasm (noted by prominence of paraspinal muscles on one side or flattening of lumbar lordosis) (Fig 17–2).

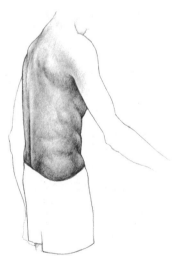

FIG 17–2. A patient with an organic back problem will often have the lower lumbar curve obliterated. Unilateral paravertebral muscle spasm on one side elevates the iliac crest. This is most commonly seen with a root lesion.

    b. List or curvature: the patient often leans away from the site of the pain and the scoliosis becomes more prominent as the patient tries to bend forward.

    c. Any palpable mass or tenderness along the vertebral column (including percussion of the flanks looking for kidney disease and percussion over the spinous processes with a tendon hammer) (Fig 17–3).

    d. Range of motion in flexion, extension, and sideways bending: often the patient will keep the spine rigid and do the flexion at the hip.

    e. Dimples, birthmarks, abnormal patches of hair (clues to congenital malformation or tumors).

▶ 3. Straight leg raising test is the *key to identifying nerve root irritation.* With the patient supine, passively raise the extended leg until pain occurs (Fig 17–4); normally an 80-degree movement can be made with little discomfort; if the pain is only in the back of the thigh, it is likely to be due to hamstring tightness and not to nerve

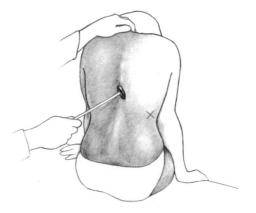

FIG 17–3. Percussion of the spinous processes will often cause more discomfort over the involved vertebrae. Be certain also to percuss the costovertebral angle in search of renal disease.

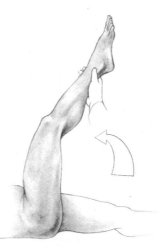

FIG 17–4. Straight leg raising: With disc disease, raising the affected leg will often cause pain in the distribution of the affected root. This pain is centered in the buttocks at the sciatic notch and radiates down the leg. Pain at the knee from tight hamstring muscles does not constitute a positive straight leg raising test.

root tension, irritation, or compression. If the pain radiates to the back as well as to the leg, it often indicates nerve root involvement. When in doubt, use one or more of the following maneuvers to confirm a positive straight leg raising test.

a. The straight leg is brought down until the pain just disappears when an attempt is made to suddenly dorsiflex the ankle; genuine root pain will be reproduced by this maneuver.

b. Have the patient sit up in bed with the legs extended at the knee or repeat the test with the patient in the sitting position with the legs dangling over the edge of the table (Fig 17–5). When the leg is extended

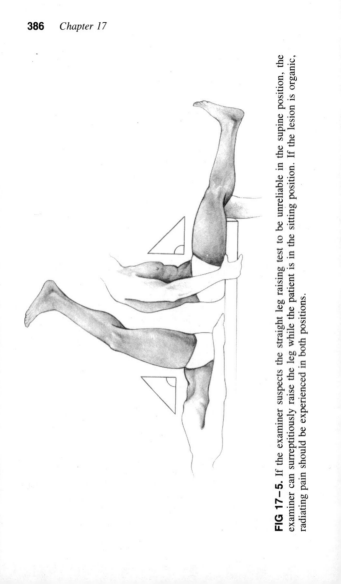

FIG 17–5. If the examiner suspects the straight leg raising test to be unreliable in the supine position, the examiner can surreptitiously raise the leg while the patient is in the sitting position. If the lesion is organic, radiating pain should be experienced in both positions.

at the knee, the patient should complain of pain and lean backward to produce the same angle as for the straight leg raising test in the lying position. If the patient experiences no pain in the sitting position, a previous positive straight leg raising test in the lying position probably suggests a nonorganic basis.

c. The patient may be asked to kneel on a chair; in this position the hamstrings are relaxed and the tension on the sciatic nerve is reduced; reluctance to bend forward while in this position is suggestive of a false-positive straight leg raising test.

4. While performing the straight leg raising test, hip joint mobility should also be evaluated. This is done by passive rotation of the leg at the hip (Fig 17–6). A patient with pathologic spinal changes will have no pain or re-

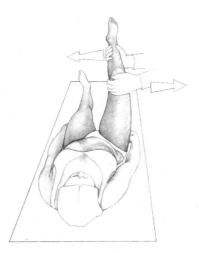

FIG 17–6. Hip rotation: with the hip and knee flexed, inward rotation of the lower leg with the knee flexed will cause pain if there is hip joint disease.

striction on rotary movements of the hip, but the patient with hip disease (who may present as a back pain problem) will show a marked aggravation of the pain when the hip is rotated internally or externally.

Caveat: Disease at the L5–S1 intervertebral disc space may present as hip pain.

5. Concentrate on those aspects of the neurologic examination that may be helpful in confirming nerve root compression:
   a. Unilaterally absent or diminished patellar (L4), internal hamstring (L5), or Achilles (S1) tendon reflexes localize an involved nerve root with reasonable accuracy. Be aware of the occasional patient who may show hyperactive reflexes in the presence of acute back pain owing to keeping the lower extremity muscles tense; in such a patient the plantar response will remain flexor.
   b. Absent cremasteric reflexes suggest an upper lumbar root or conus medullaris lesion (Fig 17–7).

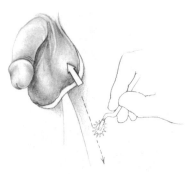

FIG 17–7. Cremasteric reflex: A light stroke downward on the inner surface of the thigh produces an upward movement of the testicle.

c. Unequal superficial abdominal reflexes may suggest a thoracic lesion from T9 to the T12 level (Fig 17–8).
d. A dermatomal sensory loss, if typical, is useful in localizing the root involved.

   Caveat: Never make a diagnosis on the basis of sensory loss alone.

e. Motor weakness demonstrated by specific muscle testing may confirm a motor root lesion. Muscle testing may also demonstrate involvement of multiple roots.
f. Bilateral simultaneous muscle testing is a valuable method of detecting hysterical weakness. The pa-

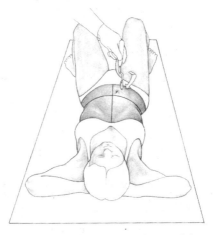

FIG 17–8. Abdominal reflex: a light stroke toward the umbilicus will normally cause muscle contraction with movement of the umbilicus toward the stimulus. The pinwheel is a more effective and reliable stimulus than a sharp stick.

tient is unable to coordinate hysterical "giving way" between both extremities (Figure 17–9).

6. The physical examination should also include abdominal palpation, palpation of the lower extremity pulsations, and listening for a bruit over the aorta, the iliac arteries, and the femoral arteries.

7. A rectal examination is quite important in evaluating patients with persistent back pain or back and leg pain to detect pelvic pathologic changes and sphincter involvement. The anal reflex, which is often lost in conus medullaris and cauda equina lesions, should also be tested (Fig 17–10).

E. **Clinical investigations.** The history and physical findings should narrow the differential diagnosis. The investigations are chosen on the basis of the most likely diagnoses. When evaluating the investigations keep in mind the false-positive and false-negative results for each:

1. Plain radiographs of the lumbar and sacral spine: Anteroposterior (AP), lateral, and oblique views are done to look for abnormalities in the vertebral bodies, intervertebral disc spaces, and intervertebral foramina, and for any abnormal shadows.

   Caveat: Asymptomatic bony abnormalities are not uncommon and do not always correlate with neurologic deficit.

2. A computed tomography (CT) scan–myelogram (CT scan of the spine following instillation of contrast material into the subarachnoid space) of the lumbar spine is highly useful, particularly in disc lesions, to obtain good visualization of the vertebral body, spinal cord, nerve roots, intervertebral disc, neural arch, zygapophyseal joints, and intervertebral foramina.

   Caveat: The CT scan is most useful if on neurologic examination the physician can identify the level of the lesion.

3. Magnetic resonance imaging (MRI) is a useful adjunct, but is most helpful in thin patients under age 50 years.

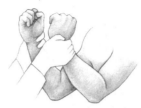

FIG 17–9. Test comparable muscle strength simultaneously if there is a suspicion of nonorganicity. It is very difficult to give way with one muscle while maintaining strength in another.

4. Radionuclide bone scans are particularly useful when metastatic disease is suspected as a cause of low back pain. It is also often positive in inflammatory diseases of the spine and in fractures.
5. Electromyography (EMG): Function of the nerve root should be assessed by EMG and nerve conduction studies; CT-myelography and MRI show only the anatomy. In experienced hands it provides accurate localization of the root involved. It is useful in identifying periph-

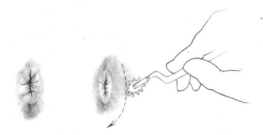

FIG 17–10. A light stroke with a pinwheel in the perianal area normally causes the anus to pucker.

eral neuropathies which may confuse the picture of root involvement.

6. When metabolic bone disease or metastases are suspected, erythrocyte sedimentation rate (ESR), calcium, phosphate, and alkaline and acid phosphatase assays may be done. When disc space infections or inflammatory disease is suspected, ESR, antinuclear antibodies, and rheumatoid factor assays need to be done. When myeloma is suspected, radiographic studies of other parts of the skeleton, examination of the urine for Bence Jones protein, serum protein electrophoresis, and a bone marrow examination are necessary.

II.   PROTRUDED INTERVERTEBRAL DISC.
A.   Clinical features.

▶ 1. *The most important diagnostic feature* is the onset of low back pain followed by radiation down one lower extremity.

Caveat: All such pain is not due to disc prolapse; any condition that afflicts the nerve root can present similarly.

2. The initial attack may be provoked by an identifiable precipitating event (often lifting a weight or a twisting movement). The pain may be described as severe enough to "take the breath away" and cause the patient to be completely immobilized.

3. The area of pain is usually well localized, and the extension can be traced with a finger. There is a feeling of associated tingling in the distal extension of the pain.

4. During subsequent episodes, which may again be precipitated by physical activity, the pain is often less severe and may disappear within a few days; less severe attacks are usually precipitated by movement and may be relieved by change of posture or rest.

5. The pain is improved by flexion of the thigh and the knees; individual patients may be worse at night or during the day; activity relieves pain in some patients but

more commonly aggravates symptoms. The patient will often move about gingerly for fear of aggravating the pain.

6. The patient may complain of extremity weakness, numbness, and paresthesias in localized areas of the leg or foot. Infrequently, there may be interference of bowel, bladder, or sexual function; these symptoms are more common in midline disc herniation, involving the sacral nerve roots of both sides.

B. **Physical examination.** The physical examination reveals one or more of the following:

1. The patient often stands in a listed position and tends to walk with the affected leg slightly flexed at the knee and at the thigh. There may be difficulty standing in an upright position with the leg fully extended.

2. There may be difficulty supporting weight on the toes or heels. Walking on the heels often acutely aggravates the pain.

3. Hopping is often difficult to perform, but if performed, a tendency for the knee to buckle suggests quadriceps weakness and the possibility of an L3 or L4 root lesion.

4. Examination of the back shows paravertebral muscle spasm with limitation of bending forward or backward. Bending forward is more often limited in ruptured disc at the L5–S1 interspace; bending backward is often limited in ruptured disc at the L3–4 or L4–5 interspaces. Frequently a scoliosis with convexity toward the symptomatic side may be seen.

5. Percussion over the spine may produce radiation of the pain into the affected leg.

6. The straight leg raising test is positive on the symptomatic side. Occasionally there is a positive crossed straight leg raising test with pain extending into the leg opposite the one being raised (this is suggestive of an extruded fragment).

7. The patient will flex the knees and thighs and roll with legs flexed in the process of turning over or getting out of bed.

8. Over 90% of ruptured lumbar discs with nerve root compression affect either the L5 or S1 roots producing the following neurologic alterations:
   a. S1 root lesion (Fig 17–11):
      1) Diminished or absent Achilles tendon reflex (ankle reflex).
      2) Sensory deficit in the lateral aspect of the heel and the lateral aspect of the sole of the affected foot.
      3) Difficulty standing on tiptoe on the affected extremity (suggests calf weakness).
   b. L5 root lesion (Fig 17–12):
      1) Trouble supporting weight on heel or presence of foot drop; the patient may complain that his toes get caught on carpet.

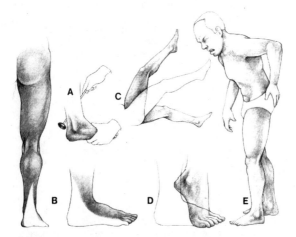

FIG 17–11. Summary of an S1 root lesion: diminished Achilles reflex **(A)**, sensory disturbance over the lateral aspect of the heel and toe **(B)**, positive straight leg raising **(C)**, difficulty standing on tiptoe **(D)**, pain worse bending forward **(E)**.

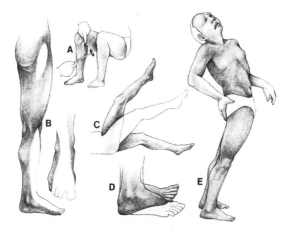

FIG 17–12. Summary of an L5 root lesion. Diminished internal hamstring reflex (**A**), sensory disturbance over dorsum of foot and great toe (**B**), positive straight leg raising (**C**), footdrop (**D**), pain worse bending backward (**E**).

2) Sensory deficits over the anterolateral aspect of the affected leg below the knee and extending to the dorsum of the foot and the big toe.
3) Diminished or absent internal hamstring tendon reflex.

c. L4 root lesion:
1) Diminished or absent patellar tendon reflex.
2) Weakness in the quadriceps muscle of the affected leg.
3) Sensory deficit extending from the knee down the medial aspect of the lower portion of the affected leg as well as the medial malleolus.

Caveat: Sensory deficits must be interpreted very carefully, taking into account an intuitive assessment of patient reliability and the examiner's experience.

C. **Other investigations.**

1. The routine laboratory and plain spinal radiographs in protruded lumbar intervertebral discs seldom show diagnostic abnormalities. Electromyography (EMG) may provide objective evidence of denervation due to damage to ventral (motor) root. The dorsal (sensory) root function can be evaluated by doing H-reflex and dermatomal somatosensory evoked potential studies.

2. MRI of the lumbar spine is frequently useful in evaluating patients with lumbar disc prolapse, but in elderly patients CT-myelography is often more useful than MRI.

D. **Management.**

1. In acute disc prolapse, at least 10 days of conservative treatment should be tried unless there is a rapidly progressive neurologic deficit. This includes:

a. Strict bed rest (except for bathroom privileges); the bed should be firm (firm mattress or bed board) and flat. The fetal position with a pillow placed between the thighs is comfortable for most patients.

Caveat: Elderly people tolerate bed rest less well than younger patients because of the development of venous thromboses and disuse atrophy.

b. Anti-inflammatory agents, mild analgesics, and mild antidepressant medications are helpful during the period of bed rest: high-dose aspirin (325 mg every 2–3 hours), diazepam 5 mg q8h, and amitriptyline 25 mg qhs is a suggested regimen. Heating pads delivering both heat and massage are now available. Transcutaneous electrical nerve stimulation (TENS) is useful in patients with acute low back pain and in those with low back pain and radicular pain.

c. After recovery from the acute attack, a concerted program of back exercises should be undertaken for at least 6 weeks.

d. A lumbar roll (hand towel rolled into a 4-in. roll secured by rubber bands) in situations where prolonged sitting is necessary (e.g., an automobile) helps prevent recurrences.

2. Failure to respond to conservative treatment may result from noncompliance with strict bed rest, incorrect diagnosis, persistent or worsening nerve root compression, unstable spine, secondary gain, litigation, or other psychosocial factors. A comprehensive evaluation is needed at this stage to determine the reason for nonimprovement. In some metropolitan areas, referral to rehabilitation facilities specializing only in low back problems may be useful.

3. Surgical intervention should be considered with the greatest skepticism; extruded disc fragments, spinal cord compression, and progressive objective neurologic deficit are some of the reasons for early surgery. Surgery is successful more often in older patients.

III.   SPRAIN OR FRACTURE.
A.   Clinical features.
▶ 1. Paravertebral muscle spasm is one of the commonest causes of acute low back pain. *The most important clue to the diagnosis* is pain specifically related to an injury that reaches a crescendo (quickly or over a period of days) and gradually tapers to a plateau that may persist for weeks to months.

2. The pain is described as diffuse backache with associated stiffness, spasm, and limitation of motion. Stiffness may extend up to the neck and down to the pelvis and legs.

3. Extension of the pain is vague unless a fracture has produced nerve root compression. In the facet syndrome (due to tearing of the capsule of the facet joint) the pain may extend to the buttock and posterior thigh of the involved side.

4. The pain is relieved somewhat by reclining, changing position, analgesics, and heat. Massage or manipulation often gives temporary relief, but may be dangerous in an unsuspected fracture. There is no relationship of the pain to the time of day or night.

5. Temporary ileus or difficulty in initiating urination may occur in the acute phase of pain.

6. Damage or compression of the spinal cord or nerve root by fracture may produce deficits in motor, sensory, bowel, bladder, or sexual function, individually or severally.

B.   Physical examination.

1. The gait *should not* be tested during the acute phase until x-ray examination has excluded the presence of an unstable vertebral fracture.

2. Initially there may be palpable swelling or hematoma. Palpation of the back usually reveals an area of focal tenderness over the spinous processes in the region of the injury. Reversal of the spinal curve may be palpable at the level of the compression fracture.

3. Because a common site of fracture is the T12 vertebra, examination of sensation in the perianal area is mandatory to exclude injury to the conus medullaris without simultaneous nerve root injury. There may be loss of bowel and bladder function, sexual dysfunction in the male, and loss of anal reflex or a patulous anal sphincter.

4. In all patients careful documentation of reflex, motor, and sensory function is important in the acute phase so that comparison can be made with follow-up examinations.

C.   Radiographic studies.

1. In the case of low back sprain, spinal films reveal few changes other than obliteration of the normal spinal curvature resulting from paravertebral muscle spasm.

2. In the case of spinal fracture, spinal films are the diagnostic tool for identifying the lesion.

   Caveat: Unsatisfactory films or films taken too low or too high in the spine result in many fractures being missed.

D.   Management.

1. Back sprain is treated like a lumbar disc herniation, both in the acute and chronic phases.

2. Spinal fracture requires absolute bed rest on a flat, firm surface (bed board) and consideration of surgical treat-

ment by decompression laminectomy or surgical stabilization, or both.

IV. STRUCTURAL BONY LESIONS.
A. Clinical features.

1. The conditions that may lead to low back pain due to structural bony abnormalities include osteoporosis, old fracture, congenital bony abnormalities such as partially sacralized lumbar vertebrae, unilateral pedicle defect, spondylolisthesis, facet asymmetry, and spinal stenosis.

2. Most of these conditions present with chronic low back pain of long duration; the patient may trace the onset to injury.

3. The major feature is chronic, nagging, and centrally located back pain without radiation to the lower extremities; the notable exceptions are spondylolisthesis and spinal stenosis in which radicular pain spreading to the lower extremities may occur.

4. Pain is precipitated or aggravated by lifting, standing, or prolonged forward bending, and is aggravated by work, sexual, physical, and recreational activity; the pain is often relieved by sitting or lying down; it is seldom troubling at night.

▶ 5. An important clue to the diagnosis is that the pain is least troublesome on arising from bed, but increases with activity during the day.

6. No complaints of motor, sensory, bladder, bowel, or sexual dysfunction occur except in cases of spinal stenosis or spondylolisthesis with nerve root involvement.

B. *Physical examination* shows normal gait, with ability to walk on heels and toes, a negative straight leg raising test, and normal reflexes, muscle strength, and sensory perception. The abnormality is easily identified by spine radiographs. The CT scan or MRI is of immense help in locating and characterizing the defect.

C. **Treatment.** Acute back pain resulting from a structural bony abnormality should be treated like an acute herniated disc. Excessive weight in the abdominal area (potbelly) should be eliminated by a weight reduction program (Fig 17–13).

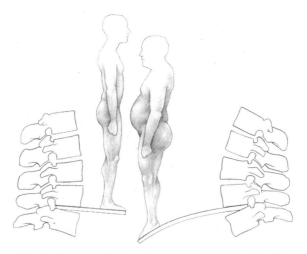

FIG 17–13. A potbelly increases stress on the lumbar spine. The length of the springboard is proportional to the distance between the navel and the spine.

V.   LUMBAR STENOSIS.
A.   Clinical features.
1. Although this is also a structural abnormality, it is mentioned separately since the clinical presentation is somewhat typical. There is narrowing of the nerve root foramina and spinal canal resulting in compression of the lumbosacral nerve roots. A congenitally narrow canal with acquired factors such as hypertrophy of vertebral bone and interspinal ligamentous tissue, as well as displacement of the intervertebral discs, may result in lumbar stenosis.

▶ 2. *The most important diagnostic clue* is the occurrence of symptoms suggestive of *bilateral lumbosacral radiculopathy,* either acutely following minor trauma or insidiously.

3. Typical features include claudication (pain usually involves the lower extremities, is provoked by exertion, and relieved by sitting), postural aggravation of symptoms (exacerbation of radiating leg pain, paresthesia, numbness or weakness when standing erect or bending backward; the patient may complain of sudden onset of severe pain in the legs on reaching for objects overhead, which is quickly relieved by bending forward). A typical patient will be one with bilateral sciatica who enters the examining room hunched over and walking with a short cane.

4. The diagnosis is confirmed by MRI or CT scan of the lumbar spine. The treatment is surgical and consists of wide laminectomy with bilateral foraminotomy.

VI. INFLAMMATORY DISEASE AFFECTING THE SPINE.

A. **Ankylosing spondylitis.** Persistent low back pain may be caused by inflammatory disease of the spine, such as ankylosing spondylitis. This condition is estimated to occur in about 1% of the population. The characteristic features include:

1. Onset between ages 20 and 40 years, more often in men.

2. Insidious onset of chronic low back pain without sciatica.

3. Feeling of stiffness and pain aggravated by maintaining one position for a long time and improved by mild activity.

4. Absence of motor or sensory abnormalities; the straight leg raising test is negative.

5. Discomfort may be present on hip rotation with general reduction in movements of the lumbar spine in all directions.

6. The diagnosis is confirmed by CT scan or MRI (involvement of sacroiliac joints, and calcification of anterior and posterior spinal ligaments) and elevated ESR.

B. *Rheumatoid arthritis* may lead to persistent low back pain. The most useful diagnostic features include involvement of other joints and laboratory data supporting the diagnosis.

C. Infection.

1. Both acute and chronic infection of the spine may present with back pain.

2. Disc space infection, which may occur following surgery or as a complication of systemic infection, presents with severe back pain, local spinal tenderness, and paraspinal spasm. Spinal radiographs, bone scan, CT scan, and blood studies are often diagnostic.

3. Involvement of the spine may also occur in conditions such as tuberculosis, brucellosis, and typhoid. Spinal tuberculosis may present with pain and spinal deformity (gibbus) in the lower thoracic area; cold abscess may form and compress the spinal cord and produce acute or subacute onset of paraplegia. The radiologic appearance is characteristic, showing rarefaction and often collapse of the adjacent vertebrae with paraspinal mass.

VII. INTRASPINAL OR SPINAL NEOPLASM.

A. Clinical features.

1. Intraspinal or spinal neoplasms occur with metastatic prostatic or breast carcinoma and primary tumors such as meningioma, neurofibroma, or ependymoma.

▶ 2. *The most important diagnostic clue is steady relentless progression* of symptoms (as opposed to static or intermittent pain noted with most other causes).

3. With a progressive increase in the severity and constancy of the pain the patient may describe radicular extension of the pain (often with motor and sensory deficits).

4. Pain is aggravated by activity and unrelieved by any therapeutic measures; there is slight improvement on reclining with the knees flexed; prolonged lying aggravates the pain and may wake the patient at night. With arousal and ambulation pain may lessen. Pain may be increased by the Valsalva maneuver (which, however, does not necessarily differentiate this cause of pain from other causes of back pain).

5. Progression of the lesion often results in impairment of bowel and bladder control and sexual dysfunction in the male.

B. **Physical examination.**
  1. Evidence of a spinal lesion is manifested by:
     a. Muscle spasm.
     b. Area of focal tenderness.
     c. Reflex alterations.
     d. Sensory deficits.
     e. Motor group weakness.
  2. Examination of the breast or prostate may lead to diagnosis of the underlying metastatic neoplasm in a high percentage of cases.

C. **Laboratory studies.**
  1. Primary intraspinal neoplasms have no characteristic laboratory abnormalities.
  2. Metastatic spinal neoplasms may exhibit laboratory findings of malignancy such as anemia, elevated ESR, and elevation of alkaline phosphatase or acid phosphatase levels, or both.

D. **Imaging studies.**
  1. Spinal films may be negative; CT scan or MRI may show widening of the spinal canal, erosion of the pedicles, or scalloping of the vertebral bodies. Metastatic neoplasms may show erosion of elements of the vertebral body or osteoblastic changes.
  2. A bone scan may show evidence of metastatic lesions when the plain films are negative. Pain usually precedes radiographic changes by several weeks.

E. **Treatment.**
  1. Early diagnosis may obviate the need for neurosurgical treatment and may avoid serious neurologic sequelae in cases of metastatic lesions.
  2. Late diagnosis usually necessitates immediate neurosurgical decompression.
  3. In almost all cases of malignant neoplasms intensive anticancer chemotherapy and radiotherapy are necessary. Short-term corticosteroid therapy is useful when there is cord compression.
  4. Early surgical treatment of benign intraspinal tumors such as neurofibroma and meningioma leads to excellent results.

VIII. RETROPERITONEAL LESIONS.
A. Clinical features.
▶ 1. *The most important diagnostic clue* is the pain, which is described as deep and burning and which radiates from the abdomen through to the back. When the nerve plexus is involved, there is usually acute neuralgic pain, or burning paresthesia, which may radiate from the abdomen to the back, groin, or the lower extremities.

2. The pain may be related to ingestion of food and may be aggravated by lying flat, by emptying the bladder, or by moving the bowels; pain may occur related to menstrual flow.

3. Activity has little or no effect on the pain.

B. Physical examination.
1. The back examination and neurologic examination are normal, unless the lumbosacral plexus has been affected.

2. Percussion of the costovertebral angle may produce pain (this maneuver does not produce pain in other causes of back pain).

3. Hyperextension of the leg at the thigh may produce pain if there is psoas muscle irritation.

4. Rectal examination may reveal a presacral or pelvic mass.

5. Evidence of lumbosacral plexus involvement may be present.

C. Other studies.
1. Laboratory studies may show evidence suggesting inflammatory or neoplastic disease.

2. Routine spinal radiographs are seldom helpful; a CT scan of the abdomen is often highly useful in identifying the lesion.

3. Special studies, such as a gastrointestinal (GI) series or intravenous pyelography (IVP) may be of value in the diagnosis.

4. EMG studies may be useful in determining the extent and severity of lumbosacral plexus involvement.

5. Treatment must be directed toward the primary disease process.

IX.   EMOTIONAL DISORDER.
A.   Diagnosis.
▶ 1. *The most important diagnostic clue* is that the patient is inconsistent with regard to the chronological history, description of pain, factors affecting the pain, and relationship of the pain to the time of day or night. If the pain is injury-related, the circumstances of the injury are usually presented in explicit detail in contrast to the vague description of the nature of the pain problem.

2. The history may be misleading if the patient has had previous exposure to leading questions by other examiners.

3. Sometimes the patient may purposely mislead the examiner.

4. Examination.

a. The patient exhibits overreaction to the examiner's physical contact.

b. The patient reacts to palpation in a manner disproportionate to the lack of objective findings in the examination.

c. The patient frequently exhibits an oscillatory giveaway weakness on muscle testing and exhibits vague, indefinite, and unphysiologic sensory alterations.

d. The appearance and attitudes of the patient may vary from inappropriate cheerfulness to indifference and apathy, inappropriate distress, or hostility.

e. Simultaneous muscle testing (see Fig 17–9) or an inappropriate straight leg raising test (see Fig 17–5) may be clues to an underlying emotional disorder.

5. Do not be misled by nonspecific laboratory and radiographic findings.

B.   Treatment. Appropriate management of the underlying emotional problem is often indicated without denying the distress the patient is experiencing from the problem.

BIBLIOGRAPHY

Blumer D: Psychiatric and psychological aspects of chronic pain. *Clin Neurosurg* 1978; 25:276–283.

Condon RH: Modalities in the treatment of acute and chronic low back pain, in Finneson BE (ed): *Low Back Pain,* Philadelphia, JB Lippincott, 1981, pp 204–232.

Donelson RG: Identifying appropriate exercises for your low back pain patient. *J Musculoskeletal Med* 1991; 8(12):14–29.

Frymoyer JW: Back pain and sciatica. *N Engl J Med* 1988; 318:291–300.

Hall S, Bartleson JD, Onofrio BM, et al: Lumbar spinal stenosis. *Ann Intern Med* 1985; 103:271–276.

Hardy RW, Plank NW: Clinical diagnosis of herniated lumbar disc, in Hardy RW Jr (ed): *Lumbar Disc Disease,* New York, Raven Press, 1982, pp 17–28.

Kelsey JL, White HH, Pastides H, et al: The impact of musculoskeletal disorders on the population of the United States. *J Bone Joint Surg [Am]* 1979; 61:959–964.

Mills K, Page G, Siwek R: *Color Atlas of Low Back Pain.* Philadelphia, FA Davis, 1990.

Nakano K: *Neurology of Musculoskeletal and Rheumatic Disorders.* Boston, Houghton Mifflin, 1979.

Ponte DJ, et al: A preliminary report on the use of the McKenzie protocol versus Williams protocol in the treatment of low back pain. *J Orthop Sports Physic Ther* 1984; 6:130–139.

Shields CB, Williams PE Jr: Low back pain. *Am Fam Physician* 1986; 33:173–182.

CERVICAL SPINE DISEASE   *18*

The grave implications of quadriparesis from spinal cord involvement or the severe disability of an arm from nerve root damage make it imperative that symptoms relating to the neck be thoroughly investigated. Otherwise, management of cervical spine disease usually consists of treating a "pain in the neck." However, this chapter is titled "Cervical Spine Disease" rather than "Neck Pain" because a number of conditions affecting the cervical spine may occur without any symptomatic neck pain. Cervical spine disease may be classified as follows:

I.   CLASSIFICATION.
A.   With neurologic involvement.
1. Acute spinal cord trauma.
2. Tumor.
3. Protruded disc.
4. Spinal canal stenosis.
5. Infection.
B.   Without neurologic involvement.
1. Meningeal irritation.
2. Sprain, strain, or fracture.
3. Degenerative or inflammatory disease.
4. Lesions of the vertebrae.
5. "Tension" or emotional disturbances.

II.   DIAGNOSIS.
A.   History. Patients with neck pain should be interviewed with particular attention to neurologic dysfunction. In most respects the same types of questions should be used to assess the patient with cervical spine disease as in the patient with

low back pain (see Chapter 17, section I. B). In addition, the following information may be specifically important in disease of the cervical spine:

1. As in other pain syndromes, information should be gathered through nonleading questions, e.g., "What happens when you bend your head forward?" If the patient has shocklike feelings in the legs or arms on flexion or extension of the neck, Lhermitte's sign is present.

2. If the patient volunteers sensory or motor symptoms, obtain specifics, as in low back pain (see Chapter 17, section I. B).

3. Part of the examination must include careful observation of the patient during the history taking. Such observation often gives clues to the extent of the disability. Particular attention should be paid to a patient's facial expression during head movements (a patient who freely moves the head without evidence of pain during the history taking, but complains of pain during examination is suspect). Pay attention to the manner in which the patient changes position (e.g., the neck will be held stiffly during head movements in the patient with painful organic spine disease).

B.   Examination.

1. Hyperactive tendon reflexes in the lower extremities (patellar and Achilles reflex) combined with upgoing (extensor) plantar responses (Babinski reflexes) suggest spinal cord involvement.

2. Hyperactive tendon reflexes in the lower extremities and upgoing (extensor) plantar responses (Babinski reflexes) associated with hypoactive or absent reflexes in the upper extremities (biceps, triceps, or brachioradialis) localize the lesion to the cervical spinal cord. This could occur with:

   a. An extrinsic lesion involving both nerve roots and spinal cord (extramedullary lesions as in meningioma or bony tumors).

   b. Lesion involving the central portion of the spinal cord (intramedullary lesion as in syringomyelia).

3. Presence of a sensory level is highly suggestive of spi-

nal cord involvement. This may best be demonstrated by having the patient run fingers up the trunk until sensation changes (Fig 18–1). In lesions of the central portion of the spinal cord there is selective loss of pain and temperature sensations in the arms and trunk with sparing of the sacral region (Fig 18–2).

4. Brown-Séquard syndrome indicates pathologic changes in the lateral half of the spinal cord:
   a. Weakness, hyperreflexia, Babinski reflex (extensor plantar response), and loss of position and vibration sensation in the lower extremity on one side, associated with a deficit in pinprick and temperature sensation in the other leg
5. Diminished deep tendon reflex in one arm associated with a normal reflex in the other suggests unilateral nerve root involvement and is usually accompanied by

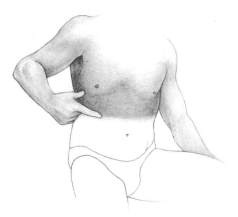

FIG 18–1. The cooperative patient may be able to outline a sensory change with his own finger more accurately than an examiner with multiple pinpricks.

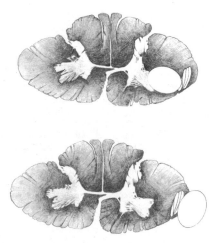

FIG 18–2. In the spinothalamic tract, the sacral pain fibers are more lateral than cervical pain fibers; destructive lesions in the center of the cord may spare the sacral fibers and sacral sensation. An extrinsic lesion may damage the sacral fibers first and produce a sensory disturbance in the sacral area as well as a bladder disturbance.

other motor and sensory deficits in the distribution of that nerve root (Table 18–1).

6. Examination of the neck should be carried out with the patient in the sitting position and with the patient's hands folded in a relaxed position on the lap.
   a. Palpate the cervical and occipital muscles for spasms or masses.
   b. Palpate the posterior cervical triangle for masses or tenderness (Fig 18–3).
   c. Assess the bulk and strength of the sternocleidomastoid muscles.
   d. Palpate and percuss the spinous processes for abnormalities or tenderness.

TABLE 18–1.
Localizing Findings in Cervical Radiculopathy

Nerve Root	Muscle Involved	Motor Weakness	Sensory Loss	Reflex Abnormality
C5	Deltoid Supraspinatus	Shoulder abduction	Lateral upper arm	Biceps
C6	Biceps	Elbow flexion	Thumb and index fingers	Biceps
	Extensor carpi radialis	Wrist extension		Brachioradialis
C7	Triceps	Elbow extension	Middle and index fingers	Triceps
	Flexor carpi radialis	Wrist flexion		
C8	Flexor digitorum	Finger flexion	Little and ring fingers	Finger flexor
T1	Interossei	Abduction and adduction of fingers	Medial forearm and medial upper arm	

    e. The examiner should determine the passive range of motion in flexion, extension, side bending, and rotation of the neck.

    f. Radicular pain caused by nerve root compression may be reproduced by the following maneuvers:

      1) Spurling's maneuver: hyperextend and tilt the neck to the affected side and apply downward pressure over the vertex; this may cause pain in the affected root.

      2) A light blow to the patient's forehead in the previous position (Fig 18–4) will often cause pain when hyperextension and tilting do not.

      3) A light blow to the top of the head with the neck in the normal position may also cause pain in the distribution of the affected root.

        Caveat: Do not perform these tests in suspected cervical spine trauma or instability.

    g. Lhermitte's sign: flexion of the neck produces

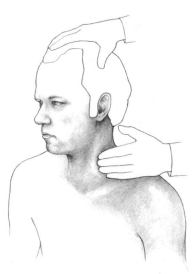

FIG 18–3. Palpation posterior to the sternocleidomastoid muscle may reveal masses and tenderness of the roots or upper brachial plexus.

shocklike sensations down the back or arms; indicates probable meningeal or dorsal column abnormalities.

7. Horner's syndrome (ptosis, miosis, decreased sweating) may occur in diseases that affect the cervical cord or the T1 root.

8. Examination of sensation over the posterior part of the head can reveal sensory impairment from a lesion involving the second and third cervical roots (Fig 18–5).

9. Hyperabduction and external rotation of the shoulder will obliterate the pulse in a thoracic outlet syndrome (also see Chapter 15, section II. B. 1) or will cause severe pain in periarthritis of the shoulder (Fig 18–6).

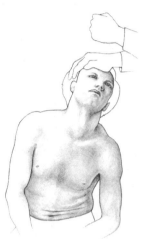

FIG 18–4. Spurling's maneuver: extension and tilting of the neck toward the affected arm may reproduce the pain by further compressing a nerve root in its exit from the foramen. Light percussion on the head may accentuate this phenomenon.

III. ACUTE SPINAL CORD TRAUMA.

A. Evaluation and management.

    1. In a patient with acute cervical trauma, evaluation and management must be carried out simultaneously.

        Caveat: Until a thorough evaluation has been carried out, the neck must be immobilized as completely as possible with sandbags, wraparound collar, or head-halter traction, and with the head and shoulders supported on a board.

    2. Adequate suctioning, administration of oxygen, and the maintenance of a good airway are important if the patient presents with paralysis.

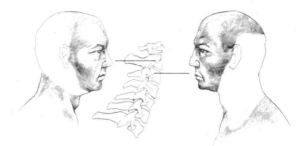

FIG 18–5. A fracture of the upper cervical vertebrae may result in a sensory loss in the distribution of C2 or C3. Failure to detect this sensory loss in upper cervical spine fractures may lead to dislocation of upper cervical vertebrae and severe quadriparesis or death. *Remember:* The C1 root innervates the meninges and has no cutaneous representation, and the root of C2 exits above the vertebral body of C2.

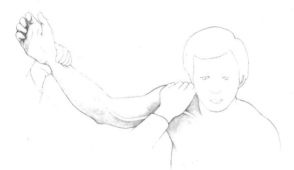

FIG 18–6. Rotation of the shoulder posteriorly when the arm is held in the position shown here may obliterate the radial pulse at the wrist and be a clue to the thoracic outlet syndrome. As the shoulder is rotated posteriorly, the pulse should be obliterated in the affected arm sooner than in the normal arm.

Caveat: Under no circumstances should the head be hyperextended for insertion of an endotracheal tube. It is safer to do a tracheostomy if no other means of maintaining a good airway is possible.

3. Circulatory stability must be maintained since acute cervical cord injury often results in peripheral vasodilation and shock; volume expanders are usually not necessary; vasopressors are usually indicated (see Chapter 13).
4. An indwelling urinary catheter should be inserted to prevent overdistention of the bladder.
5. The level of spinal cord injury can be best evaluated by determining the sensory level utilizing pinprick, beginning in an anesthetic area and extending upward to the area in which sensation is perceived. Do not forget to examine sensation in the arm and hand beginning with the lower dermatome in the axilla (T2) and ending with the higher dermatome over the deltoid (C4).
6. If paralysis or cervical fracture is not present, muscle function should be assessed by testing the ability of the patient to perform antigravity movements in the legs and by testing the strength of elbow flexion and extension, wrist extension, grip, and finger extension.
7. Deep tendon reflexes should be tested; in the acute phase these reflexes may be diminished or absent (spinal shock).
8. An accurate history of the details surrounding the injury should be obtained as soon as possible. The history is most reliable immediately after the injury.
9. The patient should be examined carefully for associated injuries, especially fractures of the long bones, rupture of abdominal organs, and injury to the chest or lungs.

Remember: The patient with paralysis and sensory loss may not be able to feel the pain of a broken bone or ruptured viscus below the level of the lesion.

10. Radiographic examination should be performed after the patient's vital functions have been stabilized.
    a. If the patient has paralysis from a cervical spine injury, a single good lateral radiograph will usually re-

veal the pathologic changes. In order to visualize adequately *all cervical vertebrae and the top of the first thoracic vertebra,* the shoulders must be depressed by pulling the arms toward the feet during the process of taking the radiograph. If the radiograph is normal but a neurologic deficit is present, a computed tomography (CT) scan or myelogram is indicated.

b. If the patient does not have paralysis or neurologic dysfunction, lateral views as described previously and AP cervical spine radiographs should be obtained. Views of the odontoid (through the mouth) are important to rule out a fracture through the base of the odontoid. If no fracture is demonstrated, then oblique views, flexion-extension views, and occasionally tomograms or CT scan should be done to evaluate suspicious areas.

B.   Treatment.

1. For the patient with paralysis or severe spinal fracture, referral to an appropriate specialist is indicated. The patient should always be transported with the neck immobilized, preferably in head-halter traction.

   Note: Beneficial effects have been reported with a regimen of continuous high-dose intravenous methylprednisolone started within 8 hours of the injury.

2. The patient having cervical pain with no fractures or neurologic deficit probably has neck strain or sprain. Such a patient should be treated with:

   a. Bed rest with the patient lying flat with the neck flexed 30 degrees; the neck should be stretched using head-halter traction with no more than 1.5 kg of weight.

   b. Treat the pain with medication on demand and a muscle relaxant around the clock (combination of diazepam 2–5 mg with aspirin 650 mg tid may be effective).

   c. During the ambulatory phase, the patient's neck can be supported with a soft, wraparound cervical collar.

      d. Remove the collar after 1 to 2 weeks and begin an intensive program of physical therapy consisting of heat, massage, and range-of-motion exercises to restore mobility to the cervical spine.

IV.   **TUMOR.**

A.   Tumors of the cervical spine may be primary bone tumors, primary intraspinal tumors, or secondary tumors such as multiple myeloma, lymphoma, or metastatic carcinoma (common primary sources include breast, prostate, lungs, and kidneys). Spinal cord damage may occur either from compression by metastatic tumor in the epidural space (more commonly) or by direct invasion of spinal cord parenchyma.

  ▶ 1. *The most important diagnostic clue* is a relentless progression of pain or neurologic deficit (as opposed to static or intermittent pain noted with other causes).

    2. Initial symptoms may vary with the location of the tumor:

      a. A bone tumor (tumor involving the vertebrae) usually presents with neck pain later progressing to radicular pain (pain in the arm).

      b. A neoplasm within the spinal canal may present with progressive neurologic deficit and radicular pain (pain extending into the arm) or Lhermitte's sign.

    3. The examination may show:

      a. A stiffly held neck.

      b. Palpable masses, commonly in the posterior triangle or over the paraspinal areas.

      c. Areas of focal tenderness over the cervical spine.

      d. Fasciculations and atrophy of muscles of the upper extremities with hyperactive tendon reflexes in the lower extremities and Babinski reflexes suggest compression of the spinal cord by an extrinsic or intrinsic tumor (Table 18–2).

    4. Cervical spine radiographs may be negative (with tumors growing within the spinal cord itself) or may show destruction (as a result of bony or metastatic tumors) or erosion (from pressure effects by intraspinal tumors).

    5. CT scan with contrast or magnetic resonance imaging (MRI) is mandatory in a patient with suspected spinal tumor.

TABLE 18–2.
Differential Diagnosis of Combination of Atrophy of Arm Muscles and Spasticity of Legs

Disorder	Age of Onset	Diagnostic Features	
		Clinical	Investigative
Spondylitic myelopathy	>50	Progressive spasticity and sensory ataxia with fasciculations restricted to one or two myotomes in the upper extremities	Spondylitic changes often with narrowing of foramina or spinal canal on plain radiographs, CT scan, MRI, or myelography
Amyotrophic lateral sclerosis (ALS)	>40	Generalized fasciculations (including bulbar muscles) with hyperactive tendon reflexes even in atrophic muscles and lack of sensory symptoms or signs	Normal radiographs, CT scan, and myelogram; electromyelogram (EMG) findings diagnostic
Cervical syringomyelia	<40	Dissociated sensory loss (absent pain and thermal sensation with intact touch) in the upper extremities and trunk with sacral sparing; fasciculations limited to a few myotomes of upper extremities	Widening of cord on myelogram and CT scan; best seen on MRI
Extramedullary tumor	Any age	Radicular pain and paresthesia, with loss of touch and pain below the level of compression	Typical appearance on myelogram; CT scan and MRI valuable

6. Bone scan is often helpful in identifying abnormalities, especially when multiple metastatic lesions are suspected.

7. Primary neoplasms of the cervical spine have no characteristic laboratory abnormalities, but secondary neoplasms may exhibit laboratory findings of malignancy such as anemia, elevated erythrocyte sedimentation rate (ESR), and elevation of serum alkaline or acid phosphatase.

B.   Treatment.

1. Acute or subacute signs of spinal cord compression constitute a neurologic emergency. Immediate referral to an appropriate specialist is necessary if the diagnosis is suspected. A cerebrospinal fluid (CSF) sample should be obtained if contrast material is injected into the subarachnoid space.

   Caveat: If bone erosion is present, support the neck in a collar (preferably a Philadelphia hard collar).

2. Immediate management of spinal cord compression from a metastatic lesion consists of dexamethasone 100 mg intravenously (IV) immediately followed by 24 mg qid for 3 days, and then 20 mg for 3 days.

V.   PROTRUDED CERVICAL DISC.
A.   Clinical features.

▶ 1. *The most important diagnostic clue* is the patient frequently awakening with pain in the neck followed within hours or days by development of pain radiating in the distribution of the affected nerve root. (This is in contrast to tumor in which there is a longer duration of cervical pain prior to radicular involvement.)

2. A protruded cervical disc may present with or without a history of trauma.

3. The pain is usually aggravated by the patient's assuming an upright position and is often relieved by lying supine with the arm abducted at the shoulder.

4. The Valsalva maneuver often exacerbates the pain.

B.   Examination.
   1. Examination may show:
      a. Limitation of range of neck motion.
      b. Positive Spurling's maneuver.
      c. Neurologic deficits in the distribution of the affected nerve root. About 80% of all ruptured cervical discs compress either the C6 or C7 nerve roots. The salient features are given in Table 18–1 and in Figures 18–7 and 18–8.
   2. Cervical spine radiographs may show narrowing of the

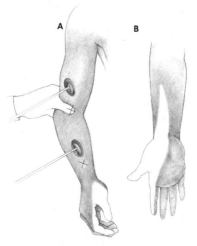

FIG 18–7. C6 root lesion: The sensory disturbance is primarily over the thumb and the lateral aspect of the index finger (**A**); this sensory disturbance is most easily appreciated on the palmar surface of the hand. Decreased biceps and brachioradialis reflexes (**B**) and weak flexion of the elbow (**C**) and weak extension of the wrist (**D**) may also be present.

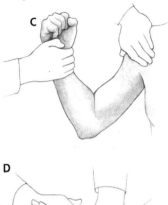

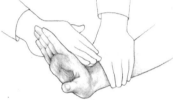

FIG 18-7 (cont.).

intervertebral disc space at the site of disc protrusion. The oblique views (which should be done in all patients) may show encroachment on the intervertebral foramen.

3. CT scan with contrast or MRI is valuable for demonstrating narrowing of the intervertebral foramen and disc protrusions.

4. EMG provides objective evidence of denervation and identifies the ventral root or roots that are affected.

C. **Treatment.**

1. Cervical traction is an effective treatment for protruded cervical disc with or without mild neurologic deficits:

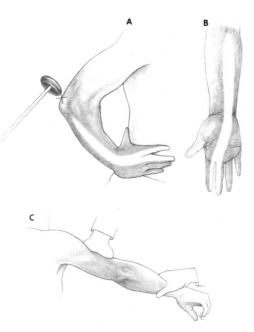

FIG 18–8. C7 root lesion: The sensory disturbance occurs in the index and middle fingers (**A**) and this is also most easily appreciated on the palmar surface of the hand. A decreased triceps reflex (**B**) and weak extension of the elbow (**C**) may also be present.

    a. If the patient is in bed, the head should be in a head halter and the neck flexed 30 degrees (Fig 18–9).
    b. Traction should be applied continuously. More than 1.5 kg of weight often is irritating to the jaw.
  2. Once the patient has improved, upright traction may be used intermittently. An over-the-door head-halter traction apparatus using 5 to 7 kg of weight for a period of 20 minutes two or three times daily (Fig 18–10) is often effective. However, staring at a blank door does not

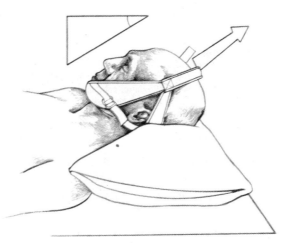

FIG 18–9. Cervical traction in the supine position: the direction of pull is 30 degrees upward from the horizontal.

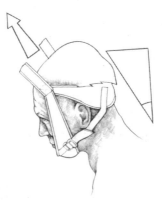

FIG 18–10. Cervical traction in the sitting position: note the head is flexed 30 degrees, and the direction of pull is 30 degrees from the vertical.

promote compliance, and we suggest modification of the over-the-door traction (Fig 3–1).

3. High-dose aspirin (at least two 325-mg tablets every 4 hours) usually will control pain and relieve inflammation. Other nonsteroidal anti-inflammatory drugs may be used instead.

4. For very severe pain, a short course of corticosteroids (such as dexamethasone in the Decadron Dose PAK) is often effective.

5. Persistent or progressive neurologic deficit indicates the need for neurosurgical evaluation.

VI.   INFLAMMATION AND INFECTION.

A.   **Inflammation and infection** typically occur with rheumatoid arthritis or spondylitis, hypertrophic osteoarthritis, gouty arthritis, disc space infection, tuberculosis, or Paget's disease.

▶ 1. *The most important diagnostic clue* is an insidious onset with exacerbations and remissions, although acute disc space infection may have a rapid onset with no remissions. The history of exacerbations and remissions helps to differentiate chronic inflammation from tumor.

2. The patient experiences a feeling of general stiffness aggravated by movement and by maintaining one position for a long period ("jelling effect"), such as after spending the night in bed, and pain that may be worse in the late afternoon or evening, especially after an active day.

3. Radicular symptoms are rare, but the pain may extend into the trapezius muscles.

4. There may be a history of related pain in other joints.

5. Examination shows:

   a. Stiffly held neck and evidence of pain on extremes of motion in all directions.

   b. Tightness but not spasm in the cervical, occipital, and trapezius muscles.

   c. Normal reflexes, muscle strength, and sensation.

6. In the early phases, cervical spine radiographs may be normal. In the late stages, degeneration of the intervertebral discs and facet joints becomes apparent. In tuberculosis of the spine there is often collapse of adjacent vertebrae.

7. The ESR may be an important diagnostic clue, but an elevated ESR is not diagnostic, and a normal ESR does not exclude certain inflammatory processes such as gouty arthritis or Paget's disease.

8. Other valuable studies for inflammatory disease include a complete blood count (CBC), rheumatoid factor testing, antinuclear antibody studies, serum uric acid levels, serum calcium and serum alkaline phosphatase determinations, *Brucella* agglutination tests, and tuberculosis skin tests.

9. Treatment.

   a. Specific treatment for the underlying inflammatory process is necessary.

   b. In acute disc space infection, immobilization of the cervical spine is mandatory. The patient should be in bed with head-halter traction until infection has subsided, then placed in a halo brace or Philadelphia hard collar. In tuberculosis of the spine, apart from immobilization, appropriate antibiotic treatment is instituted. Surgical treatment is needed if there is spinal cord compression.

   c. In inflammatory arthritis, physical therapy such as diathermy and ultrasound, anti-inflammatory drugs, and temporary immobilization with a soft cervical collar may relieve the pain.

VII. STRUCTURAL BONY ABNORMALITIES.

A. **Structural bony abnormalities** typically include degenerative arthritis, osteoporosis, facet asymmetry, nonunion of the odontoid, absence of bony structure, Klippel-Feil disease, and spinal canal stenosis (cervical spondylosis or cervical bars).

1. Cervical spondylosis. Cervical spondylosis is a degenerative process involving the cervical spine and constitutes a common cause of cervical pain. The degenerative changes begin in the intervertebral space, leading to narrowing of the disc space, and protrusion of the disc with calcification and bar formation at multiple levels, most prominently at the C4–5, C5—6, and C6–7 levels. The clinical features are as follows:

▶ a. *The most important diagnostic clue* is the occurrence of chronic, nagging, centrally located cervical pain, which may radiate to the occipital areas, arms, or chest; the pain is least troublesome on arising from bed, but increases with activity during the day. Recurrent episodes of neck pain with limitation of neck movement and bouts of upper extremity, infrascapular, or shoulder pain are characteristic.

b. Onset is usually after age 50 years.

c. The symptoms are of relatively long duration (there may be a history of injury preceding the onset of symptoms).

d. With spinal canal stenosis, the patient describes progressive weakness and wasting of muscles of the arms with a feeling of stiffness and difficulty in controlling movements of the legs.

e. Dizzy spells related to neck rotation may occur in those patients in whom the degenerative changes encroach on the vertebral artery foramen.

f. Dysphagia may occur with anterior bars compressing the esophagus.

g. Minor neck trauma may precipitate major neurologic deficit in patients with cervical spondylosis, particularly when there is significant narrowing of the spinal canal.

h. Physical findings:

  1) Cervical muscle spasm and limitation of neck movement.

  2) When radiculopathy is the main feature, signs of nerve root compression are seen.

  3) When there is an accompanying spinal cord involvement (spondylitic myelopathy) due to compression by bony bars or ischemia, the patient may show muscle atrophy, fasciculations, and decreased tendon reflexes in the upper extremities with hyperreflexia, spasticity, and Babinski reflexes (extensor plantar responses) in the lower extremities. Myelopathy occurs more often when there is a spinal canal stenosis. The differential diagnoses of spondylitic myelopathy include

amyotrophic lateral sclerosis (ALS), syringomyelia, and extramedullary compression (see Table
18–2).

   i. EMG studies are often necessary to distinguish between spondylitic myelopathy and ALS.

   j. Investigations:

      1) Radiographs of the cervical spine will reveal
bars, narrowing of foramina, and the extent of
narrowing of the spinal canal.

      2) CT scan with contrast or MRI clearly demon-
strates spinal stenosis with spinal cord compression, nerve root entrapment, and osteophytes.

   k. Treatment.

      1) Treatment must at first be conservative except
when progressive neurologic deficit occurs. During the acute phase analgesics and muscle relaxants are given. A combination of aspirin (650
mg) and diazepam (5 mg) may be useful.

      2) A soft cervical collar to limit neck movements
may be helpful in the acute phase.

      3) Surgical management (decompression of roots
and spinal cord) is indicated in patients with persistent radicular pain or increasing neurologic
deficit.

VIII. MENINGEAL IRRITATION.

A. **Meningeal irritation** typically occurs with hemorrhage or
infection in the subarachnoid space.

   1. The symptoms of cervical pain begin acutely or sub-
acutely.

   2. The pain is associated with nonthrobbing occipital headache.

   3. The patient complains of stiffness of the neck and a
pulling sensation in the lower back with forward flexion of the neck.

   4. Examination shows:

      a. An ill-appearing patient.

      b. Hyperextension of the neck.

      c. Guarding of the neck against forward flexion. Flex-
ion increases the cervical pain and may produce pain
between the scapulae.

d. No aggravation of pain with rotatory neck movements.

e. An elevated temperature.

f. Kernig's and Brudzinski's signs (See Figs 14–1 and 14–2).

5. Patients with either hemorrhage or infection in the subarachnoid space may show elevation of the peripheral white blood cell count with a shift to the left.

6. Abnormal CSF often confirms the diagnosis (be sure to culture the CSF).

B.   Treatment.

1. Appropriate antibiotic therapy in the case of meningitis (see Chapter 14).

2. Treat subarachnoid hemorrhage with analgesics, and sedation if necessary, limiting visitors, and enforcing absolute bed rest with no bathroom privileges. Neurosurgical consultation is indicated.

IX.   ENTRAPMENT OF THE GREATER OCCIPITAL NERVE.

A.   The C-2 nerve root is almost wholly sensory and after exiting the intervertebral foramen becomes the greater occipital nerve which innervates the scalp. Common causes of irritation include cervical muscle spasm from emotional stress and work-related circumstances (such as a secretary holding the head in a fixed position while working at a word processor for a prolonged period of time), whiplash injuries, and osteoarthritis.

1. Pain radiates to the sternocleidomastoid muscles, the occiput, and over the top of the forehead.

2. Because the condition is chronic and responds poorly to treatment, the patient often is anxious, despondent, angry, or hostile.

3. Examination shows:

a. Tense and tender paracervical and trapezius muscles.

b. Resistance to passive movement of the neck in all directions.

c. Tenderness to percussion in the high cervical area and altered sensation in the scalp.

> *Caveat:* Do not be misled by nonspecific laboratory and radiographic findings. Cervical spine films in most patients over age 40 years show some degenerative changes.

B. Treatment.
1. Cervical traction and aspirin or other nonsteroidal antiinflammatory medication should be tried first.
2. Injection of corticosteroids and anesthetics into the occipital area may provide immediate but transient relief.
3. Simple measures such as courses in stress reduction, altering placement of the word processor up and down and right and left at regular intervals, and heat and massage to the cervical area often make the symptoms tolerable.
4. For extremely severe chronic pain, surgical sectioning of the greater occipital nerve may be considered.

BIBLIOGRAPHY

Bracken MB, et al: A randomized controlled trial of methylprednisolone or naloxone in the treatment of acute spinal cord injury. Results of the second national acute spinal cord injury study. *N Engl J Med* 1991; 322:1405–1411.

Brain WR, Baron J, Wilkinson M: *Cervical Spondylosis and Other Disorders of the Cervical Spine.* Philadelphia, WB Saunders, 1976.

Caillied R: *Neck Arm Pain,* ed 3. Philadelphia, FA Davis, 1991.

Hoppenfeld S: *Orthopedic Neurology: A Diagnostic Guide to Neurologic Levels.* Philadelphia, JB Lippincott, 1977.

Jenkins DG: Differential diagnosis and management of neck pain. *Physiotherapy* 1982; 68:252–255.

Patchell RA, Posner JB: Neurologic complications of systemic cancer. *Neurol Clin* 1985; 3:729–750.

Schmidek HH: Cervical spondylosis. *Am Fam Physician* 1986; 33:89–99.

Walker MD: Acute spinal cord injury. *N Engl J Med* 1991; 324:1885–1887.

THE PATIENT WITH A HEAD INJURY

19

Head trauma is the most common cause of brain damage in the young adult and the leading cause of death under age 24 years. Some of this damage is avoidable if prompt management is undertaken soon after the injury. However, many physicians feel apprehensive and insecure in managing the unconscious head-injured patient. This chapter outlines the initial evaluation and treatment, which should be carried out before transfer to a tertiary care center.

Remember: Evaluation and management of the patient must be carried out simultaneously.

I. ACUTE MANAGEMENT OF THE HEAD-INJURED PATIENT.

A. **Following a head injury,** the patient may present to the emergency room in an alert state or arrive in a state of coma. While the alert patient will need only a computed tomography (CT) scan and careful observation, the comatose patient needs urgent measures.

  1. Initial management.

    Caveat: Potentially reversible lesions may become permanent secondary to hypoxia and hypotension.

    a. Stabilizing vital functions.

      1) A good airway and adequate blood oxygenation must be maintained.

        a) Insert an oropharyngeal airway; suction adequately to remove secretions. Insert an endotracheal tube if the patient is comatose. It is important to do this procedure rapidly and without causing any distress since even short periods of hypoxia and hypercarbia may increase the brain edema and initiate herniation. A tracheostomy is needed urgently only in cases of severe maxillofacial and neck injuries.

b) In the patient with respiratory distress, for whatever reason, oxygen in high concentration must be administered.

Note: Prompt endotracheal intubation and hyperventilation sufficient to drop partial pressure of arterial carbon dioxide ($PaCO_2$) to less than 28 mm Hg (torr) may have contributed to the decreasing morbidity and mortality following head injury.

2) Circulatory stability must be maintained.

Note: Head trauma does not cause hypotension, but head trauma may cause bradycardia and hypertension (Cushing's reflex).

a) Intravenous (IV) fluids should be held to a minimum in patients with cerebral edema or possible brain herniation.

b) The patient with a low blood pressure and rapid pulse may have reduced circulating blood volume (blood loss). The source of hemorrhage may not be apparent since the comatose patient cannot complain of pain or exhibit typical signs of bleeding (e.g., rigidity of abdominal wall with intraperitoneal hemorrhage). An IV line must be established and treatment aimed at maintaining adequate cerebral circulation by replacing blood loss and administering vasoconstrictors. A hemogram and type and crossmatch should be obtained as soon as possible. Partial pressures of oxygen (PaO_2) and carbon dioxide ($PaCO_2$) should be carefully monitored.

2. Immediate management.
    a. Once the vital functions are stabilized, there must be an ongoing determination of the level of consciousness and neurologic function (refer to Chapter 13, section I. A) by determining:
        1) The level of consciousness: The most important criterion in the initial evaluation and follow-up of patients with head injury is the level of consciousness. The Glasgow Coma Scale (based on eye opening, best motor response, and verbal response; see Table 13–1) is simple enough for repeated recording by nurses, paramedical personnel, and physicians and has been shown to provide a reliable indication of prognosis. In one study 87% of patients with a score of more than 11 in the first 24 hours had good recovery, while 87% of those with scores of less than 5 remained in a vegetative state or were dead.
        2) Pupillary size and reaction to light are highly useful in detecting impending herniation. With uncal herniation through the tentorial notch, the ipsilateral pupil dilates, and becomes poorly reactive to light, followed by similar changes in the contralateral pupil. In a large study, 50% of patients with intact pupillary reaction made good recovery while 91% with nonreactive pupils (in the first 24 hours after coma) either died or remained in a vegetative state.
        3) Any focal deficit as evidenced by asymmetry of tendon reflexes or plantar response or movements in response to painful stimulation.
    b. An indwelling urinary catheter should be inserted to obtain a urine specimen for analysis, to evaluate urinary output, and to avoid overdistention of the bladder.
    c. Insert a nasogastric tube attached to suction to prevent abdominal distention and vomiting.
    d. Hyperthermia should be treated by placing the patient on a cooling blanket or by applying ice water and alcohol to the skin.
    e. Seizures should be controlled with IV anticonvulsants (see Chapter 11, section IX).
    f. Extreme restlessness may be treated with lorazepam (Ativan) 1 to 5 mg q2h.

Caveat: The most important clinical criterion in a comatose patient is the level of consciousness; it is not
possible to assess this properly if sedatives are administered to the patient. Hence, never use morphine, and
give sedatives only sparingly to a patient with head injury.

g. Rapidly appraise associated injuries to identify intrathoracic or intraabdominal hemorrhage, fractures, or lacerations with excessive blood loss. Appropriate management of such problems must be instituted immediately.

h. It is not sufficient to assume that the unconsciousness
has resulted solely from the head injury. It may be the
result of shock, alcohol or drug intoxication, adrenal
insufficiency, stroke, diabetic acidosis, insulin shock,
or other metabolic disturbances (see Chapter 13). Do
the relevant blood studies.

i. Elevating the patient's head by 30 degrees can aid in
reducing intracranial pressure.

j. As soon as the vital signs are stable all patients with
severe head injury should undergo CT scan of the head
and radiographs of the skull.

(Note: Fractures clearly evident on one study may not
be readily apparent on the other.)

Radiographs of the spine, chest, abdomen, or other areas should be done depending on the clinical presentation. In a comatose patient, fractures of the extremities
or pelvis can be easily missed since the patient will not
complain of pain.

Caveat: Always suspect a cervical spine injury until
excluded by lateral cervical spine radiographs (see
Chapter 18, section III. A. 10).

k. A description of the nature and mechanism of injury
from any available sources of information should be obtained. Appropriate consultations with neurosurgery,
general surgery, cardiopulmonary surgery, or orthopedic surgery staff should be requested as the need for

specialized care is identified. Transfer to a specialized center may be necessary.

3. When the patient's condition has been stabilized, a more complete neurologic examination should be performed (see Chapter 13, section I. B). This examination should include the following:

   a. State of consciousness.

   b. Respirations: Slow, deep, or irregular respirations suggest serious intracranial abnormalities, while shallow and rapid respirations are more commonly associated with pathologic changes extrinsic to the nervous system, such as shock related to blood loss.

   c. The degree of paresis of extremities: Early complete flaccid paralysis occurring unilaterally suggests marked damage to the opposite cerebral hemisphere, while spasticity of all four extremities suggests severe brainstem or cervical spinal cord injury.

   d. The presence of peripheral cranial nerve palsies is suggestive of a basilar skull fracture.

   e. Spinal fluid draining from the ear or nose is diagnostic of a skull fracture.

   Caveat: Basilar skull fractures may be missed on routine CT scans or skull radiographs.

II. CLASSIFICATION AND MANAGEMENT OF CRANIAL INJURY (Table 19–1).

A. Injuries to the scalp.

1. Abrasions should be treated by careful cleaning with soap and sterile water; hair need not be removed; particles embedded in the scalp should be removed with a surgical brush to avoid the tattoo effect of retained particles. The area may be left either exposed to the air or covered with a sterile nonadherent dressing.

2. Contusions (bruises) may be treated by cold compresses.

3. Lacerations should be closed by suturing after the hair has been shaved from around the area and the area has been carefully cleaned. If a laceration extends through the galea, it is desirable to close the galea with absorbable suture *separately* from the closure of the skin.

TABLE 19–1.
Risk Groups of Patients With Head Trauma

Risk Group	Clinical Features
Low	Asymptomatic
	Dizziness
	Headache
	Scalp hematoma, laceration, contusion, or abrasion
	No moderate-risk or high-risk criteria
Moderate	Alteration in level of consciousness either at time of injury or later
	Amnesia
	Basilar skull fracture
	Drug abuse or alcohol intoxication
	Multiple trauma or facial injuries
	Possible depressed or compound skull fracture
	Posttraumatic seizure or vomiting
	Progressive headache
	Unreliable or inadequate history of injury
High	Depressed or compound skull fracture
	Focal neurologic signs
	Stupor or coma (not due to alcohol, drugs, metabolic disorder, or seizures)

4. Avulsions constitute a serious problem and in all cases the avulsed scalp should be preserved in normal saline. Microvascular surgical anastomoses of the vessels to restore circulation to the avulsed tissue are necessary.

B. Injuries to the skull.

1. Linear skull fractures (particularly if they occur in the base of the skull) are often difficult to identify on routine skull radiographs and may be confused with vascular markings or suture lines. Skull fractures should be suspected when there is:

   a. Blood behind the eardrum or Battle's sign (black-and-blue discoloration over the mastoid) suggests a basilar skull fracture.

   b. Raccoon eyes (ecchymoses around the eyelids) suggest a frontal skull fracture.

2. Stereoscopic radiographs of the skull are the most helpful studies for evaluating linear skull fractures. Obtaining skull

films in minor head trauma may not be necessary, but remember that skull fractures can occur without loss of consciousness. A patient with a skull fracture that crosses a venous sinus or a branch of a meningeal artery should be hospitalized and observed with hourly cranial checks for 24 hours (see Chapter 12, section VI, A. 1).

3. A patient with a compound comminuted skull fracture should be treated with debridement and neurosurgical reconstruction.

4. Depressed skull fractures should be surgically elevated.

C. **Injuries to the dura and leptomeninges.**

1. Injuries to the dura and leptomeninges are usually associated with a skull fracture.

2. An injury to the dura and leptomeninges over the paranasal sinuses or mastoid allows admission of air and infection to the intracranial contents and escape of cerebrospinal fluid (CSF). Unless contraindicated for other reasons, patients with CSF leakage should be placed in a position with the head elevated to a 45-degree angle. This minimizes retrograde infection into the cranial cavity and encourages tamponade of the brain into the fistula tract. Prophylactic use of a broad-spectrum antibiotic in a therapeutic dose should be considered. Watch for signs of meningitis (see Chapter 14). The patient should be instructed to avoid blowing the nose. Neurosurgical consultation is advisable.

3. Intracranial hemorrhage may occur in skull fractures with meningeal involvement from injury to the blood vessels:

   a. *Extradural (epidural) hematoma* (bleeding from damage to a dural artery, most commonly the middle meningeal artery):

      1) Progressive drowsiness may follow a lucid interval, or the patient may remain unconscious from the time of the initial trauma.

      2) Progressive headache may be a presenting symptom.

      3) A dilating pupil on the side of the hemorrhage is highly suggestive of extradural hemorrhage (due to herniation).

      4) A hemiparesis opposite to the side of the hemorrhage may be present.

5) A focal motor seizure in the extremities opposite the side of the hemorrhage may occur.

6) A slowing of the pulse and respirations and an increase in blood pressure are late and ominous signs. Progressive hemiparesis occurring on the same side as the dilated pupils suggests brainstem involvement and indicates a grave prognosis.

Caveat: This condition represents one of the most acute of all emergencies. Prompt neurosurgical evacuation of the clot usually results in complete functional recovery; delayed intervention results in permanent brain damage or death. If a diagnosis extradural hematoma is suspected, immediate neurosurgical consultation is indicated. The diagnosis can be confirmed by CT scan or magnetic resonance imaging (MRI).

b. *Acute subdural hematoma* usually results from damage to the venous sinuses or to the veins communicating between the cortex and the venous sinuses. Patients may show a variety of neurologic findings such as seizures, progressive deepening coma, progressive headache, progressive hemiparesis, confusional state, and signs of increased intracranial pressure.

Caveat: Although the progressive deterioration in the patient with acute subdural hematoma is not usually as rapid as that in extradural hematoma, prompt neurosurgical treatment is still necessary. As with extradural hematoma, the diagnosis can be confirmed by CT scan or MRI.

D. Injuries to the brain.

1. *Cerebral concussion* may be defined as a temporary impairment of cerebral neuronal function resulting from a blow to the head and may be divided into the following categories:

   a. Mild concussion—impaired neurologic function lasting less than 5 minutes.

   b. Moderate concussion—impaired neurologic function lasting more than 5 minutes but less than 3 hours.

    c. Severe concussion—impaired neurologic function lasting more than 3 hours.
2. There are no demonstrable structural abnormalities in cerebral concussion. Patients with concussion recover completely, although sometimes a postconcussional syndrome consisting of headache, dizziness, and personality changes may occur.
3. Treatment.
    a. The patient with either mild or moderate cerebral concussion can be managed at home if someone is available to observe the patient's responsiveness, pupillary size, and ability to move the extremities on an hourly basis for 24 hours.
    b. If the patient is hospitalized, hourly evaluation of the level of consciousness and the pupillary reactions should be performed (see Chapter 12, section VI. A. 1).
4. *Cerebral contusion* is an impairment of neuronal function resulting from structural damage ("bruised brain"). Focal contusions occur under the site of impact or more often in the undersurface of the frontal or the anterior part of the temporal lobes from impact against the lesser wing of the sphenoid (the lesser wing of the sphenoid has been called the "dashboard" of the cranial cavity). Clinical findings include focal neurologic abnormalities and loss of consciousness.
    a. Treatment: The patient should be hospitalized with at least hourly neurologic evaluations (see Chapter 12, section VI. A. 1) during the acute phase. Supportive care should be provided based on the degree of neurologic impairment.

    Note: For medical, legal, and prognostic purposes, concussion and contusion may be differentiated by CT scan or MRI and serial electroencephalograms (EEGs). In the case of cerebral concussion, the EEGs show only temporary changes, whereas in the case of cerebral contusion, they show persistent abnormalities. CT scan or MRI usually shows blood at the site of a cerebral contusion and is normal with a concussion.

5. *Cerebral lacerations* are secondary to depressed skull fractures or penetrating wounds.

a. Treatment: Lacerations require immediate (within 6 hours) neurosurgical treatment. Emergency management should include control of hemorrhage from the scalp at the site of the injury and application of a sterile dressing. Accompanying scalp lacerations should not be sutured until after neurosurgical reconstruction has been performed.

6. *Traumatic subarachnoid hemorrhage* should be suspected when the patient presents with headache and stiff neck with or without other neurologic signs. Subarachnoid hemorrhage may also be present in the patient with coma and stiff neck. The diagnosis can be confirmed by CT scan or MRI.

a. Treatment: Support of vital functions, elevation of the head to approximately 30 degrees, and careful observation with at least hourly neurologic evaluations (see Chapter 12, section VI. A. 1) are required. Lumbar puncture should be deferred for 72 hours or longer if the patient is unstable. Symptomatic improvement may be obtained by removal of bloody CSF with repeated lumbar punctures. CSF will be xanthochromic and under elevated pressure. The amount of fluid removed should only be the volume necessary to reduce the spinal fluid pressure to one half of the initial reading.

7. *Traumatic intracerebral hematoma* is suggested by increased intracranial pressure, progressive focal neurologic deficits, and a deteriorating state of consciousness. The presence of blood can be readily demonstrated by CT scan or MRI. Neurosurgical consultation is indicated.

III. COMMON COMPLICATIONS.

A. **Increased intracranial pressure.** Increased intracranial pressure following head trauma is common. It may be due to simple causes such as airway obstruction with accompanying hypoxia and hypercarbia, or the presence of an intracranial hematoma, or sometimes no specific cause is demonstrable on CT scan or MRI. Edema of the brain following injury may account for the increased pressure.

1. Treatment: Increased intracranial pressure has a deleterious effect on the outcome, and prompt treatment should be undertaken depending on the cause. It is common practice now to monitor the intracranial pressure using an epidural, subdural, or intraventricular pressure monitor. Such procedures can be done only in a neurosurgical unit. The measures used in such centers include:
   a. Hyperventilation: Hyperventilation is an effective way of reducing intracranial pressure rapidly. The ventilatory rate should be adjusted such that the $PaCO_2$ is around less than 28 mm Hg (torr). The effect achieved on intracranial pressure is by reduced intracranial blood volume and perhaps by decreased CSF formation.

      Caveat: Lowering the $PaCO_2$ below 25 mm Hg (torr) may result in areas of cerebral ischemia.

   b. Infusion of hyperosmolar agents such as 20% mannitol: Use only after neurosurgical consultation unless the patient is in a state of impending herniation.
   c. Corticosteroids: There is no consensus as to the efficacy of corticosteroids in posttraumatic cerebral edema.
   d. In children with posttraumatic cerebral edema (with no surgically treatable cause), induction of barbiturate coma is undertaken in some centers.
B. **Posttraumatic epilepsy.** While seizures may occur early in the course of a head injury, late posttraumatic epilepsy is one of the most frequent delayed complications. It occurs in about 5% of all patients admitted to hospitals after nonmissile head injury. The risk of epilepsy is higher when there has been intracranial hematoma or a compound depressed skull fracture or when there has been an early seizure (in the first week after injury). The onset is most common during the first 2 years although it has been reported even after 10 years.
   1. Treatment: See Chapter 11.
C. **Postconcussional syndrome.**
   1. Following head trauma, 30% to 80% of patients have been reported to develop one or more of the following symptoms:

      a. Chronic posttraumatic headache: a constant, dull, non-throbbing headache often described as a tight band around the head, sometimes associated with local area of tenderness or pain, especially if a scar is present; rarely intermittent throbbing headaches may also occur. May last for several weeks to months or sometimes years.

      b. Dizziness, either intermittent or chronic, may be a major symptom (see Chapter 4, section I).

      c. Amnesia, poor concentration, and learning difficulties in children.

      d. Emotional lability: irritability, aggressiveness, and hyperkinesis.

2. The syndrome may occur following open and closed head trauma. There is no consistent correlation with duration of unconsciousness, posttraumatic amnesia, skull fracture, or blood in the CSF.

3. Preexisting psychiatric problems (e.g., depression) and pending litigation are believed to be predisposing factors.

4. Treatment: Amitriptyline hydrochloride 50 to 100 mg daily over a period of several weeks to months has been found to be effective, especially for the chronic posttraumatic headache. Reassure the patient and, if necessary, institute psychotherapy.

BIBLIOGRAPHY

Changaris DG, et al: Correlation of cerebral perfusion pressure and Glasgow Coma Scale to outcome. *J Trauma* 1987; 27:1007–1013.

Jennett B, Teasdale G: *Management of Head Injuries*. Philadelphia, FA Davis, 1981.

Master SJ, McClean PM, Arcarese MS, et al: Skull x-ray examinations after head injury: Recommendations by a multidisciplinary panel and validation study. *N Engl J Med* 1987; 316:84–91.

Muizelaru JR, Marmarou A, Ward JD, et al: Adverse effects of prolonged hyperventilation in patients with severe head injury: A randomized clinical trial. *J Neurosurg* 1991; 75:731–739.

Vogel HB: Trauma of the head, spine and peripheral nerves, in Earnest MP (ed): *Neurologic Emergencies,* New York, Churchill Livingstone, 1983, pp 177–217.

White RJ, Likvec MJ: The diagnosis and initial management of head injury. *N Eng J Med* 1992; 327:1507–1511.

NEUROLOGIC EMERGENCIES

20

The word *emergency* is used to mean those conditions which, if not treated immediately, may result in death or permanent nervous system damage. There are conditions, such as the excruciating pain of trigeminal neuralgia, that may require immediate treatment but which are not included here because lack of treatment will not result in permanent damage. What is "neurologic" is also open to discussion; delirium tremens, threat of suicide, and acute glaucoma are ordinarily not considered neurologic problems, although clearly they are emergencies and if untreated may lead to permanent nervous system damage. Table 20–1 lists neurologic conditions that we consider emergencies with a brief statement of just why we consider them so. The remainder of this chapter is devoted to evaluation of symptoms we consider emergencies.

I.   COMA (see Chapter 13 for examination, differential diagnosis, and management).
A.   Immediate measures for all comatose patients include the following:
     1. Determine the need for cardiopulmonary resuscitation (CPR).
     2. Stabilize the patient:
        a. Establish and maintain a clear airway; provide ventilatory assistance, if necessary.
        b. Establish access to the circulation with an intravenous (IV) line, drawing blood at the same time for hematology and biochemistry tests.
        c. Maintain blood pressure by elevation of legs and ad-

TABLE 20–1.
Neurologic Conditions Considered to be Emergencies

Process	Reason for Emergency
Coma	Many causes of coma such as drug overdose, hypoglycemia, or expanding cerebral mass may cause irreversible brain damage if not treated immediately
Transient ischemic attacks	Cause of attacks may be treatable (e.g., embolus); untreated, permanent brain damage may occur
Stroke	Cause of paralysis could be reversible, such as a subdural hematoma, instead of the overused diagnosis of intracerebral atherosclerosis
Bacterial meningitis	Delayed treatment results in irreversible brain damage or death
Spinal cord compression	Unless pressure on the cord is relieved within a few hours, permanent paralysis will result
Status epilepticus	Prolonged seizures may result in brain damage or death
Fracture of the spinal column	Inappropriate movement of the patient may permanently sever the spinal cord
Thiamine deficiency	Delayed treatment results in an irreversible organic brain syndrome
Temporal arteritis	The process may spread to intracranial arteries and cause cerebral infarction or blindness
Severe muscle spasms	These are usually caused by severe hypoglycemia or tetanus, both of which are treatable
Myasthenia gravis	Respiratory failure in a crisis may occur suddenly and without warning
Guillain-Barré syndrome	Respiratory failure may occur suddenly without warning in a patient who is not severely weak

ministration of volume expanders (blood or plasma, normal saline, lactated Ringer's solution).

   d. Administer glucose (after blood for glucose assay has been drawn) in the form of 25 g in a 50% glucose solution.

3. Determine the cause of the coma.

II. **STATUS EPILEPTICUS.**

A. **Convulsive status epilepticus** is a medical emergency because of the respiratory compromise and subsequent hypoxic brain damage that may occur. Nonconvulsive status epilepticus should be terminated in a timely manner, but is not as dangerous as convulsive status epilepticus because no respiratory compromise occurs. See Chapter 11, sections X and XI, for management.

III. **HEAD TRAUMA (see Chapter 19, section I for management).**

IV. **FRACTURE OF THE SPINAL COLUMN AND SPINAL CORD COMPRESSION.**

A. **Cervical spine fracture** must be suspected following any neck trauma from falls, being thrown from a car, or blows to the neck. If a patient is also comatose, cervical spine fracture must be ruled out by lateral cervical spine radiographs *before* undue manipulation of the neck occurs. If there is a neurologic deficit and plain radiographs are normal, computed tomography (CT) scan of the spinal column and cord or myelogram is indicated. For management, see Chapter 18, section III. Spinal cord emergencies present with acute paralysis of the legs, and with varying involvement of the trunk and upper extremities, depending on the level of the compression. There is a sudden and rapidly progressive onset of sensory or motor loss, or both, of function in the trunk and extremities below the level of the lesion.

Remember: If decompression laminectomy can be performed or radiation therapy initiated (for malignancy) before all neurologic function (below the level of the lesion) has been lost, complete recovery of function is possible. High-dose IV corticosteroids initiated immediately (within 8 hours) may produce improvement. See Chapter 17, section III, for management.

B. **If pain occurs,** it is often radicular from involvement of the sensory spinal nerves at the level of the spinal cord lesion; pain seldom involves the trunk or extremities below the level of the lesion.

C. **The causes** of spinal cord emergencies include the following:
1. Sudden compression of the spinal cord during trauma, usually secondary to a compression fracture or fracture-dislocation of the spine.
2. Collapse of a vertebra from involvement by infection (tuberculosis, osteomyelitis) or neoplasm (metastatic carcinoma, multiple myeloma).
3. Protruding intervertebral disc.
4. Ischemia of the spinal cord from:
   a. Aortic occlusive disease.
   b. Progressive compression by a neoplasm, primary or metastatic, intraaxial or extraaxial.
   c. Thrombosis of anterior spinal artery.
5. Spontaneous hemorrhage into the spinal cord from a vascular malformation.
6. Acute or subacute infection (subdural empyema) or inflammation of the spinal cord (transverse myelitis).

D. **Findings.**
1. Motor deficits resulting from lesions of the spinal cord may be identified by hyperactive reflexes in the lower extremities combined with Babinski reflexes (extensor plantar responses). In acute spinal cord damage there is often a temporary flaccid paralysis with absent deep tendon reflexes in the lower extremities from "spinal shock."
2. A sensory level is an important clue to spinal cord involvement.
   a. Begin sensory testing in an anesthetic area and work toward an area of normal sensation (usually a pin is used).
   b. Test for sensory level on the back, as well as on the chest and abdomen.
   c. With a high thoracic or cervical lesion, examine sensation in the arms and hands beginning with the lower dermatome in the axilla (T2) and ending with the higher dermatome over the deltoid (C4).
3. Beevor's sign can help determine a motor level over the trunk, particularly the abdomen. Place your index fin-

ger at the level of the umbilicus and ask the patient, who is lying flat, to look at the finger. If the umbilicus moves up, the level of the lesion is at T10 or below: the normally strong upper abdominal muscles will contract, while the lower abdominal muscles (below the umbilicus, or T10) will not, pulling the umbilicus up toward the head.

4. Spinal cord involvement localized to one half of the spinal cord will result in a Brown-Séquard syndrome:

   a. The leg on the same side will show weakness, hyperreflexia, a Babinski reflex, and loss of sensation to position and vibration.

   b. The opposite leg will show a deficit to pinprick.

5. A central cord injury of the cervical spinal cord may result in a flaccid paralysis of the muscles of the arms with absent deep tendon reflexes in the arms (due to damage involving the anterior horn cells), and hyperactive reflexes with Babinski reflexes in the lower extremities (due to damage involving the corticospinal tract).

6. Management.

   a. In the patient with acute spinal column trauma associated with spinal cord injury, the spinal column must be kept immobile (see Chapter 17, section III). These same principles should also be followed in cases showing acute involvement of the spinal cord from other lesions.

   b. Administration of high-dose IV corticosteroids (methylprednisolone) has been shown to be beneficial if instituted within 8 hours of the acute spinal cord injury.

   c. Adequate blood pressure must be maintained, since acute spinal cord damage often results in peripheral vasodilation and shock.

      1) Elevate the legs.

      2) Administer peripheral vasoconstrictive agents (see Chapter 13, section II. E).

   d. An indwelling catheter should be placed as soon as practicable to prevent overdistention of the bladder.

e. If respiratory insufficiency is present consider the following:
   1) Suctioning and the administration of oxygen.
   2) Intubation with a soft-cuff endotracheal tube or tracheostomy.
f. Patients with acute spinal cord compression must be referred for emergency neurosurgical management.

V. **TRANSIENT ISCHEMIC ATTACKS (See Chapter 12, section II. A. 1. d).**
A. **Transient ischemic attacks (TIAs)** are episodes of temporary central nervous system (CNS) dysfunction, usually lasting minutes, but always lasting less than 24 hours. Approximately one third of patients with TIAs go on to develop stroke.

Caveat: Transient dysfunction today could be a permanent dysfunction tomorrow.

Many of the causes are treatable.
   1. Thromboemboli from the heart (atrial fibrillation, valvular heart disease, or postmyocardial infarction).
   2. Platelet emboli from an ulcerated carotid plaque.
   3. Carotid or vertebral stenosis.
   4. Hypoglycemia.
B. **Treatment.** Adequate treatment depends on adequate diagnosis and this almost invariably includes the following:
   1. CT scan or magnetic resonance imaging (MRI) of the brain, mainly to rule out hemorrhage.
   2. A Doppler duplex scan of the carotid arteries aids in identifying carotid stenosis.
   3. Four-vessel cerebral angiography aids in the diagnosis of carotid stenosis, arteritis, emboli, and aneurysms.

Caveat: All TIAs are not "ischemic" and anticoagulation of the patient whose transient dysfunction was caused by bleeding could be disastrous.

VI. **STROKE IN PROGRESSION.**
A. **The only way to be certain of the diagnosis of stroke in progression** is to actually observe the patient deteriorating

over time. Since deterioration may be stuttering in temporal profile, this is a difficult judgment to make. If the neurologic deficit is progressive, it is imperative to determine first whether bleeding is occurring, as in hypertensive hemorrhage, subarachnoid hemorrhage secondary to aneurysm or arteriovenous malformation, or hemorrhage into a tumor. An emergency CT scan of the brain is the procedure of choice. Barring that, if there are no contraindications (such as increased intracranial pressure or evidence of supra- or subtentorial mass), lumbar puncture may reveal bleeding. If there is no evidence of subarachnoid, parenchymal or intraventricular hemorrhage, occlusive disease (i.e., thrombosis or embolus) is the most likely cause. Within the first 24 hours or so, the CT scan may not show any decreased densities or evidence of infarct. Short-term anticoagulation may be considered (see Chapter 12, section VI. A. 9).

1. There is universal agreement that anticoagulation with heparin first, and then oral anticoagulants later, is indicated for cardiogenic emboli. If the deficit is massive and the infarct is hemorrhagic, one may need to wait a week or more to initiate anticoagulation.

2. If there is evidence of progressive stroke and no evidence of either cardiogenic emboli or hemorrhage, use short-term anticoagulation beginning with heparin sodium, 1,000 units/hr through a pump and adjust dosage in order to maintain the activated partial thromboplastin time (PTT) 1.5 to 2.0 times normal.

3. Subsequently, decisions can be made as to whether to institute long-term anticoagulation using warfarin compounds or aspirin (or aspirin plus dipyridamole). Carotid endarterectomy for high-grade stenosis has been proved beneficial.

VII. STROKE (for evaluation, see Chapter 12, section I).

A. A stroke is the sudden occurrence of a neurologic deficit, usually due to vascular disease, but some of the other causes of stroke are curable. The preceding remarks under TIAs are appropriate for stroke. **DO NOT** assume that all strokes are caused by intracerebral atherosclerosis.

VIII. FEVER AND CENTRAL NERVOUS SYSTEM SYMPTOMS (see Chapter 14, section I).
A. **Meningitis.**
   1. Consider the possibility of bacterial meningitis in any patient with fever and even minimal mental or neurologic symptoms.
   2. Whenever the diagnosis is suspected, a lumbar puncture must be performed and bacterial cultures obtained. When the cerebrospinal fluid (CSF) is abnormal, tuberculous and fungal cultures should also be obtained.
   3. Prognosis depends on the interval between the onset of the illness and institution of therapy.
   4. Treatment.
      a. If the CSF examination is suggestive of bacterial meningitis (increased nucleated cells, particularly neutrophils, and low sugar) and after cultures have been sent, the patient must be started on IV antibiotics. The choice of antibiotics depends on the patient's age and medical history (see Chapter 14, section II), and the results of the Gram stain of the CSF. The antibiotic regimen can be modified later when culture and sensitivity results are known.
      b. Management of complications may be necessary (see Chapters 11, 13, and 14, section VI).

IX. ENCEPHALITIS.
A. **If severe headache, stiff neck, and Brudzinski's and Kernig's signs are absent,** mental symptoms are prominent, and the CSF shows normal sugar value, a low number of cells, or predominantly a mononuclear pleocytosis (lymphocytosis), encephalitis must be suspected. It is important early in the course of the illness to recognize or suspect herpes simplex encephalitis since it has now been shown that acyclovir instituted early, and even without brain biopsy confirmation, has decreased the morbidity remarkably. Patients with herpes simplex encephalitis classically present with an acute onset of mental and behavioral symptoms, often with an amnestic syndrome, and may have lateralized findings, such as mild hemiparesis or aphasia. They have an electroencephalogram (EEG) with focal slowing

over the temporal lobe and (at some point during the course) periodic lateralizing epileptiform discharges (PLEDs). The CT scan shows decreased density and swelling of the involved temporal lobe.

    1. Treatment: For herpes simplex encephalitis begin acyclovir immediately at 10 mg/kg/day IV q8h for at least 10 days; in some cases, brain biopsy may have to be performed for confirmation.

X.   GUILLAIN-BARRÉ SYNDROME (see Chapter 15, section II. D. 3. a).

A.   Treatment.

    1. Respiratory function initially must be closely monitored with frequent (at least hourly) bedside forced vital capacity (FVC) and inspiratory force measurements. Respiratory function must be closely monitored even in patients with no apparent respiratory involvement, since rapid progression over several hours may lead to respiratory failure. If FVC falls below 1,400 mL in the 70-kg patient, tracheostomy or insertion of a soft-cuff endotracheal tube must be very seriously considered. An inspiratory force (a direct reflection of respiratory muscular strength) of less than 25 cm H_2O also indicates the probable need for tracheostomy. The frequency of monitoring of respiratory function may be reduced as the patient shows signs of clinical improvement.

    2. Respiratory insufficiency may have causes other than muscle weakness:

        a. Aspiration pneumonia from inability to swallow properly.

        b. Pulmonary embolism from venous stasis of immobilized legs.

        c. Pneumonia from decreased cough and hypoventilation.

    3. *Early* institution of plasmapheresis hastens recovery and reduces morbidity.

XI.   MYASTHENIA GRAVIS (MYASTHENIC OR CHOLINERGIC CRISIS) (see Chapter 15, section II. C. 1).

A.   The patient with myasthenia gravis may present as a neurologic emergency or crisis in which there is rapidly progressive respiratory insufficiency. Crisis usually occurs in a patient with known myasthenia during added stress such as infection, anesthesia, surgery, or medication changes; occasionally a patient with undiagnosed myasthenia gravis will present primarily with respiratory failure. Crises are of two types:

1. Myasthenic crisis—an increase in severity of the disease relative to the treatment (i.e., undertreatment).
2. Cholinergic crisis—an excess of anticholinergic activity (usually from anticholinesterase drugs) relative to the severity of the disease (i.e., overtreatment).

B.   **It is difficult or impossible to differentiate these two types of crises** at the time of presentation with imminent respiratory failure. Sometimes the evidence of excessive acetylcholine effect, such as abdominal cramps, sweating, lacrimation, bradycardia, miosis, muscle cramps, and fasciculations, may suggest that the patient is in a cholinergic crisis; however, caution is necessary, since such signs may be absent in definite cholinergic crisis or present in a myasthenic crisis.

1. Treatment.
   a. Maintain ventilation initially with an Ambu bag and later with a soft-cuff endotracheal tube or a tracheostomy. The soft-cuff endotracheal tube may be left in place for up to a week without serious risk or distress to the patient.
   b. Withdraw all medications used to treat myasthenia and all drugs with a curare-like action (such as antibiotics that end in "-mycin").
   c. After 24 hours, gradually reintroduce antimyasthenic medication.
   d. Plasmapheresis will result in marked improvement in patients with either cholinergic or myasthenic crises.

   Remember: (1) Myasthenia is a disease characterized by muscle fatigability; artificial ventilatory support will temporarily restore respiratory strength, which will then gradually decline; (2) respiratory failure may occur in the presence of normal arm and leg strength; (3) myasthenia kills only by respiratory failure.

XII. **WERNICKE'S ENCEPHALOPATHY – THIAMINE DEFICIENCY (see Chapter 8, section II. A).**

A. **The presentation is of a patient with an acute confusional state** (characterized by disorientation and an amnestic syndrome) accompanied by extraocular muscle paralysis and evidence of polyneuropathy. Although it occurs primarily in nutritionally deficient alcoholics, it may occur in other settings, such as the hospitalized patient receiving IV feedings without thiamine supplements or persons who are on diets deficient in thiamine.

    1. Treatment: Thiamine 100 mg IV (preferable) or orally immediately, followed by 50 mg bid maintenance dose.

XIII. **ACUTE PARALYSIS OF EXTRAOCULAR MOVEMENT THAT MAY HAVE EMERGENCY IMPLICATIONS.**

A. **Botulism** presents as paralysis of extraocular muscles rapidly progressing to involvement of swallowing, generalized weakness, and respiratory failure. It is most commonly associated with eating improperly home-canned non-acidic foods (such as green beans), and the diagnosis should be strongly suspected when several members of a family acquire symptoms.

    1. Treatment: Antitoxin should be administered immediately. Contact the local poison control center for a supply of antitoxin. Respiratory failure should be treated with mechanical ventilatory support.

B. **Myasthenia gravis** (see Chapter 15, section II. C. 1): Paralysis of extraocular movement in ocular myasthenia may occur acutely, but presents no immediate danger, and there is no long-term danger if weakness is confined to those muscles. However, if generalized myasthenia develops, respiratory failure may result.

C. **Cavernous sinus thrombosis** presents with paralysis of extraocular muscles and a painful bulging red eye; it is often associated with sinus infection. Four-vessel cerebral angiography may be necessary to establish the diagnosis.

    1. Treatment: Blood and CSF cultures must be obtained; skull radiographs with sinus radiographs, CT scan, or MRI may reveal the source of infection. Massive doses

of IV antibiotics, as if treating meningitis, should be given (see Chapter 14).

D. **Carotid-cavernous fistula:** The patient usually has suffered a recent head injury and presents with extraocular palsies and a painful bulging red eye, which pulsates synchronously with carotid pulsation. A bruit may be heard over the eye. Cerebral angiography will establish the diagnosis.

　1. Treatment: Neurosurgical intervention is usually necessary.

E. **Posterior communicating artery aneurysm:** The patient often presents with third cranial (oculomotor) nerve palsy; the affected eye is turned down and out and the pupil is dilated. The ocular palsy occurs most often when the aneurysm ruptures and the patient develops severe headache and stiff neck. Unlike the acute third cranial nerve palsy of diabetes in which pupillary reactivity is intact, in the case of an aneurysm the pupil is dilated and poorly reactive to light on the side of the palsy. The diagnosis is established by four-vessel cerebral angiography.

　1. Treatment: Neurosurgical consultation is mandatory, and surgical intervention is necessary if the aneurysm has a neck that can be clipped.

XIV. TEMPORAL ARTERITIS AND SUDDEN LOSS OF VISION.

A. **Clinical features.**

　▶ 1. In an elderly person, a firm, tender temporal artery associated with an elevated erythrocyte sedimentation rate (ESR) suggests a diagnosis of temporal arteritis.

　2. Temporal arteritis is often heralded by diffuse arthralgias and myalgias. Sudden onset of monocular blindness or infarction associated with damage to other intracranial arteries is a serious complication.

　3. An edematous retina with optic disc pallor may be visualized by ophthalmoscopy, when a visual disturbance is present.

B. **Treatment.**

　1. With headache as the only symptom, immediate treatment with prednisone 60 mg/day PO is recommended (see Chapter 3).

2. If monocular visual loss has occurred, in order to prevent visual loss in the other eye, administer immediate
IV corticosteroids, either methylprednisolone 120 to
500 mg IV followed by 120 mg/day, or dexamethasone
30 to 125 mg IV followed by 30 mg/day. This should
be continued until ESR is normal, when the patient can
then be switched to oral prednisone.

Caveat: The ESR is normally higher in elderly persons.

3. Temporal artery biopsy should be performed within 2
to 3 days to confirm the diagnosis.

C. **Differential diagnosis of sudden visual loss.** The sudden
loss of all or part of visual function is a potential neuro-
ophthalmologic emergency.

1. The type of visual loss suggests the location of the disease.
   a. Monocular visual loss suggests disease of the optic
   nerve or globe.
   b. Partial loss in both eyes suggests CNS disease behind the optic chiasm.

2. Eye pain is associated with glaucoma, infection, or optic neuritis.

3. Transient visual loss in one eye associated with paralysis on the opposite side suggests emboli from an ulcer-
ating plaque in the carotid artery (see Chapter 12, section I. C. 2).

4. Prodromal phenomena (zigzag lights, stars, etc.) are
seen both in CNS infarction and migraine.

5. A firm globe to palpation (tonometry is much more accurate) suggests a diagnosis of glaucoma.

6. An unreactive pupil or a Marcus-Gunn pupil (see Fig
10–1) suggests disease anterior to the optic chiasm.

7. With unilateral blindness, the cause can often be diagnosed with the ophthalmoscope:
   a. Intraocular hemorrhage.
   b. Retinal detachment.
   c. Emboli.
   d. Retinal infarction.
   e. Infection.

8. A bruit over the neck raises the possibility of the carotid artery being a source of embolus to the ophthalmic artery.

9. Conditions requiring immediate treatment.

   a. Retinal artery or branch occlusion: A monocular defect is found in the visual field corresponding to an ischemic retina with reduced or absent arterial blood flow evident on ophthalmoscopy. Occasionally, an embolus can be visualized on ophthalmoscopy; small retinal hemorrhages and retinal edema may also be seen. If the blindness is transient and associated with a contralateral hemiparesis, the diagnosis of carotid artery stenosis or ulceration is strongly suggested.

      1) Treatment: Anticoagulants (heparin) to prevent further embolization while looking for site of origin of emboli.

   b. Optic or retrobulbar neuritis: Subacute (over hours) unilateral or bilateral visual loss with patient complaining of eye pain with eye motion; the ophthalmologic examination may be normal; Marcus-Gunn pupil (see Figure 10–1) may be demonstrated. Unilateral optic neuritis is almost always associated with multiple sclerosis, while bilateral optic neuritis is most often associated with a toxic disturbance, such as methyl alcohol poisoning.

      1) Treatment: Treatment of optic neuritis due to multiple sclerosis with corticosteroids may increase the risk of long-term disability.

10. Conditions requiring referral to an ophthalmologist.

    a. Acute glaucoma: Usually the globe is hard (increased tension) with an unreactive dilated pupil and enlarged optic cup. Assess intraocular tension by palpation or preferably by tonometry. Sudden blindness may occur secondary to vascular occlusion due to the raised intraocular pressure.

       1) Treatment: Instillation of cholinergics (pilocarpine in sufficient dose to constrict the pupil); referral to an ophthalmologist to consider paracentesis of the eye.

b. Retinal detachment: Monocular visual loss in field corresponds to the area of retinal detachment; detachment is visible on ophthalmoscopic examination.

1) Treatment: Avoid excessive head or eye movement. Refer to ophthalmologist for photocoagulation or surgery to prevent progression of the detachment to completion.

c. Intraocular hemorrhage: Monocular visual loss with blood is visible on ophthalmoscopic examination.

1) Treatment: Ophthalmologic evaluation to determine cause of the bleeding and consideration of ocular paracentesis to reduce pressure.

d. Intraocular infection: Monocular visual loss with purulent material is evident on ophthalmoscopic examination; eye pain is common.

1) Treatment: Ophthalmologic evaluation with paracentesis for culture, and immediate antibiotic treatment similar to that used for meningitis (see Chapter 14).

11. Neurologic conditions that may not require emergency treatment

a. Migraine: A transient hemianopic field defect may occur, as well as transient monocular blindness. Headache is not invariably present, especially if this is the first presentation of migraine. The ophthalmologic examination is normal. The diagnosis is suggested by the presence of a strong family history of migraine, use of birth control pills, or subsequent development of a unilateral throbbing headache.

1) Treatment: Acute treatment may not be necessary (see Chapter 3, section III. B. 2).

b. Occipital lobe damage presents as a binocular visual field defect, most commonly a hemianopsia from occlusion of the posterior cerebral artery; the remainder of the neurologic examination may be normal. Bilateral occipital lobe damage presents as cortical blindness.

1) Treatment: see Chapter 12, section VI.

XV. SEVERE INCAPACITATING MUSCLE SPASMS.
A. Tetanus.

1. Patient has a fixed smile with teeth clenched (trismus). Remainder of muscles are in constant contraction.
2. Appears 1 to 54 days (in more than half of cases within 14 days) after a puncture or lacerating wound (but may appear without a demonstrable wound); especially common in older adults who have not been reimmunized for many years.
3. Autonomic disturbances may occur, resulting in cardiac arrhythmias and wide fluctuations in blood pressure.
4. Treatment
   a. Penicillin G should be given IV at a dose of 10 to 20 million units/day.
   b. Tracheostomy should be performed in all but very mild cases. Continuous artificial ventilation is needed.
   c. Analgesics should be used to relieve the pain from muscle contractions.
   d. Toxin should be neutralized with human tetanus immune globulin (TIG-H) 3,000 to 10,000 units intramuscularly (IM) at several sites, including the area of the presumed injury (infection).
   e. Diazepam 80 to 230 mg/day is often effective in reducing spasms.

B. Hypocalcemic tetany.

1. Hypocalcemic tetany may be distinguished from tetanus by a milder degree of muscle spasm and by the presence of carpopedal spasm, Chvostek's sign (unilateral facial muscle spasm precipitated by tapping the facial nerve near the ear), and Trousseau's sign (carpal spasm precipitated by brief inflation above systolic pressure of a blood pressure cuff on the arm).
2. Most commonly seen in infants on cow's milk. It is important to recognize this disorder in infants because of the possible respiratory compromise and associated seizures.
3. Tetany in adults may be associated with hyperventilation syndrome (see Chapter 4, section II. A).

4. Diagnosis is established by low serum calcium and high serum phosphate.
5. Treatment: Slow IV administration of calcium gluconate (10% solution) should be given in severe cases (up to 10 mL in children and 30 mL in adults). Oral calcium gluconate or a change to commercially prepared formula feeding in the infant may be adequate treatment in milder cases.

BIBLIOGRAPHY

Bracken MB, et al: A randomized controlled trial of methylprednisolone or naloxone in the treatment of acute spinal cord injury. Results of the second national acute spinal cord injury study. *N Engl J Med* 1990; 322:1405–1411.

Orland MJ, Saltman RJ (eds): *Manual of Medical Therapeutics,* ed. 25. Boston, Little, Brown, 1987.

Graef JW, Cone TE Jr: *Manual of Pediatric Therapeutics.* Boston, Little, Brown, 1984.

Hyman SE: *Manual of Psychiatric Emergencies.* Boston, Little, Brown, 1984.

O'Doherty DS, Fermaglich JL: *Handbook of Neurologic Emergencies.* Flushing, NY, Medical Examining Publishing, 1977.

Samuels MA: *Manual of Neurologic Therapeutics,* ed.2. Boston, Little, Brown, 1982.

CONSIDERATIONS IN THE CARE OF THE PATIENT WITH SEVERE AND IRREVERSIBLE NERVOUS SYSTEM DAMAGE $\mathit{21}$

Advances in medical technology have provided clinicians with the means of preserving life at the expense of a great deal of unnecessary pain and suffering by patients. The decisions with regard to neurologic patients should be governed by the same general principles as those used in other disciplines of medicine. Usually, these problems have a way of providing their own solutions without the aid of complicated rules, regulations, and fancy machines. For example, cardiac resuscitation in patients with severe brain damage is rarely successful.

I. GENERAL PRINCIPLES.
A. The following are a few important principles in handling patients with severe and irreversible nervous system disease:
1. Always keep the family and loved ones fully informed about the patient's condition. Avoid technical jargon such as,

"The cerebral angiogram showed bilateral cerebral hemisphere infarction"; a preferable statement would be, "When we injected dye into the arteries of the brain, we found that no blood is reaching those parts of the brain which control movement and thought. Without blood, brain tissue dies and does not have the capability of ever recovering."

2. Families relate better to one physician than to a team, which can seem (to the family) to be giving conflicting information.

3. Families and patients must be involved in the decision-making process. The physician has the responsibility to provide clearly and simply the facts that are necessary to make a decision. Often it is appropriate to give the family advice as to what action to take in a particular situation. The wishes of the patient and the family take precedence over the physician's preference.

4. Consider the quality of life *before* the current neurologic disability, e.g., the patient with a clearly documented severe dementia who develops a sudden left hemiparesis may not need more than fluid and nutritional support.

5. Consider the quality of life *after* the neurologic disability, e.g., most physicians do not provide respiratory support to patients with end-stage amyotrophic lateral sclerosis (ALS) or muscular dystrophy. A patient with ALS on a respirator faces the prospect of consciously watching the body wither away until the person becomes little more than a "living uncommunicative brain in a fishbowl."

6. All discussions and decisions must be carefully documented in the medical record.

7. The physician should promote the use of traditional patient and family support systems such as clergy, close friends, and fraternal organizations during times of severe stress.

8. Cases of suspected homicide, assault, child abuse, and the like require that the physician use special care in the decision-making process, and it is always wise to seek additional (including legal) opinions.

II. BRAIN DEATH.

A. Once artificial life support systems have been instituted
and irreversible coma or brain death is suspected, state or lo-

cal hospital criteria for discontinuing respiratory support should be followed. These criteria often include recommendations from multiple consultants (medical and sometimes clergy and legal). Human death is the irreversible loss of the capacity for consciousness and the capacity to breathe. Guidelines have evolved since the late 1960s for the determination of brain death:

1. Brain death is defined as the *irreversible cessation* of all clinically ascertainable functions of the entire brain, including the brainstem (but not necessarily including the spinal cord).
2. Cessation of brain function is interpreted as both:
   a. Cerebral unreceptivity and unresponsivity.
   b. Absent brainstem reflexes.

   Note: Spinal cord activity (reflexes) and peripheral nervous system activity may persist after brain death.

3. Minimal accepted clinical neurologic findings are:
   a. No spontaneous movement and no movement elicited by painful stimuli to the face or trunk (see Chapter 13, section I. A. 6. b).
   b. Pupils fully dilated or in midposition and totally unreactive to light (examine under magnification with a bright light in a darkened room).
   c. Absence of oculocephalic (doll's-eye) and oculovestibular (caloric) responses (see Chapter 13, section I. B. 1. e), absent corneal reflex, absent pharyngeal reflex (insertion and removal of a nasopharyngeal suction tube should not produce a cough or gag), and absent cough reflex (after suctioning or irrigation of the endotracheal tube). There should be no spontaneous blinking (eye opening) or swallowing.
   d. No spontaneous respirations (apnea) after the arterial carbon dioxide partial pressure ($PaCO_2$) has reached a level that provides maximal respiratory stimulus, which is about 60 mm Hg (torr). Apnea testing should be performed with a protocol that permits pretest hyperoxygenation, exposure of the tracheobronchial tree to oxygen during the test, and monitoring of arterial $PaCO_2$

levels, which rise an average of 4 mm Hg (torr)/min during apnea.

4. Irreversibility is interpreted to mean:

   a. The *cause* of the coma is established, is sufficient to account for the coma, and is not a reversible condition.

      Caveat: The frequent reversible conditions of meta-
      bolic or drug (sedative) intoxication, hypothermia, neu-
      romuscular blockade, and shock must be excluded.

   b. The possibility of recovery of any brain function is excluded. Demonstration of a lack of blood flow to the
   brain is confirmation of irreversibility.

      Caveat: Conventional cerebral angiography can falsely
      demonstrate flow in a brain-dead patient owing to ex-
      cessive injection pressure forcing dye into the intracra-
      nial vessels, or injection with the head in a dependent
      position allowing contrast material to leak into vessels.

   c. The cessation of all brain function persists for an adequate observation period (6 hours with confirmatory
   tests, 12–24 hours in the absence of confirmatory tests).

5. Confirmation of electrocerebral silence by electroencephalography (EEG) performed at least 6 hours after loss of
   clinically ascertainable brain function is desirable when
   confirmatory documentation is needed to substantiate the
   clinical findings, but an EEG is not legally required.

   Caveat: EEG tracings must be carried out utilizing the
   technical guidelines established by the American Electroencephalographic Society. These guidelines have been established to insure that tracings for electrocerebral silence
   are not artifactual and that all measures to maximize recording of minimal cerebral electrical activity have been performed. Usually, if everything has been done by a registered EEG technologist (REEGT), and interpreted by an experienced electroencephalographer, this is assurance
   enough that the guidelines have been followed.

   a. Electrocerebral silence tracings may be seen in the potentially reversible situations:

      1) Barbiturate intoxication.

      2) Hypothermia.

      3) Premature or full-term infant who is not brain-dead.

   b. Brainstem auditory evoked responses may also be used in the diagnosis of brain death. It is known that brainstem auditory evoked responses can be present while an EEG shows electrocerebral silence, but may finally disappear when medullary function ceases.

6. Before respiratory support is discontinued, the family must be carefully informed of the situation.

7. Guidelines for the determination of brain death in children under the age of 5 years are still in the process of development. Clinical criteria similar to those in use for patients over age 5 years have been found to be applicable to infants and term newborns (>38 weeks gestational age) older than 7 days of age. It has been recommended that two EEG tracings be performed in children under 1 year of age with these EEG tracings separated by an interval of 48 hours in infants 7 days to 2 months of age and by an interval of 24 hours in infants 2 months to 1 year of age. Beyond 1 year of age, laboratory tests are not necessary if an irreversible cause exists and clinical criteria for brain death are met.

BIBLIOGRAPHY

A definition of irreversible coma: Report of Ad Hoc Committee of the Harvard Medical School to Examine the Definition of Brain Death. *JAMA* 1968; 205:337–340.

American EEG Society: Minimum technical standards for EEG recording in suspected cerebral death, in Klass DW, Daly DD (eds): *Current Practice of Clinical Electroencephalography*. New York, Raven Press, 1979, pp 492–496.

Black PMcL: Brain death. *N Engl J Med* 1978; 299:338–344, 393–401.

Goldie WD, Chiappa KH, Young RR, et al: Brainstem auditory and short-latency somatosensory evoked responses in brain death. *Neurology* 1981; 31:248–256.

Guidelines for the determination of death: Report of the Medical Consultants on the Diagnosis of Death to the President's Commission for the Study of Ethical Problems in Medicine and Biomedical and Behavioral Research. *JAMA* 1981; 246:2184–2186.

Kaufman HH, Beresford R, Bernat JL, et al: Brain death. *Neurol Neurosurg Update Ser* 1986; 6:1–8.

Moshé SL, Alvarez LA: Diagnosis of brain death in children. *J Clin Neurophysiol* 1986; 3:239–249.

Rowland TW, Donnelly JH, Jackson AH: Apnea documentation for determination of brain death in children. *Pediatrics* 1984; 74:505–508.

Ruank JE: Initiating and withdrawing life support. *N Engl J Med* 1988; 318:25–31.

Schwartz JA, Baxter J, Brill DR: Diagnosis of brain death in children by radionuclide cerebral imaging. *Pediatrics* 1984; 73:14–18.

Silverstein MD, et al: Amyotrophic lateral sclerosis and life-sustaining therapy: Patient's desires for information and participation in decision making and life-sustaining therapy. *Mayo Clin Proc* 1991; 66:906–913.

Sundram JC: Informed consent for major medical treatment of mentally disabled people. *N Engl J Med* 1988; 318:1368–1373.

Task Force for the Determination of Brain Death in Children: Guidelines for the determination of brain death in children. *Ann Neurol* 1987; 22:616–617.

Youngner SJ, Bartlett ET: Human death and high technology: The failure of the whole-brain formulations. *Ann Intern Med* 1983; 99:252–258.

HEAD CIRCUMFERENCE CHARTS* AND DENVER DEVELOPMENTAL TEST†

A

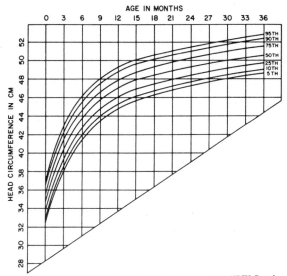

Boys head circumference by age percentiles: ages birth-36 months

*Growth charts courtesy of National Center for Health Statistics: NSCH Growth Charts, 1976. Monthly Vital Statistics Report, Volume 3, Supplement (HRA) 76-1120 Health Resources Administration, Rockville, Maryland. Used by permission.

†From William K. Frankenburg, MD, and Josiah B. Dodds, PhD, University of Colorado Medical Center. Used by permission.

Girls head circumference by age percentiles : ages birth - 36 months

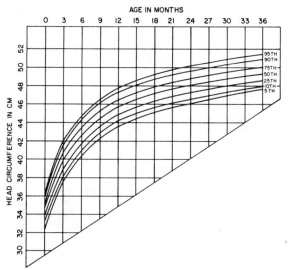

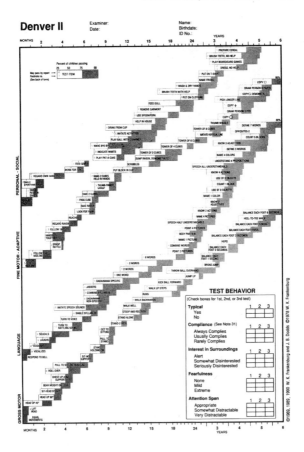

DIRECTIONS FOR ADMINISTRATION

1. Try to get child to smile by smiling, talking or waving. Do not touch him/her.
2. Child must stare at hand several seconds.
3. Parent may help guide toothbrush and put toothpaste on brush.
4. Child does not have to be able to tie shoes or button/zip in the back.
5. Move yarn slowly in an arc from one side to the other, about 8" above child's face.
6. Pass if child grasps rattle when it is touched to the backs or tips of fingers.
7. Pass if child tries to see where yarn went. Yarn should be dropped quickly from sight from tester's hand without arm movement.
8. Child must transfer cube from hand to hand without help of body, mouth, or table.
9. Pass if child picks up raisin with any part of thumb and finger.
10. Line can vary only 30 degrees or less from tester's line. ╱
11. Make a fist with thumb pointing upward and wiggle only the thumb. Pass if child imitates and does not move any fingers other than the thumb.

12. Pass any enclosed form. Fail continuous round motions.

13. Which line is longer? (Not bigger.) Turn paper upside down and repeat. (pass 3 of 3 or 5 of 6)

14. Pass any lines crossing near midpoint.

15. Have child copy first. If failed, demonstrate.

When giving items 12, 14, and 15, do not name the forms. Do not demonstrate 12 and 14.

16. When scoring, each pair (2 arms, 2 legs, etc.) counts as one part.
17. Place one cube in cup and shake gently near child's ear, but out of sight. Repeat for other ear.
18. Point to picture and have child name it. (No credit is given for sounds only.)
    If less than 4 pictures are named correctly, have child point to picture as each is named by tester.

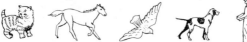

19. Using doll, tell child: Show me the nose, eyes, ears, mouth, hands, feet, tummy, hair. Pass 6 of 8.
20. Using pictures, ask child: Which one flies?... says meow?... talks?... barks?... gallops? Pass 2 of 5, 4 of 5.
21. Ask child: What do you do when you are cold?... tired?... hungry? Pass 2 of 3, 3 of 3.
22. Ask child: What do you do with a cup? What is a chair used for? What is a pencil used for?
    Action words must be included in answers.
23. Pass if child correctly places and says how many blocks are on paper. (1, 5).
24. Tell child: Put block **on** table; **under** table; **in front of** me, **behind** me. Pass 4 of 4.
    (Do not help child by pointing, moving head or eyes.)
25. Ask child: What is a ball?... lake?... desk?... house?... banana?... curtain?... fence?... ceiling? Pass if defined in terms of use, shape, what it is made of, or general category (such as banana is fruit, not just yellow). Pass 5 of 8, 7 of 8.
26. Ask child: If a horse is big, a mouse is __? If fire is hot, ice is __? If the sun shines during the day, the moon shines during the __? Pass 2 of 3.
27. Child may use wall or rail only, not person. May not crawl.
28. Child must throw ball overhand 3 feet to within arm's reach of tester.
29. Child must perform standing broad jump over width of test sheet (8 1/2 inches).
30. Tell child to walk forward, ⚬⚬⚬⚬⚬⚬➤ heel within 1 inch of toe. Tester may demonstrate. Child must walk 4 consecutive steps.
31. In the second year, half of normal children are non-compliant.

OBSERVATIONS:

THE SYMPTOM-ORIENTED NEUROLOGIC EXAMINATION

B

William H. Olson, Vasudeva Iyer, Abdulsalam A. Al-Sulaiman, and Roger A. Brumback

This appendix is written to assist with the mastery of the neurologic examination. Each phase of the examination is divided into three parts: (1) step-by-step directions on how to proceed, (2) common problems facing the beginner, and (3) common abnormalities.

The first sections comprise the "routine examination." With a cooperative patient, an experienced examiner can perform this in less than 15 minutes. However, with *each* patient, the examiner must individually modify the "routine examination" according to the chief complaint, age, degree of cooperation, and other individual factors. The neurologic examination is never exactly the same, even for patients with the same age and complaint. The most important part of the neurologic evaluation is the *history taking;* it is during the interview that the examiner forms *hypotheses* concerning the nature of the complaints. The examiner then tailors the examination to gather objective data to verify these hypotheses. In this appendix, attention is given only to the form in which the history should be recorded. The *art* of gathering this history is the same as in other specialties of medicine.

It is important to emphasize that there are many correct ways to do a neurologic examination. What is presented here certainly is not the only "right" examination, but simply one which has worked for us over a period of many years. The astute physician will ultimately adopt those techniques that work best for him or her.

I. PATIENT RECORD.

A. **The general principles of interviewing and examining the patient with a neurologic complaint** are no different from those of interviewing and examining the patient with any medical illness; only the emphasis is different. In every patient encounter, the physician must form *hypotheses* as to the cause of the patient's distress; these hypotheses are strengthened or discarded according to the facts that emerge during the interview and examination. This section is a general framework for recording the illness of a patient with a neurologic complaint. Obviously, such a framework emphasizes a neurologic review of systems and the neurologic examination. The purpose of preparing such a record is to communicate information concerning the patient's illness in an *organized, succinct,* and *legible* manner. The uniqueness of each patient encounter cannot be overemphasized. Thus, it is impossible to present a "cookbook" that outlines precisely how to proceed. For example, it is useless to spend much time taking a history and review of systems from a patient with a severe memory deficit; information in such circumstances is best gathered from other sources. If the physician performs a "routine" neurologic examination on every patient, important data will be routinely missed. For example, palpation of the temporal arteries and a careful search for early papilledema are important in the elderly patient with the complaint of headache, but tests usually reserved for the patient complaining of low back pain (such as straight leg

TABLE B–1.
Steps in Arriving at a Neurologic Diagnosis

Process	Concepts	Skill	Knowledge
History	Anatomic and pathologic concept of the disorder *[A]*	Interrogative skill	Basic neuroscience and neuropathology
Physical signs	Anatomic and functional localization *[B]*; confirm or refute *[A]*	Clinical examination	Interpretation of physical signs to localize and to assess dysfunction
Differential diagnosis			
Investigations	Confirm or refute *[A]* or *[B]*	Discriminative	Knowledge of sensitivity and predictability of tests
Final diagnosis			

raising, abdominal reflexes, cremasteric reflexes, and internal hamstring reflexes) will yield little useful information. The problem-oriented approach to neurologic examination necessitates individualization (Table B–1).

II. THE OUTLINE OF THE MEDICAL RECORD OF THE PATIENT WITH A NEUROLOGIC COMPLAINT

A. History.

1. Chief complaint.
2. Present illness.
3. Allergies.
4. Previous illnesses.
5. Drug history: current and past drugs, including tobacco, alcohol, caffeine, illegal drugs.
6. Social history: marital status, family structure, employment.
7. Family history: hypertension, diabetes, heart disease, paralysis, seizures, mental illness, mental deficiency.
8. Review of systems.
   a. General: fatigue, appetite change, fever, sleep disturbance.

      b. Skin: rashes, bruises, change in texture or color.

      c. Endocrine: temperature intolerance, abnormal menses, fertility, excessive salt intake, excessive change in shoe or hat size.

      d. Respiratory: cough, shortness of breath, hemoptysis, sinusitis.

      e. Heart and blood vessels: chest pain, palpitation, edema, claudication.

      f. Breast: masses, tenderness.

      g. Gastrointestinal: nausea, abdominal pain, diarrhea, constipation, melena, incontinence.

      h. Genitourinary: urinary burning, frequency, incontinence, sexual dysfunction, venereal disease.

      i. Neurologic:

         1) Mental status: memory loss, occupational difficulties, moodiness, hallucinations, speech difficulty, confusion.

         2) Cranial nerves: visual disturbance, diplopia, facial numbness, difficulty chewing or swallowing, change in auditory acuity, dizziness, voice change.

         3) Coordination: difficulty with skilled tasks, tendency to fall, clumsiness, unsteady gait, slurred speech.

         4) Sensation: numbness, tingling, painless cuts or burns, difficulty ambulating in the dark.

         5) Motor: difficulty climbing stairs, abnormal movements, sore muscles, weakness, cramps, stiffness.

         6) Episodic: seizures, alteration of consciousness, headaches.

B. Physical examination.

    1. Vital signs: blood pressure lying and standing, temperature, pulse rate, respiratory rate, height, weight, head circumference (in children and adolescents)

    2. Skin: bruises, rash, lesions, color, texture.

    3. Lymph nodes: cervical, supraclavicular, axillary, inguinal.

    4. Head, eyes, ears, nose, throat (HEENT): head size and shape, evidence of trauma or inflammation, sclerae, tympanic membranes, pharynx.

5. Neck: thyroid, masses, deformity, carotid palpation, carotid bruits, suppleness.
6. Breasts: masses, tenderness.
7. Chest: percussion, auscultation, respiratory pattern.
8. Heart: heart sounds, percussion, venous distention.
9. Vascular: peripheral pulses, bruits, temperature of extremities.
10. Abdomen: organomegaly, tenderness, masses.
11. Genitourinary and rectal: external genitalia, rectal examination, sphincter tone, prostate, discharges, pelvic.
12. Extremities: joints, deformities.
13. Neurologic examination:
    a. Mental status: alertness, orientation, memory (immediate, recent, remote), fund of knowledge, abstract thinking, calculations, constructional testing, affect, behavior; Mini-Mental State Test
    b. Language: spontaneous speech, fluency, comprehension, repetition, naming, reading, writing, handedness.
    c. Cranial nerves:
       II: visual fields to confrontation and double simultaneous stimulation, funduscopy, visual acuity in each eye.
       III, IV, VI: extraocular movements, nystagmus, pupillary size, shape and reactivity to light and accommodation, asymmetry of palpebral fissures; red lens test (if indicated).
       V: corneal reflexes, facial sensation, jaw muscles.
       VII: facial movements, eye closure, expression, strength, taste.
       VIII: auditory acuity
       IX, X: pharyngeal reflex, phonation, palatal sensation, palatal movements.
       XI: sternocleidomastoid and trapezius muscles.
       XII: tongue position, atrophy, fasciculations, strength.
    d. Motor examination: individual muscle strength testing if indicated, fasciculations, atrophy, alteration in tone, involuntary movements, drift test.
    e. Reflexes: muscle stretch (tendon) reflexes (activity and symmetry), plantar reflex, release signs (snout,

suck, glabellar); abdominal and cremasteric reflexes, if indicated.

f. Coordination: finger-to-nose and heel-shin tests, rapid alternating movements, speech articulation and melody, fine movements.

g. Gait: spontaneous gait, posture, walking on heels, toes, and sides of feet, deep knee bend, tandem walking.

h. Sensory examination: light touch, pinprick, vibration, passive movement, two-point discrimination, object identification, double simultaneous stimulation.

C.   Assessment.

1. Summary:

2. Discussion: anatomic localization, pathophysiology, diagnostic considerations

3. Differential diagnosis:

4. Pertinent diagnostic tests:

D.   Comments.

1. Referring physician: Since most neurologic disease is chronic, a majority of medical care is provided by primary care physicians and therefore it is essential to obtain his or her name and address so that copies of the records can be properly forwarded.

2. Chief complaint: This is not necessarily what the patient states, but may be a general statement of the patient's major problem, e.g., "On a routine screening ophthalmologic examination, Dr. James noted early signs of bilateral papilledema," or "Mr. Thurber was found unconscious with a stiff neck and brought to the emergency room." Information regarding the duration or date of onset of the complaint should be stated.

3. Present illness: This should be an organized description of events leading to the present admission or consultation, including pertinent negatives as well as positives and any disease processes which may be directly related to the disability. For example, a history of diabetes, hypertension, or sickle cell anemia is relevant to a patient suffering from the stroke syndrome. Family history would be part of the present illness in a patient suffer-

ing from a possible hereditary disorder. Current and past treatment for the condition should be summarized, e.g., all drugs used for a seizure disorder, giving dose, response, and reason discontinued.

4. Allergies: Any medication allergy should be clearly flagged on the chart.

5. Previous illnesses: This includes events not related to the present illness and may be briefly stated.

6. Drug history: This should include dose, length of time taken, and name of prescribing physician. Include over-the-counter medications, illicit drugs, and tobacco and alcohol use. Many neurologic disabilities are medication-related.

7. Social history: Occupation, family situation, hobbies, and sexual preference are all items which may be included in the social history. This information may be useful in suggesting a diagnosis, in planning for future care, and in making the patient feel like a "person."

8. Family history: A detailed family history is necessary when there is a possible relationship between the family history and the present illness. Occasionally, examination of a family member is important, as in a doubtful case of myotonic muscular dystrophy.

9. Review of systems: The review of systems must be modified to fit the specific case, and depending on the chief complaint, much of this information will be included in the present illness.

10. Neurologic examination: The outlined examination is the routine "complete" examination, recognizing that there is really no such thing as a complete examination. The examination should be expanded in areas where there is reason to believe a pathologic condition exists. When time is severely limited, e.g., in a busy outpatient setting, the examination may be shortened by abbreviating the less pertinent parts, but at a minimum, the functional integrity of *all* major areas of the nervous system must still be established by some screening test. In an inpatient setting, the examination should never be any less complete than outlined, within the limits of the patient's ability to cooperate. Whatever the examination

performed, it is important to state in the written record exactly what was tested (e.g., it is inappropriate to record: "cranial nerve II normal"; instead, the statement should be: "visual acuity, visual fields to confrontation, and funduscopic examination were normal," and if there are visual complaints, more detailed testing is required and should be so stated, such as numerical visual acuity by chart with and without correction in each eye; size and color of test object used for visual fields, etc.). It will be assumed that any test not specifically mentioned in the record was not performed.

11. Summary: A brief summary statement should be made that includes the patient's age and sex; the nature and duration of symptom development (i.e., abrupt, gradual, insidious, etc.); and the salient findings on examination. Use conclusive terms, such as "dementia," "hemiparesis," or "aphasia," rather than repeating the signs already detailed. For example, "This 59-year-old man with a 12-year history of hypertension had the sudden onset of right-sided weakness and difficulty speaking two days ago. Examination shows a mild right hemiparesis, mild nonfluent aphasia, and no sensory abnormality."

12. Discussion: The differential diagnosis of neurologic problems begins with an assessment of the anatomic location of the abnormality. For example, "The patient has a peripheral polyneuropathy because of the bilateral distal loss of sensation and tendon reflexes." When localizing a disease process, it is often helpful to go through the following checklist mentally:

   a. Does the problem involve the central or the peripheral nervous system?

   b. If peripheral nervous system, is muscle or nerve primarily involved?

   c. If central nervous system (CNS), is the lesion above or below the foramen magnum?

   d. If above the foramen magnum, is it above the tentorium cerebelli (anterior or middle cerebral fossae) or below (posterior fossa)?

   e. If above the tentorium, is it in the right or left hemisphere? Is it gray matter or white matter disease?

   f. Are multiple systems involved?

     This should be followed by a discussion of the pathophysiological process involved. For example, sudden onset of symptoms suggests vascular occlusion; slow progression, positive family history, and multiple system involvement suggest a degenerative process. Then discuss the possible diagnoses and the reasons for considering them and for excluding other conditions. For example, in a patient with a peripheral neuropathy: "Because the patient has insulin-dependent diabetes mellitus for 8 years and the neuropathy is primarily sensory, the most probable diagnosis is diabetic peripheral polyneuropathy. However, because of the history of a gastrectomy 12 years ago and possible recent exposure to lead, subacute combined degeneration of the spinal cord (combined systems disease) and lead intoxication must also be considered possibilities."

13. Differential diagnosis: This should be a list, in order of probability, of all diseases that reasonably account for the clinical picture. Specific diseases should be listed, not generalities such as "some kind of degenerative disease." The differential diagnosis serves as a guide to proper evaluation, because appropriate tests will be chosen to confirm or exclude each condition listed.

14. Pertinent diagnostic tests: In the example above of the patient with a peripheral neuropathy, indicated tests would include an electromyogram (EMG), nerve conduction velocity (NCV) studies, glucose tolerance test (GTT), serum vitamin B_{12} level, red blood cell smear for morphologic evaluation, and urinary screening for heavy metals. "Routine" studies (e.g., complete blood count [CBC], urinalysis, serum chemistry panel, electrocardiogram [ECG], chest radiographs, etc.) need not be repeated, unless specific tests are critical in confirming or excluding one of the differential diagnoses. Table B–2 lists commonly ordered diagnostic tests.

TABLE B–2.
Diagnostic Tests in Neurologic Disorders

Test	Anatomic/Physiologic Basis	Most Useful In
Electroencephalogram (EEG)	Spontaneous electrical activity of cerebral cortical neurons	Seizure disorders Metabolic encephalopathy Tumors Infectious encephalopathy Dementia Brain death determination
Visual evoked potentials (VEPs)	Arrival of electrical signals at the visual cortex through the visual pathways, when the retina is stimulated	Multiple sclerosis Disorders of optic nerve Lesions of optic tract, radiations, or occipital cortex
Brainstem auditory evoked potentials (BAEPs)	Passage of electrical signals through auditory nerve, auditory nuclei, lateral lemniscus, and inferior colliculus to auditory cortex	Acoustic neurilemmoma (neuroma) Brainstem tumor Brainstem infarct Multiple sclerosis
Somatosensory evoked potentials (SSEPs)	Passage of electrical signals through peripheral nerves to central somatosensory pathways (including dorsal columns, medial lemnisci, thalamus, thalamocortical pathways) and arrival at sensory cortex	Multiple sclerosis Spinal cord tumors Myelopathy
Nerve conduction studies	Conduction of electrical signals through myelinated nerve fibers (motor or sensory)	Peripheral neuropathy Nerve trauma Nerve compression (e.g., carpal tunnel syndrome) Denervating disease (e.g., amyotrophic lateral sclerosis)
Needle electromyography (EMG)	Electrical activity of muscle during rest and voluntary contraction	Muscular dystrophy Polymyositis

Test	Basis	Disorders diagnosed
Repetitive nerve stimulation test (Jolly's test)	Neuromuscular transmission	Myasthenia gravis Lambert-Eaton (myasthenic) syndrome
Muscle biopsy	Morphology and histochemistry of muscle fibers	Muscular dystrophy Polymyositis Metabolic disorders
Nerve biopsy	Quantitative morphology of axons and myelin	Peripheral neuropathy
Cerebrospinal fluid (CSF) study	CSF pressure, biochemistry, cell count, serology, microbiology	Meningitis Encephalitis Subarachnoid hemorrhage Multiple sclerosis CNS syphilis
Myelogram	Radiopaque contrast in subarachnoid CSF space outlines spinal canal and its contents (may be combined with CT scan)	Cervical or lumbar disc herniations Spinal cord tumors
Magnetic resonance imaging (MRI)	Protons in various tissues and compartment of nervous system have different responses to high-intensity magnetic fields, providing basis for computerized imaging	Multiple sclerosis Tumors (especially in posterior fossa) Spinal cord lesions Infarcts Malformations
Computed tomographic (CT) scan	Various tissues and compartments within nervous system have different x-ray absorption coefficients, providing basis for computerized imaging	Hemorrhage Infarct Tumor Hydrocephalus Dementia Head trauma

III.   THE MEDICAL BAG OF A NEUROLOGIST.
A.   The medical bag of the neurologist might contain many of the following tools.

1. Ophthalmoscope: This instrument should have a bright light source (good batteries, quartz-halogen bulb), a light aperture that can be adjusted to provide various sizes and colors of light beam, multiple lenses calibrated in a range of diopters, and an otoscope head (with removable ear speculum) for examining small or irregular pupils under magnification.

2. Reflex hammer: There are at least 20 varieties available; three of the most common are:
   a. The Queen's Square hammer: This is favored by us because the long flexible handle greatly simplifies elicitation of reflex activity.
   b. The Trommer hammer: The rigid short handle makes this instrument more compact, but at the same time more difficult to use.
   c. The standard hammer (also known as the "red rubber hatchet" or "tomahawk"): This instrument is inexpensive, portable, and found at almost any clinic or nurse's station.

3. Blood pressure cuff: The aneroid style with the hand-held gauge is preferable because it facilitates measuring postural hypotension.

4. Stethoscope: This is also useful in detecting cranial and spinal bruits.

5. Flashlight: A bright, pinpoint light source is preferable. Disposable pocket flashlights generally provide inadequate light.

6. Visual acuity test card: This handheld card tests near vision. If the patient wears corrective lenses (glasses or contact lenses), they should be worn during this test.

7. Red target on a wire (about the size of a dime): This is used to detect visual field defects. A red-headed hatpin may also be used.

8. Opticokinetic tape: Testing for opticokinetic nystagmus may be useful in identifying a parietal lobe lesion. An easily constructed homemade cloth tape consisting of alternating 2-in.-wide light and dark stripes is all that is necessary.

9. Tape measure: Required for measuring head circumference and muscle atrophy.

10. Pin: Used for testing pain sensation. Other sharp objects are inadequate: injection needles are too sharp and diaper pins do not permit quantitation. *Caution:* The human immunodeficiency virus (HIV, the causative virus of acquired immunodeficiency syndrome [AIDS]) and hepatitis B can be spread with contaminated pins; therefore, it is mandatory that a new pin be used for each patient.

11. Key: This is the best instrument to use for plantar stimulation to elicit the Babinski reflex. Sharp or very smooth objects are ineffective.

12. Tuning forks (128 Hz and 256 Hz): Use a 128-Hz tuning fork for measuring vibratory sense; use the higher-frequency (256-Hz) tuning fork to test auditory acuity.

13. Assorted small objects for testing astereognosis (penny, dime, sandpaper, silk, key, safety pin, etc.).

14. Syringe with soft plastic catheter: Used for caloric testing with ice water.

15. Red piece of plastic or glass: Occasionally used for analysis of diplopia.

16. Cotton-tipped swabs: A wisp from the end is useful for testing the corneal reflex; can also be used to elicit the pharyngeal reflex.

17. Tongue depressor: May be necessary for depressing the tongue when eliciting the pharyngeal reflex. When broken, may also be used for eliciting cutaneous reflexes.

18. *Aids to the Examination of the Peripheral Nervous System* (Her Majesty's Stationery Office, 51 Nine Elms Lane, London, SW8 5DR, England): This compact reference provides a detailed description for the testing for peripheral nerve and muscle dysfunction.

IV. EXAMINATION OF THE CRANIAL NERVES.
A. Optic nerve (second cranial nerve, cranial nerve II).

1. Examining the optic fundus with the ophthalmoscope:
   a. The room should not be totally darkened since pupillary constriction will occur from shining the bright ophthalmoscope light into the patient's eye and the patient will not be able to see a fixation point; how-

ever, dimming the room lights may diminish glares and reflections from the cornea and iris that can be distracting and interfere with examination of the retina.

b. Instruct the patient to look at an object more than 5 ft away.

c. In general, both the examiner and the patient should remove their eyeglasses, although contact lenses (except some very darkly tinted lenses) may be left in place.

d. Ophthalmoscope light should be as bright as possible and the size of the light should be adjusted to match the size of the pupil. If the light is larger than the pupil, the fundus will be difficult to see because of light reflected from the iris.

e. The examiner should use his or her right eye to examine the patient's right fundus and the left eye to examine the patient's left fundus.

f. Systematically examine the fundus (Fig B–1).

2. Common problems:

a. Pupils too small: In selected cases where information is vital, a drop of 1% tropicamide (Mydriacil) or 2.5% neosynephrine may be used to dilate the pupils temporarily. An experienced examiner rarely needs to do this.

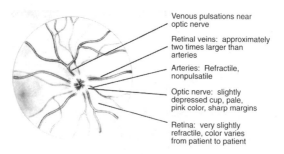

Venous pulsations near optic nerve

Retinal veins: approximately two times larger than arteries

Arteries: Refractile, nonpulsatile

Optic nerve: slightly depressed cup, pale, pink color, sharp margins

Retina: very slightly refractile, color varies from patient to patient

FIG B–1. Funduscopic examination.

Caveat: This should not be done in patients who have a history of glaucoma or have abnormally firm globes. Check pupillary reactions *before* using dilating agents. When pupillary size and reactivity may be of critical diagnostic significance (as in head trauma, subarachnoid hemorrhage, or intercerebral hemorrhage), dilating agents should *not* be used.

b. Cataracts: Unless very severe, the fundus still can be visualized. Dilation of pupils may help.

c. Absent lens (usually following a cataract operation): The fundus will appear small, but the usual features are still visible. Try using the $+10$ D ($+10$ diopters) lens on the ophthalmoscope to visualize the retina.

d. Patient uncooperative: The experienced examiner is quick and efficient; in rare cases sedation or restraints may be necessary. In children, the examination of the fundus can be upsetting and should be performed at the conclusion of the neurologic examination, often with the infant or child sitting in the mother's lap.

e. Difficulty locating the retina: Beginners having trouble locating the retina while looking through the ophthalmoscope can try identifying the red reflex through the 0 D lens of the ophthalmoscope from a distance and then move in closer.

3. Normal variations:

a. Congenital medullation of nerve fibers: White areas that fan out from the optic disc following the normal course of the retinal nerve fibers are of no pathologic significance, but may be confused with papilledema.

b. Tigroid retina: The retina tends to be pale orange in light-skinned people and darkly pigmented in dark-skinned people; the tigroid retina resembles retinitis pigmentosa, but has no pathologic significance.

c. Drusen: Whitish cobblestone-like projections near the optic disc may be mistaken for early papilledema.

4. Important abnormalities:
   a. Papilledema (Figure B–2): Elevation of the optic
      nerve head is caused by any process which impedes
      venous return from the retina (such as increased in-
      tracranial pressure or right heart failure) or any pro-
      cess which inflames the optic nerve (such as papil-
      litis). Early signs of papilledema are slight blurring
      and elevation of the optic nerve, loss of venous pul-
      sations, engorgement of the veins, an increased ra-
      tio of venous to arterial size (diameter), and a "wet"
      reflective appearance of the retina. Elevation of the
      optic nerve is measured by focusing from a high
      positive lens (such as +8 D) to a less positive lens
      (such as +1 D), until the surface of the optic nerve
      is in focus. Then, go back to the high positive lens
      (e.g., +8 D) and focus on the retina in the same
      manner. The difference in the power of the lenses
      necessary to focus on the retina and the optic nerve
      is the number of diopters of papilledema. For ex-
      ample, if the nerve is in focus at +4 D and the retina
      is in focus at +1 D, there are 3 D of papilledema
      present.
   b. Papillitis can be differentiated from papilledema by

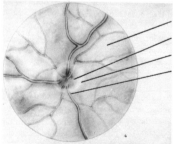

Retina appears "wet"

Elevation of optic disc

Edge of disc unclear

Veins engorged and venous
pulsations absent

FIG B–2. Papilledema.

the early, rapid loss of vision, which is not characteristic of papilledema.

5. Examining visual fields: If a *visual* field defect is *not* suspected, examine both eyes simultaneously (Fig B–3).

   a. The examiner and the patient are seated approximately 2 ft apart. The patient is instructed to look at the examiner's nose. The examiner's fingers are midway between himself or herself and the patient and at the outer limit of vision.

   b. The examiner wiggles one finger and asks the patient to point to the one that moved. Both fingers are then wiggled simultaneously. Normally, the patient will perceive all movements correctly.

   c. The process is repeated on the other diagonal.

   d. The visual field examination is concluded by the examiner placing his or her right hand over the patient's right eye. The examiner then closes his or her own left eye and instructs the patient to "look at the pupil in my right eye." The examiner brings the left finger toward the patient's nasal field on the diagonal while instructing the patient to "Tell me when you can first see my finger." Normally, both the patient and the examiner should see the finger at approximately the same time.

6. Important abnormalities:

   a. With the phenomenon of "extinction" or "neglect," the patient correctly perceives finger movement individually but not simultaneously, suggesting a contralateral parietal lobe lesion.

7. If a defect is suspected or is suggested by the screening procedure, each eye must be tested separately (Fig B–3). The patient should cover one eye (a patch may be necessary). The examiner then closes one of his or her own eyes (on the same side as the closed eye of the patient), and patient and examiner look into each other's pupils. As illustrated, the examiner then brings a finger on the diagonal toward the midline until it is perceived by the patient. In effect, the examiner is comparing his or her visual field with that of the patient. The test is

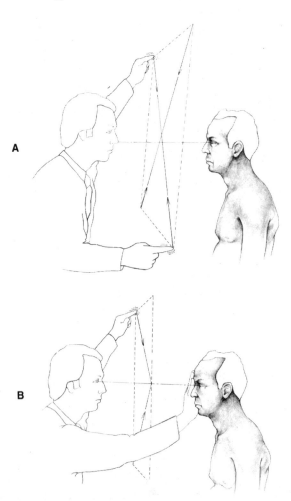

FIG B–3. A–B, visual field testing.

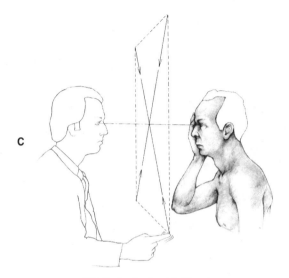

FIG B–3. C, visual field testing.

more accurate if the examiner uses a small red object, such as a 5-mm ball on a hatpin, as a target (Fig B–4).

8. Checking visual acuity (Fig B–5):
   a. Place the pocket Snellen chart approximately 14 in. (36 cm) from the eye.
   b. The room should be well-lighted, the patient should wear any corrective lenses (eyeglasses or contact lenses), and one eye should be covered.
   c. The numbers on the chart that accompany the smallest type the patient can read indicate the patient's visual acuity: for example 20/50, means that the patient can see at 20 ft what the normal person can see at 50 ft.

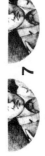

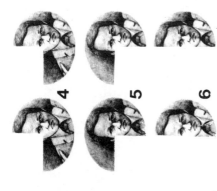

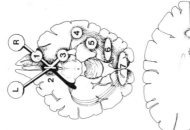

For legend see opposite page.

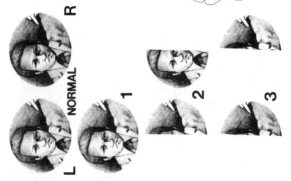

B. **Oculomotor (III), trochlear (IV), and abducens (VI).**
These cranial nerves control movement of the eyes and are tested together. The third cranial nerve also controls pupillary size.
  1. Testing ocular movement:
    a. Place one hand on patient's head (to prevent the natural tendency to turn the head as the eyes follow an object). Instruct the patient to follow the examiner's finger as it moves laterally in the horizontal plane. Continue the lateral movement until the outer edge of the iris (limbus) of the *adducting* eye (eye moving medially) just touches the punctum (the red area at the medial corner of the eye). Then test lateral movement in the opposite direction. (Fig B–6,A).
    b. Test vertical movement by having the patient look upward at the examiner's finger (Fig B–6,B) Then quickly bring the finger down (observing how quickly the lids follow) for downward gaze. Figure B–6,C shows "lid lag" suggestive of thyroid disease.
    c. Finally, ask the patient to look at his or her nose and observe for constriction of the pupils.
  2. Testing pupillary reaction to direct light: The swinging flashlight test should be performed using a bright, pinpoint source of light to determine both direct and consensual pupillary reaction. This test is used to detect the Marcus-Gunn pupil (Fig B–7,A and B).
  3. Common abnormalities:
    a. Marcus-Gunn pupil: When the sequence for testing

FIG B–4. Diagram of types of defects which may be found: Note how the various patterns are of considerable value in localizing a lesion in the brain. Formal testing with a perimeter should be performed in all patients in whom a defect is demonstrated. Note that all visual input from the left side of the patient's environment ultimately goes to the right occipital lobe, and all visual input above the horizontal goes below the calcarine fissure.

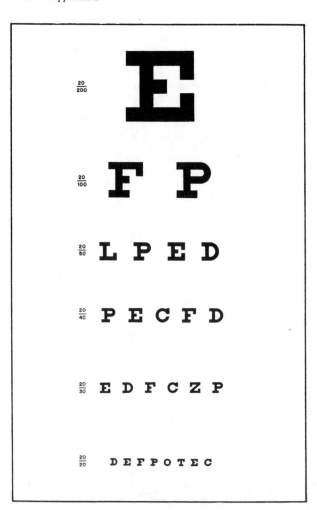

FIG B–5. Snellen chart for testing visual acuity

the pupillary reaction to direct light ("swinging flashlight test") is used, a pupil that *apparently* dilates to direct light may be observed. This phenomenon ("afferent pupillary defect") occurs with a lesion in the optic nerve anterior to the optic chiasm in which the consensual pupillary reflex is preserved while the direct reflex is impaired (i.e., the pupil dilates because there is less stimulus for pupillary constriction from light shown directly into the abnormal eye while maximal pupillary constriction occurs from the consensual reflex when light is shown in the normal eye) (Fig B–7,C).

b. Nystagmus: A rhythmic involuntary abnormal eye movement which may be present at rest or induced by eye movement and which persists after eye movement has ceased. Nystagmus can be described as slow deviation of the eye in one direction with quick jerking eye movements in the opposite direction. By convention, nystagmus is named for its quick component. The following types may be noted:

1) *End-point* nystagmus results when the normal patient gazes too far laterally. Therefore, the examiner should have the patient gaze laterally only to the point where the edge of the iris or limbus of the adducting eye meets the lacrimal punctum.

2) *Asymmetric lateral nystagmus* (absent or reduced in one direction of gaze compared to the opposite direction of gaze) suggests either central nervous system or end organ dysfunction.

3) *Nystagmus with the fast component upward (upbeat nystagmus) or with the fast component downward (downbeat nystagmus),* often most easily elicited on upward or downward gaze, usually indicates central nervous system (CNS) disease, often at the level of the brainstem.

4) *Nystagmus associated with dysconjugate eye movements or nystagmus in only one eye (monocular nystagmus)* (such as internuclear ophthalmoplegia in multiple sclerosis) would be indicative of CNS disease.

A

B

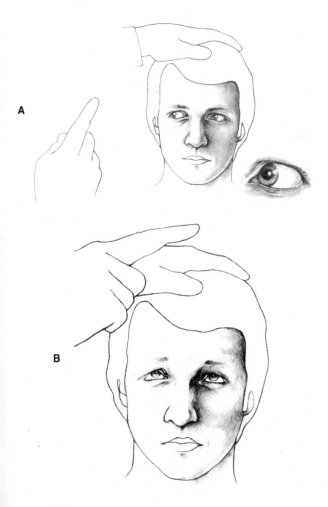

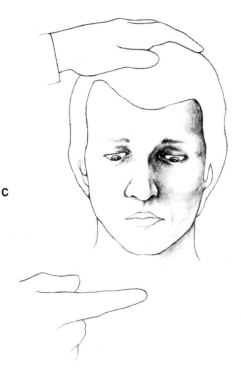

FIG B–6. A, horizontal eye movement; **B,** vertical eye movement; **C,** lid lag.

5) *Congenital nystagmus* is pendular lateral nystagmus that disappears with convergence and has a lateral movement even on upward gaze. It is usually associated with congenital bilateral visual impairment (blindness).

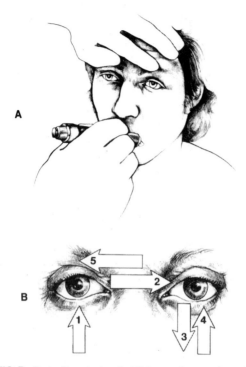

FIG B–7. A–C, swinging flashlight test: Instruct the patient to keep the eyelids open while a light is flashed in the eyes (the examiner may need to hold the eyelids open). Sequence of light movement is depicted by numbered arrows in B. Swing the light from below up to the first eye, shining the light directly into the pupil. The pupil in the tested eye should immediately constrict, as should the pupil in the opposite eye. Then quickly swing the light to the opposite eye; there should be no change in the size of either pupil. Swing the light down from the second eye; both pupils should dilate promptly; then swing the light back up to the second eye (pupils should constrict) and quickly back to the first eye (no change in pupillary size).

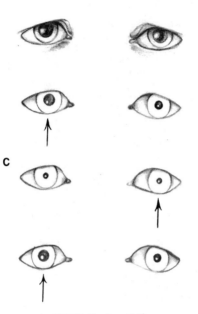

C

FIG B–7   (cont'd.).

     6) *Drug-induced or CNS nystagmus:* If nystagmus is equal in both directions of gaze, suspect a toxic or metabolic disorder; rarely brainstem dysfunction may produce similar nystagmus.

  c. Third nerve palsy: (Fig B–8,A): The oculomotor nerve (third cranial nerve) innervates all extraocular muscles (including the levator of the upper eyelid) except the lateral rectus and the superior oblique. Thus, with a complete third nerve palsy, the eye is *abducted* and deviated slightly downward, the upper eyelid droops, and the pupil is dilated and unreactive to light. Because the autonomic pupillary constrictor fibers are in the periphery of this nerve, when diabetic vascular disease affects the third nerve (by producing infarction), the pupil is frequently spared. In contrast, when the third nerve is damaged by cerebral herniation due to a temporal lobe mass causing the nerve to be compressed against the tentorium, the peripheral pupillary fibers are affected first and the pupil frequently dilates before paralysis of the extraocular muscles occurs.

d. Sixth nerve palsy: (Fig B–8,B): The abducens nerve (sixth cranial nerve) innervates the lateral rectus muscle. Therefore, with sixth nerve palsy, the eye is in an adducted position and does not move laterally beyond the midline. The pupil is not affected.

e. Internuclear ophthalmoplegia (Fig B–8,C): This abnormality superficially resembles bilateral medial rectus palsy, except that the ability to converge and look at a near object is spared. When the patient attempts to look laterally, the *abducting* eye moves laterally and develops nystagmus while the *adducting* eye does not move past the midline. The abnormality is due to a lesion of the medial longitudinal fasciculus in the central part of the pons and is often associated with multiple sclerosis.

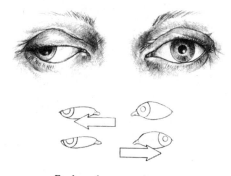

A

For legend see opposite page.

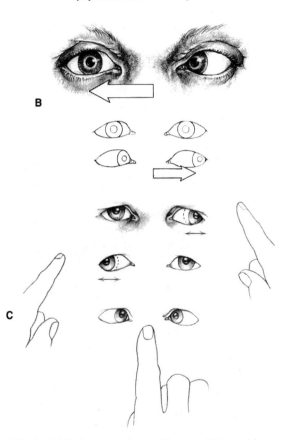

FIG B-8. Ocular nerve abnormalities. **A,** third cranial nerve palsy; **B,** sixth cranial nerve palsy; **C,** internuclear ophthalmoplegia; **D,** fourth cranial nerve palsy; **E,** Horner's syndrome.

(Continued.)

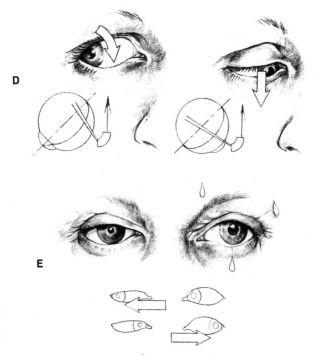

FIG B–8 (cont'd.).

f. Fourth nerve palsy (Fig B–8,D): The trochlear nerve (fourth cranial nerve) innervates the superior oblique muscle which rotates the top of the globe toward the nose in the *abducted* position and turns the globe downward in the *adducted* position. The muscle normally functions to keep the visual image upright by rotating the eye slightly during minor sideward head movements. Patients with fourth nerve palsy will complain of a vertical diplopia, especially when looking downward at relatively near objects (e.g., walking downstairs). Patients may develop a slight head tilt to prevent this diplopia. Isolated fourth nerve palsy is often due to diabetes or head trauma.

g. Horner's syndrome (Fig B–8,E): Due to damage to the sympathetic nerve supply to the eye, and not to damage to cranial nerves III, IV, or VI. The pupil is small (miotic), there is slight drooping of the eyelid (ptosis), and sweating on that side of the face is impaired (anhidrosis). Damage may occur anywhere in the course of the sympathetic pathway from the lateral medulla to the eye; some of the more common lesion sites are the cervical spinal cord, apex of the lung (affecting the sympathetic chain), and along the carotid artery (atherosclerotic damage at the carotid bifurcation).

h. Argyll Robertson pupil: An irregular small pupil that does not react to direct light but which constricts on accommodation; classically described with neurosyphilis.

C. Trigeminal nerve (V).

The fifth cranial nerve provides sensation for the face and cornea (Fig B–9).

1. Eliciting the corneal reflex in both eyes (Fig B–10).

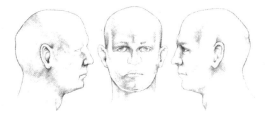

FIG B–9. Trigeminal nerve: the divisions are ophthalmic, maxillary, and mandibular.

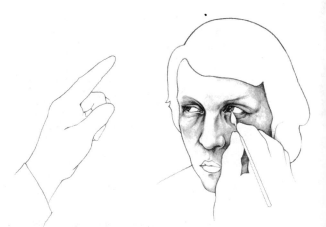

FIG B–10. Corneal reflex: Tease a wisp of cotton from the end of a clean cotton-tipped applicator. Tell the patient what will be done before the test. Ask the patient to look laterally, and lightly touch the cornea, approaching laterally from the side opposite the gaze (this avoids a threat reflex). Be certain to touch the cornea and not just the sclera. Normally, a rapid, involuntary blink will occur and both eyes blink simultaneously. Finally, ask the patient if the wisp of cotton feels the same in both corneas.

> *Caveat:* False results will be obtained if the examiner elicits a blink to threat or if the sclera rather than cornea is touched.

2. Testing facial sensation: If the patient has an abnormal corneal reflex (asymmetric or absent blink), or if the patient complains of pain, numbness, paresthesias, or other sensory disturbances about the face, check each division of the trigeminal nerve bilaterally with a wisp of cotton (light touch) and a pin (pain); for technique, see section IX.

3. Common abnormalities:
   a. If the patient has fifth cranial nerve dysfunction, the eye on that side will not blink to direct touch but will blink when the opposite cornea is touched, and the patient will report a difference in sensation between the eyes.
   b. If the patient has facial nerve (seventh cranial nerve) paralysis, the eye on that side will not blink regardless of which cornea is touched, although the patient will report sensation is the same in each eye. A partial facial nerve paralysis may be evident as a slower blink on the affected side compared with the normal side.

   Caveat: The trigeminal nerve also innervates the muscles of mastication, and if affected, the jaw will deviate *toward* the side of the lesion during jaw opening.

D. Facial nerve (VII).
   1. Observation for facial asymmetries (Fig B–11,A).
      a. On close inspection, many normal persons have slight asymmetries of the nasolabial folds and height of the palpebral fissures (size of eyelid opening). However, excessive flattening of one nasolabial fold or excessive opening of one palpebral fissure is abnormal.
   2. Observation of facial movement (Fig B–11,B):
      a. Instruct the patient to grimace ("Show me your teeth" usually communicates this movement) and to wrinkle the forehead (Fig B–11,C), observing for any asymmetry.
      b. To resolve doubt concerning weakness, instruct the patient to close the eyelids tightly; the examiner then attempts to open them (Fig B–11,D). When the eyelids are tightly closed the eyelashes are not visible. If the eyelashes are seen, there may be partial facial nerve palsy. The examiner can also instruct the patient to puff out the cheeks while the examiner taps on them; a tap on the weak side more easily expels air (Fig B–11,E).

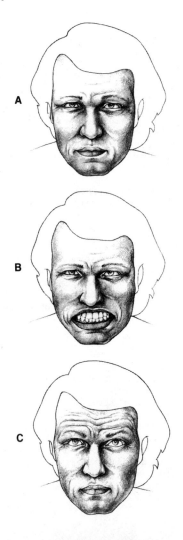

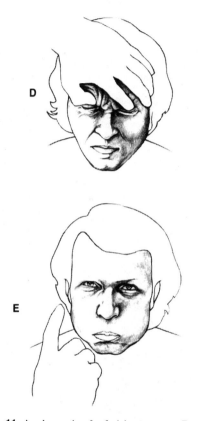

FIG B–11. A, observation for facial asymmetry; **B,** observation for facial movement (grimace and wrinkle forehead); **C,** wrinkling the forehead; **D,** forcibly opening eyes; **E,** blowing out cheeks.

3. Common problems:
   a. Absent teeth may create the impression of facial paralysis.
   b. Asymmetry of movement is a more reliable sign of abnormality than asymmetry of appearance.
   c. Patient with partial bilateral facial palsy may appear normal.
4. Common abnormalities:
   a. A patient with upper motor neuron weakness (lesion above the brainstem facial nucleus, most often in the contralateral motor cortex) will be able to wrinkle the forehead (and partially close the eyelids) but will have paresis of the remainder of the face. (Fig B–12,A).
   b. A patient with a lower motor neuron facial weakness (lesion in the brainstem facial nucleus or along the facial nerve) will have weakness of all the facial muscles (including the forehead) on the same side as the lesion (Fig B–12,B),

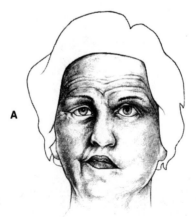

FIG B–12. A, upper motor neuron facial weakness; **B,** lower motor neuron facial weakness.

B

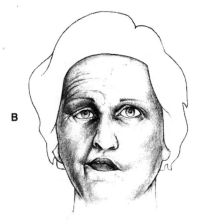

FIG B-12 (cont'd.).

E. **Auditory nerve (VIII).**
  1. Testing of auditory acuity bilaterally: Auditory acuity may be tested by lightly rubbing the fingers together several inches from the patient's ears (Fig B-13,A).
  2. Confirming a deficit in auditory acuity: If a hearing deficit is demonstrated, Weber's and Rinne tests should be performed.
     a. Rinne test (Fig B-13,B): Lightly tap a 256-Hz tuning fork, hold it for a few seconds in front of the patient's ear (air conduction), and then place the base of the fork on the patient's mastoid bone (bone conduction). Ask, "Which was louder?" The normal patient will answer "The one in front of the ear."
     b. Weber's Test (Fig B-13,C): Tap a 256-Hz tuning fork lightly, place the base of the fork on the forehead, and ask, "Is the buzzing equally loud in both ears?" The normal patient will answer "The buzzing is the same in both ears."

3. Common problems:
   a. Diminished auditory acuity is misdiagnosed because of wax or other foreign matter in the ear.
   b. A high or low frequency loss is missed because specific frequencies are not tested.
4. Common abnormalities:
   a. Conductive hearing loss (usually otosclerosis): Bone conduction is greater than air conduction (Rinne test), and the tuning fork on the forehead lateralizes to the *affected* ear (Weber's test).
   b. Sensorineural loss: Air conduction is greater than bone conduction (Rinne test), and the tuning fork on the forehead lateralizes to the *normal* ear (Weber's test).

F. **Glossopharyngeal nerve (IX) and vagus nerve (X).**
   1. Observation of soft palate: Instruct the patient to open the mouth; the arches of the soft palate should be symmetric.
   2. Observation of palate movement: Instruct the patient to say "ahh" and observe symmetric elevation of the soft palate.

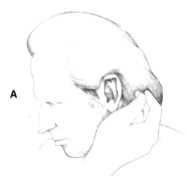

A

FIG B–13. **A,** testing auditory acuity; **B,** Rinne test. **C,** Weber's test.

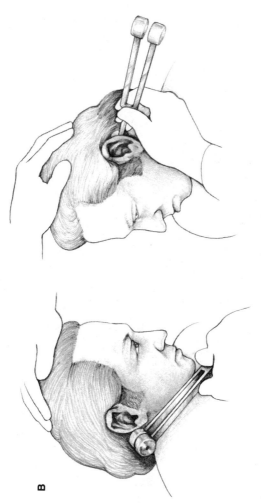

FIG B–13 (cont'd).

B

C

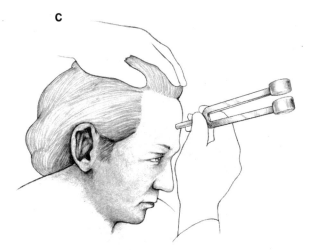

FIG B-13   (cont'd.).

3. Eliciting the pharyngeal reflex (Fig B–14): Touch both sides of the soft palate with a cotton-tipped applicator and observe the symmetric elevation of the soft palate. Ask the patient if the sensation is the same on both sides.
4. Listening to voice quality.
   a. Common problems
      1) If the tongue interferes with adequate visualization of the palate, depress with a flashlight on a wooden tongue depressor.
      2) Some normal persons may have bilateral slight or absent pharyngeal reflexes; sensation, however, remains normal. It is not necessary to make the patient gag and stimulation with a tongue depressor rather than cotton applicator is not necessary.
   b. Common abnormalities
      1) A unilateral vagal nerve (X) paresis results in

failure of the palate to move either voluntarily or to sensory stimulation. The arch will be asymmetric and the uvula will deviate toward the normal side (Figure B–15).

2) Patients with bilateral vagal paralysis will have little or no palatal movement and, in addition, will exhibit considerable difficulty in swallowing, but the uvula will be midline.

3) With palatal weakness, the voice has a nasal quality (air escaping into the nose), while with vocal cord paresis the voice is hoarse.

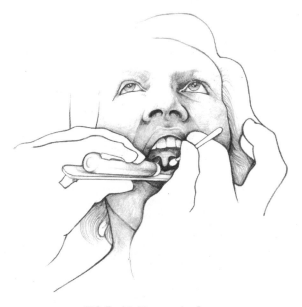

FIG B–14. Pharyngeal reflex.

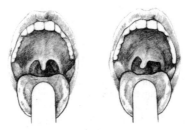

FIG B–15. Palatal deviation due to unilateral vagal nerve paralysis.

G.   **Spinal accessory nerve (XI).**
    1.   Testing the strength of the sternocleidomastoid and trapezius muscles.
        a.   Instruct the patient to turn the head to one side and keep it there. The examiner then attempts to overcome this resistance by pushing at the angle of the jaw (Fig B–16,A).
        b.   Instruct the patient to shrug the shoulders. The examiner then places both hands on the shoulders and attempts to push them down (Fig B–16,B).

A

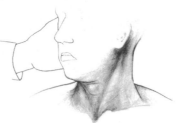

FIG B–16. A, testing sternocleidomastoid muscle function; **B,** testing trapezius muscle function.

B

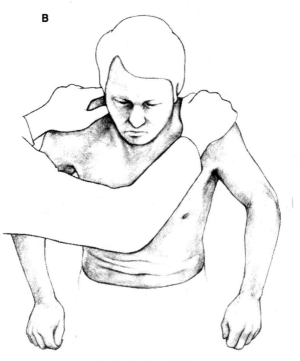

FIG B–16   (cont'd.).

2. Common problems:
   a. The examiner forgets that the left sternocleidomastoid muscle turns the head to the right.
   b. Neck pain or limitation of motion interferes with proper testing of muscle strength.
3. Common abnormalities:
   a. Weakness of these muscles is rare except when the lower motor neuron portion is injured. Cerebral le-

sions usually cause only minimal weakness.

    b. Weakness of the trapezius muscle may lead to drooping and winging of the scapula.

H.   **Hypoglossal nerve (XII).**

    1. Testing tongue movement: Instruct the patient to stick out the tongue; observe carefully for deviation, symmetry, and abnormal movements (Fig B–17,A).

    2. Common problems

       a. A patient with a facial nerve paralysis may give the illusion of having a deviated tongue. The illusion is proved false when the crease in the middle of the tongue lines up with the tip of the nose.

    3. Common abnormalities:

       a. A cerebral lesion (upper motor neuron) causes slight or no deviation of the tongue.

       b. A lesion of the hypoglossal nucleus or the 12th cranial nerve causes the tongue to deviate toward the side of the lesion and, with time, ipsilateral atrophy. Atrophy gives the tongue a wrinkled appearance (Fig B–17,B).

       c. Bona fide fasciculations are often difficult to distinguish from a "wiggly" tongue. Fasciculations are best seen at the lateral edge of a tongue which is lying quietly in the mouth.

V.   **STATION AND GAIT.**

A.   **Testing.** In an area with 20 ft of straight walking space with the patient barefooted and clothed only in underwear or hospital gown, the patient is instructed to perform a series of tasks to assess station and gait (Table B–3 and Fig B–18). By doing the station and gait testing in this manner, a skillful examiner can obtain in 1 minute a glimpse of mental status (how well the patient comprehends instructions), upper motor neuron function (posturing of arms and by gait), lower motor neuron function (muscle atrophy and weakness), muscle disease (proximal weakness), basal ganglia (abnormal posture movement), cerebellum (balance and tandem walk), and the sensory system (poor balance with eyes closed — the Romberg test). A patient who can perform all the maneuvers normally will rarely have a significant neu-

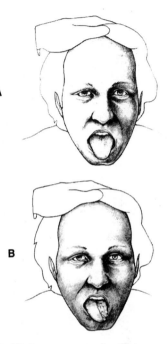

FIG B–17. A, tongue protrusion; **B,** tongue deviation.

rologic abnormality. Abnormalities noted can be more specifically tested in the remainder of the neurologic examination. For example, if station and gait testing suggests cerebellar abnormality, more specific cerebellar tests should be
performed.

B.   Common problems

1. The examiner forgets to perform the station and gait
   testing — one of the most valuable parts of the neurologic examination.

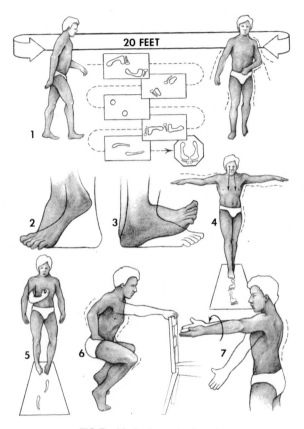

FIG B–18. Station and gait testing.

TABLE B–3.
Testing of Station and Gait

Instructions	Things to Note
Walk normally the 20-ft distance	Asymmetric arm swing, abnormal arm and hand postures, and instability of the trunk; stability of the turn
Rapidly turn around and walk on toes	Extra steps while turning around and inability to rise completely on tiptoes
Rapidly turn and walk on heels	Inability to dorsiflex the foot
Turn and walk with heels touching	Instability characteristic of midline cerebellar lesions
Turn and "walk on outsides of feet like a bowlegged cowboy" (walking on lateral aspects of feet)	This maneuver specifically brings out hemiplegic posturing of an arm from subtle or old upper motor neuron damage
Do a deep knee bend (preferably with hands on hips; if there is an obvious balance problem patient may hold onto an object, such as a chair, for stability)	Loss of balance indicates cerebellar difficulties; inability to rise indicates proximal weakness
Stand with feet together, eyes closed, arms outstretched to the front, with palms facing ceiling and fingers spread apart	Increased swaying with eyes closed would indicate either posterior column disease or peripheral neuropathy; patient with subtle hemiparesis will pronate arm which will then drift downward and outward

2. The examiner does not adequately protect the ataxic patient who may fall and be injured.
3. The examiner fixates on the patient's gait and forgets to look at the arms.
4. The female patient in hospital gown tends to use her arms to hold the gown together in the back, and thus much of the value of the test is lost; although the patient should be minimally dressed, modesty must be preserved with appropriate clothing. Many patients are reassured if the gown is closed with a safety pin or large clip.

5. The male patient in baggy hospital pants tends to trip over excessively long trouser legs or holds the pants up with his hands because of an insecure waistband. Shorts should be worn, if possible; otherwise the pants legs should be rolled up. Loose waistbands should be secured with a safety pin.

6. Uninformed examiners incorrectly interpret the Romberg test as a cerebellar sign.

VI. EVALUATION OF TENDON (MUSCLE STRETCH) REFLEXES AND PLANTAR STIMULATION.

A. Muscle stretch reflexes.

1. Technique for eliciting tendon reflexes:
   a. A muscle stretch (or tendon) reflex is the brief contraction of a muscle in response to a sudden stretch. The reflex therefore depends on:
      1) Whether the tendon is struck.
      2) How hard the tendon is struck.
      3) How quickly the tendon is struck.
   b. Reflex hammers:
      1) A hammer with a soft rubber head and flexible handle will aid the examiner in delivering a quick tap.
      2) A hammer with a long handle will aid in more accurate grading of reflexes and tapping the tendons in inconvenient positions.
      3) The authors prefer a Queen's Square style of hammer, which is available in two sizes: a small one for children and a large one for adults.
   c. Grading reflexes: Reflexes are normal, hypoactive, absent, hyperactive, or clonic. A -2 or $+4$ statement regarding reflex activity means nothing unless carefully defined in each patient's chart.
   d. Muscle contraction may be observed or felt.

2. Specific "routine" reflexes:
   a. Biceps reflex (C5 and C6 spinal roots; musculocutaneous nerve) (Fig B–19,A). The arms must be slightly flexed, relaxed, and resting on the patient's

thighs. The examiner lightly presses the biceps tendon with the thumb and taps the thumb with the hammer. Elbow flexion will be observed and contraction of the biceps tendon against the thumb will be felt.

b. Brachioradialis reflex (C5 and C6 spinal roots; radial nerve) (Fig B–19,B): With the arms positioned and relaxed as in eliciting the biceps reflex, a tap is delivered above the styloid process at the distal end of the radius. Elbow flexion and slight outward rotation of the forearm will be observed.

c. Triceps reflex (C6, C7, and C8 spinal roots; radial nerve) (Fig B–19,C): With the patient's arms resting on the hips, the examiner identifies (by palpation) the triceps tendon just above the bony prominence of the elbow (olecranon), and then delivers a tap to this tendon. Contraction of the triceps muscle will be observed along with elbow extension.

A

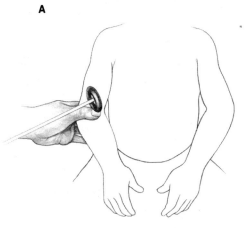

FIG B–19. A, biceps reflex; **B,** brachioradialis reflex; **C,** triceps reflex. *(Continued.)*

B

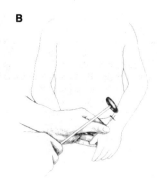

C

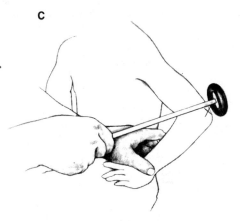

FIG B–19 (cont'd.).

      d. Patellar (knee) reflex (L2, L3, and L4 spinal roots; femoral nerve) (Fig B–20,A): The patient should be sitting with knees slightly beyond the edge of the table and legs relaxed, dangling, and not touching the floor. The patellar tendon should be palpated before it is tapped (this is especially important in obese patients or patients with bony deformity). Tapping the patellar tendon results in knee extension. In some patients with hypoactive reflexes or in whom the tendon is difficult to localize, placing the thumb on the tendon and tapping of the thumb may elicit the reflex. In addition to eliciting the patellar reflex, the examiner should also observe for contraction of the ipsilateral or contralateral adductor muscle or contralateral quadriceps (such abnormal reflex spread is seen with hyperactive reflexes) and excessive swinging of the leg back and forth (this "pendular" reflex is an indication of hypotonia).

      e. Achilles (ankle) reflex (S1 spinal root; tibial nerve) (Fig B–20,B): With the patient in the same position as for the patellar reflex, the examiner places his or her hand under the patient's foot and slightly extends the foot. The patient is instructed to apply light pressure to the palm of the examiner's hand, while the examiner strikes the Achilles tendon. The foot should move downward against the examiner's hand.

  3. Common problems:

      a. Patient is not appropriately undressed.

      b. A reflex hammer with an aged, hard rubber head is used.

      c. The patient is not relaxed or is improperly positioned.

      d. An inexperienced examiner reports a reflex as present when it is really absent (usually the inexperienced examiner does this out of anxiety that the reflex was missed because his or her technique was defective and that a more experienced examiner will find the reflex present).

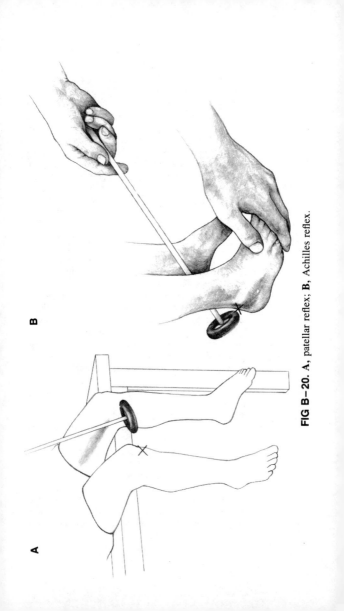

FIG B–20. **A,** patellar reflex; **B,** Achilles reflex.

Remember: There is some normal variability in reflex activity and two quite experienced examiners may find slightly different degrees of reflex activity.

e. Reflexes should be present in normal elderly patients; however, peripheral nerve dysfunction from a variety of causes is very common in elderly patients who thus have absent reflexes on the basis of a pathologic condition.

4. Common abnormalities:
   a. Hyperactive reflexes: Tense patients tend to have brisk reflexes, and there is a wide range of "normal." Hyperactive reflexes tend to have a "spread" of reflex activity, e.g. muscles distal from the one whose tendon is being tapped also contract. Hyperactive reflexes suggest an upper motor neuron lesion.
   b. Clonus may be elicited by rapidly dorsiflexing the ankle; a rhythmic alternating dorsiflexion (extension) and plantar flexion of the ankle ensues and may last seconds to minutes (Fig B–21). Clonus is often indicative of an upper motor neuron lesion.
   c. Absent reflexes suggest damage to any part of the reflex arc: muscle spindle or sensory or motor nerves. An absent Achilles (ankle) reflex has a different sound (a "thud") than that elicited with a normally active reflex.

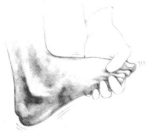

FIG B–21. Ankle clonus.

d. A slowed relaxation phase of the Achilles reflex suggests hypothyroidism.

e. The most common abnormality observed is *reflex asymmetry*, rather than absent or hyperactive reflexes. Asymmetries are best appreciated by using the *lightest tap possible* that will still elicit the reflex; many examiners strike the tendons with too much force.

B. Plantar responses.

1. Technique for eliciting the plantar response:

a. The plantar response is a complex cutaneous reflex; the type of response elicited depends on the type of stimulation used (we recommend a key), how quickly the stimulus is delivered, and the position

TABLE B–4.
Varieties of Plantar Responses

Name	Observation	Interpretation
Normal response (flexor plantar response)	First movement of great toe is flexion	Normal
Classic Babinski (classic extensor plantar response)	Extension of great toe with extension or fanning of other toes	Most often seen in upper motor neuron lesions in the spinal cord (above the L5 segment)
Babinski reflex (extensor plantar response)	First movement of great toe is extension (there may be subsequent flexion of great toe); other toes either show no movement or flexion	Seen in all types of upper motor neuron lesions (above the L5 segment)
Mute plantar response	Nothing happens	Severe sensory loss or paralysis of foot
Withdrawal	Patient pulls foot back	Often seen in metabolic neuropathies or if examiner uses excessively sharp object
Asymmetric response	Mute plantar response on side and flexor plantar response on other side	Indication of need to look for other hard signs of neurologic disease

of the patient. The key is used to stimulate the lateral aspect of the plantar surface of the foot beginning at the heel and moving up to the ball of the foot, staying lateral to the great toe. (Fig B–22 and Table B–4).

   b. Because the abnormal plantar response is such an important sign of nervous system disease, the best approach to recording the results if in doubt is to record exactly the observed movements.

2. Common problems:

   a. Too sharp a stimulus is used and a withdrawal reflex is elicited.

   b. Too light a stimulus is used and no response occurs.

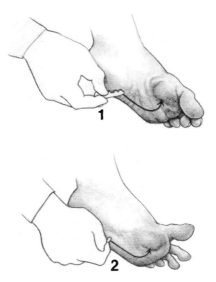

FIG B–22. Plantar stimulation.

(Continued.)

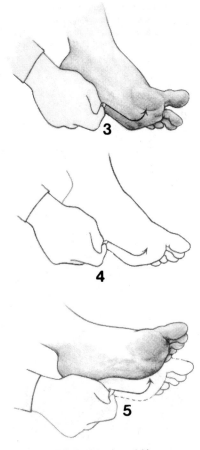

FIG B-22 (cont'd.).

c. The response may change from time to time depending on time of day, medication, and whether the patient is sitting or lying. Since the character of the plantar reflex may change with position, in a situation where the response is critical, stimulation should be done with the patient in both the lying and sitting positions.

d. The examiner brings the stimulus over the base of the big toe causing mechanical flexion of the big toe.

VII. MUSCLE APPEARANCE, STRENGTH, RANGE OF MOTION, AND INVOLUNTARY MOVEMENTS.

A. **Plan the evaluation of muscles on the basis of the history, station and gait testing, reflex examination, and coordination.**

Remember: Reflex examination and station and gait testing evaluate:

1. Distal strength (ability to walk on tiptoes and heels).
2. Proximal strength (ability to perform deep knee bends while holding arms outstretched and ability to arise from sitting position).
3. Abnormal postures and movement.
4. Abnormal muscle bulk by observation.
5. Abnormal tone (hyperactive reflexes suggest hypertonia; pendular reflexes suggest hypotonia).
6. Abnormal coordination (may be a sign of weakness as well as cerebellar disease).

B. **If the station and gait testing and reflex examination are normal and the patient does not complain of weakness, cramps, stiffness, or change in muscle bulk, specific muscle testing is rarely necessary.**

C. *Common abnormalities seen on inspection:*

1. Muscle atrophy is often best appreciated by looking at the muscle (first dorsal interosseous) between the thumb and first finger. Normally, the superficial contour in this area should be convex; with atrophy it is flat or concave as illustrated. The thenar and hypothenar areas should also have a convex surface; with atrophy they become flat (Fig B–23).

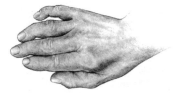

FIG B−23. Hand atrophy.

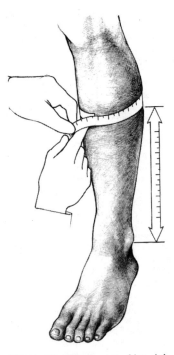

FIG B−24. Measurement of leg girth.

2. If atrophy is present in the thighs, upper arms, or forearms, the degree of wasting should be documented by measurement. For example, if atrophy of the gastrocnemius muscle is suspected, measure from a convenient landmark, e.g., the lateral malleolus to the midpoint of the muscle, and then measure the girth of the legs bilaterally at these points (Fig B–24).

3. Muscle hypertrophy is rare and is most commonly seen in the gastrocnemius muscles of boys with Duchenne's muscular dystrophy.

4. Fasciculations are seen as a brief (less than 1 second) trough-like dimpling of the skin over the muscle. They are easiest to see in the muscles of the back with the use of cross-lighting. Several light taps with a percussion hammer may precipitate a flurry of fasciculations, but clinical conclusions from fasciculations elicited in this manner should be made with caution (Fig B–25).

D. Testing muscle strength.

1. For suspected muscle weakness, first have the patient contract the muscle and allow the full normal movement of the body part to take place. Then instruct the patient

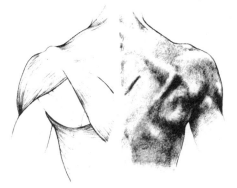

FIG B–25. Fasciculations in back muscles.

to hold that posture while the examiner attempts to return the body part to a more neutral position (Fig B–26). For example, to test the biceps muscle, the patient would be told, "Make a muscle like Popeye" (the examiner might even demonstrate the movement to the patient). Then the examiner would grasp the forearm near the elbow and tell the patient "Don't let me extend your arm," while applying force to extend the arm. Most muscles in the body can be tested in a similar manner; we recommend that examiners keep a copy of *Aids to the Examination of the Peripheral Nervous System* (see section III. A. 18) for quick reference in case complex muscle testing is required.

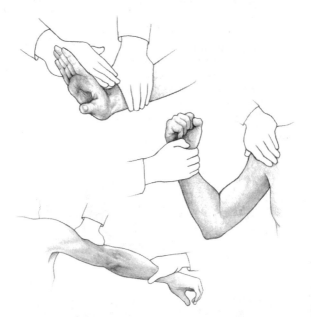

FIG B–26. Muscle strength testing.

2. Formal grading of muscle strength: The following classification of strength is most commonly used (derived by the British Medical Research Council and termed the MRC scale)

5 = normal.

4 = subjectively weak.

3 = movement possible against gravity (e.g., patient can flex supinated arm until hand touches shoulder; see Fig B–27).

2 = movement possible only when force of gravity is eliminated (e.g., with shoulder abducted, patient can flex and extend arm on the horizontal plane; see Fig B–27).

1 = contraction of muscle is seen or palpated but no movement takes place.

0 = no muscle contraction is apparent.

Caveat: As many as 60% of the muscle fibers in a given muscle may be destroyed without producing clinically detectable weakness. The majority of weak patients will fall into the 4 category, which is subjective; therefore the grading system is not perfect.

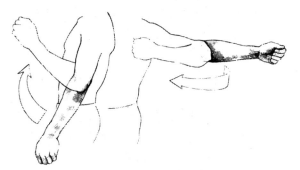

FIG B–27. MRC muscle testing.

3. Functional grading of muscle strength: In patients whose weakness may be either improving or deteriorating, it is important to test and document strength frequently. Pick a task that a patient can perform, but just barely. Suggestions include (Fig B–28):
   a. Arise from a chair with arms crossed.
   b. Raise arms above head.
   c. Extend leg from a sitting position.
   d. Hop on one foot.

E. **Testing range of movement.**
   1. If muscles are not periodically stretched, they lose their elasticity and become pathologically shortened in what is termed a *contracture*. Thus, a patient with a hemiplegia may not be able to fully extend the elbow, not because of weakness but because the length of the biceps makes it impossible to do so.
   2. Range of motion may also be limited by pain, muscle spasm, or joint deformity.

F. **Abnormal muscle tone.** Instruct the patient to relax an arm "like a rag doll"; the examiner then flexes and extends the forearm. Several abnormalities may be noted:
   1. An increased resistance to passive movement that is greater at the start of the movement and becomes less as the movement is completed is known as the "clasp-knife" phenomenon and may be seen in severe upper motor neuron lesions.
   2. Increased resistance throughout the range of movement is known as "lead-pipe" rigidity and may be seen in the parkinsonian syndrome.
   3. A severely floppy extremity is hypotonic; it is seen in severe peripheral nerve lesions and cerebellar disease.

G. **Abnormal posture and movement.**
   1. *Chorea* and *athetosis* are abnormal movements which really are repetitive assumptions of inappropriate postures. Call the movement athetosis if it is reminiscent of a ballet dance, chorea if it simulates a disco dance.
   2. *Tremor* is an involuntary, rhythmic, oscillatory movement of a body part, present at rest, and is seen in familial (senile) tremor, parkinsonian syndrome, and thyrotoxicosis.

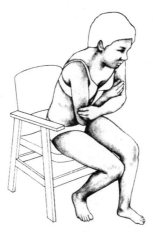

FIG B–28. Rising from a chair.

3. *Myoclonus* is a spontaneous, irregular, rapid contraction of a part of a muscle causing movement across a joint. (Commonly seen in sleeping dogs and cats.)

4. *Asterixis* is elicited by having the patient dorsiflex the wrists: brief lapses in tone make the patient appear to be waving "bye-bye" (Fig B–29).

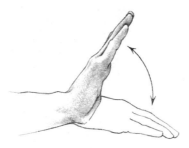

FIG B–29. Asterixis

5. Common abnormal postures include the hemiplegic posture (flexion of elbow and wrist, adduction of the shoulder, extension of the leg and feet; Figure B–30,A) and the parkinsonian posture (forward flexion of the body, shoulders internally rotated, arms at side with palms facing backward; Fig B–30,B).

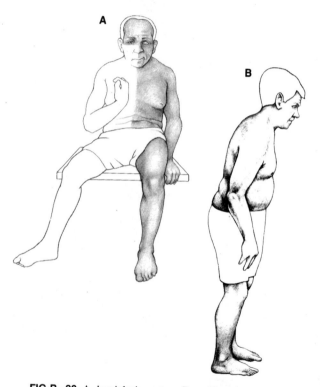

FIG B–30. **A,** hemiplegic posture; **B,** parkinsonian posture.

H. **If the patient complains of muscle stiffness or has a long thin "hatchet" face, test for the presence of myotonia (Figs B–31, B–32, and B–33).**

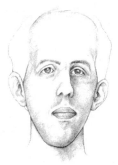

FIG B–31. Hatchet face of myotonic dystrophy.

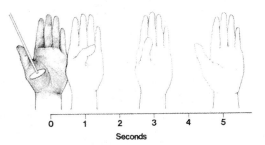

FIG B–32. Demonstration of myotonia: Percuss the thenar eminence; if myotonia is present, the thumb will make a quick, involuntary opposing movement and then slowly relax. Have the patient make a hard fist and then suddenly open it; if myotonia is present, opening the fist will be slow and laborious.

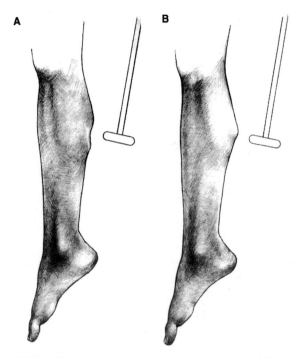

FIG B–33. Demonstration of myoedema and myotonia: with the patient prone, percuss the gastrocnemius muscles with a reflex hammer. **A,** If myotonia is present a persistent depression at the point of percussion will appear. **B,** if myoedema is present, a lump will appear.

I.   **If the patient complains of becoming fatigued easily, suspect myasthenia gravis and attempt to demonstrate fatigue** (Fig B–34).

1.   Have the patient sustain upward gaze for at least 1 minute; in patients with myasthenia gravis one or both lids may droop.

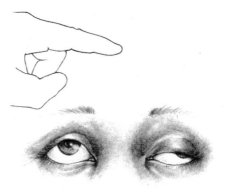

FIG B–34. Myasthenia gravis.

2. Have the patient perform some repetitive act relative to the complaint of weakness. For example, have the patient do repeated deep knee bends if the complaint is leg weakness. Have the patient repeatedly squeeze a manometer cuff if the complaint is weakness of grip. Myasthenics often gradually lose muscle power when performing such repetitive acts. The voice may lose volume during rapid loud counting.

J. **Common peripheral nerve lesions.**

1. Radial nerve (Fig B–35,A) damage produces weakness of dorsiflexion of the wrist and extension of the elbow. The lesion often is the result of compression of the nerve at the spiral groove of the humerus.

2. Median nerve damage results in weakness of opposition of the thumb and the little finger if the lesion is at the wrist (carpal tunnel syndrome). More proximal lesions in the arm result in weakness of pronation of the forearm and flexion of the radial three fingers (middle, ring, and little fingers) (Fig B–35,B).

3. Ulnar nerve injury results in weakness of abduction and adduction of the fingers, flexion of the ring and little

fingers, and ulnar flexion of the wrist. The lesion is most often the result of compression of the nerve in the ulnar groove of the elbow (Fig B–35,C).

4. Common peroneal nerve damage results in weakness of extension (dorsiflexion) and eversion of the foot. The most common site for injury is at the fibular head.

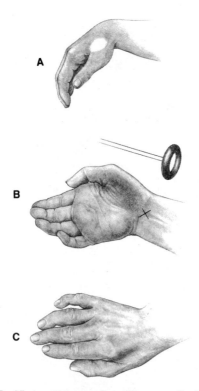

FIG B–35. **A,** radial nerve; **B,** median nerve; **C,** ulnar nerve.

VIII. TESTING OF CEREBELLAR FUNCTION.

A. **Finger-nose-finger test:** The examiner places his or her finger in front of the patient's nose at nearly the patient's arm length. The patient is then instructed, "Touch my finger and then your nose, back and forth."

B. **Rapid alternating movements:** The examiner demonstrates to the patient by alternately slapping the palm and dorsal surface of the hand on the thigh, and then requests that the patient do the same with each hand.

C. **Heel-to-toe walking:** Instruct the patient to walk a line, heel to toe (this is usually done as a part of station and gait testing).

D. **Heel-to-shin test:** In the lying position instruct the patient to run the heel of one leg smoothly up and down the shin of the other leg (Fig B–36).

E. **Common problems:**
   1. If the patient performs the finger-to-nose test too rapidly, the increase in tremor that occurs as the target is approached may be difficult for the examiner to appreciate.

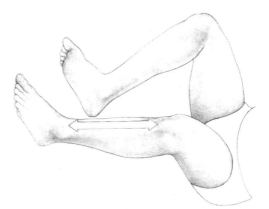

FIG B–36. Heel-to-shin test.

2. The examiner's finger must be held at arm's length to increase excursion of the patient's arm and enhance the tremor.
3. Coordination may be difficult or impossible to test in a weak or paralyzed arm.
4. Abnormal tone (such as the rigidity of Parkinson's disease or with spasticity) may significantly interfere with performance of rapid alternating movements.
5. The inexperienced examiner may not recognize that a patient with severe midline cerebellar disease can have relatively normal rapid alternating movements and finger-to-nose test.
6. Other movement disorders, such as familial tremor, may make the finger-to-nose test difficult to interpret.

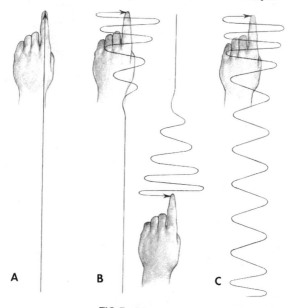

FIG B–37. Tremor.

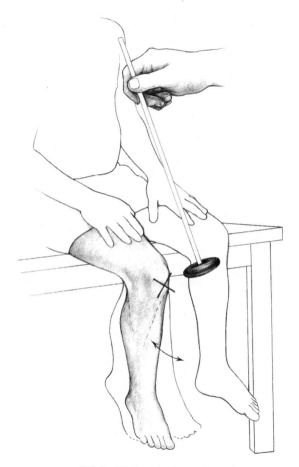

FIG B–38. Pendular knee reflex.

F. Common abnormalities.

   1. Dysfunction of a cerebellar hemisphere will cause an ipsilateral tremor notable during the finger-to-nose test. The tremor becomes worse as the target is approached and is not present in the resting hand or arm (Fig B–37).

   2. Dysfunction of a cerebellar hemisphere will cause an ipsilateral decrease in the ability to perform rapid alternating movements quickly and rhythmically.

   3. Midline cerebellar dysfunction will cause balance difficulties during heel-to-toe walking. Truncal ataxia may also be present in the sitting position.

G. Other signs of cerebellar dysfunction.

   1. Hypotonia may be manifested by a pendular knee reflex (Fig B–38).

   2. Speech melody may be disturbed and speech may become "explosive" and ataxic. This is particularly noticeable when pronouncing "tongue-twister" phrases such as "Methodist Episcopal."

   3. When a patient is flexing the arm against resistance and the examiner suddenly lets go, the patient may be unable to avoid striking his or her face. This is known as rebound. The examiner should use his or her arm to protect the patient (Fig B–39).

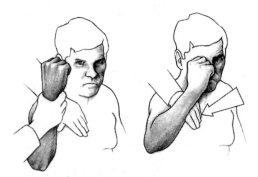

FIG B–39. Rebound.

IX. **THE SENSORY AND AUTONOMIC EXAMINATION.**
A. **Examination of peripheral sensation.** The evaluation of sensation is *subjective,* and therefore the examiner must be certain that the patient correctly interprets the procedure. Sensory testing is the *least* reliable portion of the neurologic examination, and diagnosis should rarely, if ever, be made on the basis of a sensory abnormality alone.

   1. Testing the sensation of pain (Fig B–40,A):

     a. Gently grasp the shaft of a pin (not a safety pin, ECG calipers, etc.) and test an area presumed to be normal (e.g., the neck). The pin should slide through the thumb and index finger as skin contact is made. Ask the patient, "Does this feel sharp?"

     b. To evaluate lower extremity sensation, repeat the procedure on the dorsum of the foot and ask, "Does this feel the same?" If the patient says, "No, it's not so sharp on my foot," then the examiner should prick once in a normal area saying, "If this is a dollar," and then prick once on the top of the foot saying "How much is this?" Only answers less than 70 cents are significant. The same procedure can be repeated on the dorsum of the hand to test upper extremity sensation.

     Note: Always use a fresh pin for each patient to avoid the spread of infections such as hepatitis or HIV.

   2. Testing light touch sensation. Instruct the patient to keep the eyes closed and respond whenever touched. Take a wisp of cotton or facial tissue and touch the patient on random areas of skin. Ask the patient to point to the part being touched.

   3. Testing vibratory sense (Fig B–40,B).

     a. Establish rapport with the patient by placing the shaft of a lightly vibrating 128-Hz tuning fork on a knuckle of the patient's hand and ask, "Do you feel the buzzing?" Then instruct the patient, "Tell me when the buzzing stops." When the patient says "Stop," the examiner should place the shaft of the fork on the knuckle of his or her own hand. Normally the examiner would also detect no vibration.

A

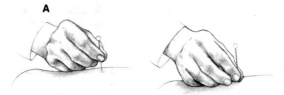

B

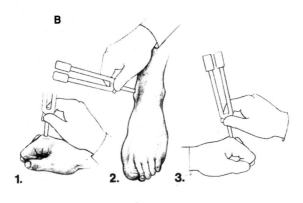

1.   2.   3.

C

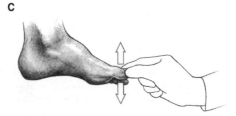

FIG B–40. A, testing for pain sensation; **B,** testing vibratory sensation; **C,** testing position sensation in the toes; **D,** testing cortical sensation; **E,** sensory self-examination.

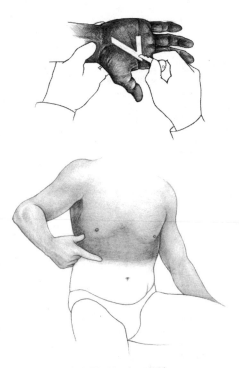

FIG B–40   (cont'd.).

b. To test vibratory sensation in the lower extremities, lightly tap the fork and place the shaft on the patient's medial malleolus, again instructing the patient, "Tell me when the buzzing stops." When the patient says "Stop," the examiner should place the shaft of the fork on the knuckle of his or her own hand. Normally, only a very slight vibration will still be felt by the examiner.

4. Testing position sense in the big toes:
   a. Establish rapport with the patient by grasping the patient's big toe *by the sides* and, with the patient observing the foot, say "When I move the toe in this direction [demonstrating] I mean up, and when I move it in this direction [demonstrating] I mean down." It is helpful to fix the proximal joints with the examiner's opposite hand (Fig B–40,C). Then with the patient's eyes closed, instruct the patient, "Tell me when I move your toe and whether I move it up or down." The examiner should move the toe unpredictably (e.g., up twice, down once). Normally, a patient will be able to detect movements of about 5 mm or less.
5. Testing for cortical sensation (Fig B–40,D):
   a. Ascertain that primary sensory modalities (pain and vibratory sensation) are intact in the hands; if sensation is not intact, this test is not valid.
   b. In order to establish rapport with the patient, have the patient watch the examiner draw a number on the patient's palm (using the dull point of an object such as a key) and ask "What number did I draw?" It is preferable to test the dominant hand first (unless a known neurologic defect exists on that side of the body) and the number should be written so that it is right side up to the patient. Then have the patient look away or close the eyes and repeat the procedure.

B. **Common problems**.
   1. The patient and examiner do not communicate adequately. The sensory examination is of limited value in patients with low intelligence, altered consciousness, aphasia, or psychiatric disturbances.
   2. The examiner tests an area of sensory disturbance with a pin, asking only, "Is this sharp or dull?" and does not compare it with a normal area; many less severe sensory disturbances are thus undiagnosed.
   3. The patient may think the response is what the examiner wants to hear; this is not necessarily malingering, but is simply a human foible of attempting to please an authority figure.

4. Posterior column disease or a cortical sensory loss cannot be demonstrated if the patient has a peripheral nerve disturbance which affects all sensory modalities.

C. Common abnormalities.

1. Patients with peripheral neuropathies (especially those secondary to diabetes, alcohol, or deficiency states) will have a symmetric sensory loss in the feet in the distribution of the socks. Often the phenomenon of summation will be present; this is tested as follows:

   a. Normally, during repeated pricking of a skin area with a pin, the patient if asked, "Does this become sharper?" will indicate that the pricks seem to be about of equal intensity.

   b. In an area of sensory abnormality, the examiner watching the patient's face will notice a sudden grimace after a dozen or so pricks if summation is present and the patient will report that the intensity of the pinprick suddenly becomes unbearably sharp.

2. Intelligent cooperative patients can often outline sensory disturbances better than the examiner can. The patient should be instructed to place a finger in an area of disturbed sensation and move the finger until an area of normal sensitivity is found (Fig B–40,E).

3. If a cortical sensory loss is suspected from the patient's inability to recognize numbers written in the palms of the hands, other tests of cortical sensation should be employed.

   a. With the eyes closed, the patient should be able to discriminate between various sizes of coins and identify common objects such as a key.

   b. With the patient's eyes closed, the examiner touches one arm, the other arm, and then both arms simultaneously. If the patient perceives the individual stimuli, but consistently neglects one stimulus during simultaneous touching, the phenomenon of *extinction* is present.

   c. Other tests of cortical sensation include tactile localization (with eyes closed, a normal patient can accurately localize the examiner's touch) and two-point discrimination (with eyes closed, the normal patient can distinguish two sharp points separated by 5 mm on the fingertips).

X.   EXAMINATION OF THE AUTONOMIC NERVOUS SYSTEM

A.   **Examine blood pressure and heart rate** in the supine and erect positions. Determine whether postural hypotension and compensatory tachycardia are present.

B.   **Instruct the patient to take a deep breath and bear down** as if having a bowel movement (Valsalva maneuver).The normal slowing of the heart associated with this maneuver can often best be appreciated with ECG monitoring.

C.   **Demonstrate the normal triple response (of Lewis)** by scratching the patient's skin with a broken throat stick; normally a white line will initially appear on the skin, followed by a red line, then reddening around the red line (flare), and finally slight elevation of the line (wheal).

D.   **Place the patient's hand in warm water** for 10 minutes or longer. The normal response is for the fingertips to become wrinkled.

E.   **Assess the pupillary size and response** (which are controlled by both sympathetic and parasympathetic innervation).

F.   **Common abnormalities.**

1.   Diabetic peripheral polyneuropathies usually cause orthostatic hypotension, loss of the finger wrinkling response, and loss of the flare in the triple response.

2.   A small pupil may be caused by sympathetic denervation of the eye (Horner's syndrome). In a darkened room, the normal pupil will dilate, while the sympathetically denervated pupil will not change in size. Failure of the pupil to dilate with instillation of a solution of 1% hydroxyamphetamine (Paredrine) suggests a lesion involving the peripheral sympathetic fibers (lesion of the third-order sympathetic neuron).

3.   A large pupil that does not constrict to bright light is the result of parasympathetic denervation as occurs with third cranial nerve palsy.

XI. EXAMINATION OF PATIENTS WITH ABNORMALITIES OF MENTATION.

A. Deciding whether a formal evaluation of mentation is necessary.

1. Consider the chief complaint and the clinical hypotheses formed during the history taking; if a CNS mass lesion, diffuse CNS dysfunction, or focal CNS damage is under consideration, formal testing of mental status is necessary.

2. Consider certain information obtained in the history as "red flags"; e.g., patients with a history of ethanol abuse should be formally tested because the conversation and appearance of a patient with Korsakoff's psychosis may be superficially normal.

3. A formal mental status examination is mandatory when friends or family report mental deterioration or where there is a history of deterioration of occupational performance.

4. Many patients with focal neurologic complaints outside the CNS, such as low back pain, muscular dystrophy, or a focal peripheral nerve paralysis, may not require formal mental status testing.

B. If CNS dysfunction is suspected and formal mental status testing anticipated, the following observations should be recorded:

1. Mood: sad, elated, withdrawn, tearful, bland.

2. Appropriateness of behavior.

3. Ability to relate the history relative to the complaint in a concise and logical manner.

4. Ability to follow directions.

5. Unusual behavior which might indicate the patient is experiencing hallucinations (such as suddenly looking at or listening to sensory stimuli which are not there).

6. The presence or absence of perseveration: this may consist of the patient continuing a motor movement (such as rapid alternating movements) for an inappropriate length of time. Another example of perseveration would be the inability to change easily from one topic of conversation to another.

7. The presence or absence of motor impersistence: this consists of the patient's inability to sustain a given motor test such as keeping the eyes closed (often noted during the sensory examination) or keeping the tongue protruded.

C. **Before starting the questioning,** reassure the patient with a statement such as, "I'm now going to ask you some questions which may sound foolish, but it is just part of the routine examination." The examiner may choose between the Mini-Mental Status Test (Six Item Orientation-Memory-Concentration Test), which is particularly useful in Alzheimer's disease and in situations where quantitative assessment of mental status is necessary, or the "standard" mental status examination used by neurologists.

1. The Mini-Mental Status Test (see Table B–5)
2. Standard mental status examination.
   a. *Memory.*
      1) *Immediate recall:* The examiner slowly and distinctly pronounces a series of random numbers and has the patient repeat them in order. Start with a series of three numbers and continue with longer series until the patient successfully repeats a series of seven numbers or the patient fails twice (e.g., if the patient fails to repeat six digits forward two times, but was able to repeat a series of five digits, record the sucess with five digits).
      2) *Recent memory:* Tell the patient three unrelated nouns (for example, "fox," "car," "blue") and have the patient repeat them. Indicate that the patient will be asked to repeat these words in approximately 3 minutes. Then distract the patient with a few other questions before asking the patient to repeat the words. Additionally, in obtaining the patient's history, questions regarding the last few hours (if the examiner can confirm the facts) are also indicative of recent memory ability.
      3) *Remote memory:* Testing of remote memory can be incorporated with obtaining family and social

TABLE B–5.
Six-Item Orientation-Memory-Concentration Test
(Mini-Mental Status Test)

This simple test, easily administered by a non-physician, discriminates between mild, moderate, and severe cognitive defects. The results correlate with Alzheimer neuritic plaque counts at autopsy and accurately predict scores on a more comprehensive mental status questionnaire. Normal subjects have a weighted score of 6 or less; scores greater than 10 are consistent with a dementing process and a completely demented patient would have a score of 28.

Item	Instruction	Maximum Error	Raw Error Score		Weighting Factor		Weighted Error Score
1	What year is it now?	1	—	X	4	=	—
2	What month is it now?	1	—	X	3	=	—
3 (memory phrase)	Repeat this phrase after me: John Brown, 42 Market Street, Chicago	1	—	X	3	=	—
4	Count backward from 20 to 1	2	—	X	2	=	—
5	Say the months in reverse order	2	—	X	2	=	—
6	Repeat the memory phrase	5	—	X	2	=	—

Score 1 for each incorrect response; maximum weighted error score = 28.

histories. Information such as the patient's age, date of birth, number and order of siblings, marriage date, and number and names of children is appropriate. The examiner may also use readily available historical facts. Ask for information that the patient should have known prior to the onset of the illness; occupational and recreational facts are much more reliable than such questions as naming Presidents or other political figures. Questions concerning a favorite television show are also useful.

b. *Ability to follow instructions* can usually be assessed during physical and neurologic examination.

c. *General information:* Rather than asking questions that are indicative of education and reminiscent of school examinations, it is as meaningful and less threatening to ask about the patient's occupation or hobbies. The patient should discuss either with interest and reasonable knowledge. Another useful line of questioning may concern a favorite television show and the plot from a recent episode. This combines recent memory with the ability to tell a story and may give insight into the patient's character as well.

d. *Mathematical ability (calculation):* Ask simple, everyday problems of calculation such as, "If a man buys 6 cents worth of stamps and gives the clerk 10 cents, how much change should he get back?," or "A newsman collected 25 cents from each of six customers. What is the total amount he collected?," or "If five apples cost a quarter, how much does one apple cost?"

Caveat: Serial-sevens (subtracting seven from 100 and continuing to subtract seven from each number obtained) is *not* a simple calculation problem. It involves not only calculation but also recent memory and ability to concentrate. Remember, that under stress even normal persons may have difficulty performing serial-sevens, and poorly educated normal persons may not be able to perform this task.

e. *Judgment and abstract thinking* are difficult to assess but may be the earliest functions to be impaired. Evidence of poor judgment often can be obtained by a history of occupational performance and daily activities. Common-sense questions can be used such as: "If you traveled to an unfamiliar city to visit a friend, what would you do to find him?," or "If you got into your car one morning to go to work and it didn't start, what would you do?" Another useful test involves similarities and differences. Ask the patient how two items are alike (what properties different objects have in common), e.g.,"What do a river and a lake have in common?"; other useful pairs of items to ask about include an orange and a banana, a dog and a lion, or a coat and a dress; the best answers would be conceptual ones such as fruit, animals, or clothing, while concrete answers may be given such as both are edible, have four legs, or have sleeves. Patients with dementia often can give differences, but not similarities.

Note: Interpretation of proverbs such as"People who live in glass houses shouldn't throw stones" or"A golden hammer breaks an iron door" is often used by physicians as a test of judgment, but may be difficult even for normal persons, especially if they are from a different cultural background.

3. Common problems in assessing mental status:
   a. The examiner records in the chart "oriented x3"; this is significant only if that is *all* the patient can do, but a patient may have a very serious impairment and still be "oriented x3."
   b. The examiner fails to take into account the patient's educational level or ethnic background.
   c. The examiner fails to appreciate that the patient is depressed or hallucinating and therefore is unable to respond correctly.
   d. The examiner asks the questions under stressful circumstances (e.g., in the presence of other physicians or patients).
   e. Aphasic patients are mistaken as being demented.
   f. The examiner fails to appreciate the difference between the patient who never, from birth, had the ability to perform well on a mental status examination and the patient who has *lost* the capacity to perform well on the examination. Dementia is a deterioration of whatever previous mental capacity the individual had.

D.   Abnormal reflexes seen in patients with generalized CNS disease.

1. Paratonic rigidity (gegenhalten) (Fig B–41,A): Request the patient to relax an arm "like a rag doll." The examiner then moves the arm quickly and unexpectedly back and forth and from side to side. The result is positive when it seems as if the patient is both not relaxing the arm and is actively trying to resist any movements (the inexperienced examiner may become impatient because of a mistaken perception that the patient is uncooperative).

2. Grasp reflex (Fig B–41,B): When the examiner strokes the patient's palm from the hypothenar eminence to the thumb and forefinger, the patient squeezes the examiner's fingers (a normal response in infants).

3. Rooting reflex (Fig B–41,C): Lightly stroking away from the corner of the patient's lips causes a movement of the lips or movement of the mouth toward the stimulus (a normal response in infants).

4. Snout reflex (Fig B–41,D): A light tap on the patient's closed lips with a reflex hammer will cause the lips to pucker.

5. Jaw reflex (Fig B–41,E): With the patient's mouth slightly open, light tapping of the examiner's thumb placed on the patient's chin results in momentary closing of the jaws. This is a tendon reflex which normally is difficult to elicit; an easily elicited reflex indicates bilateral corticobulbar tract abnormalities.

6. Common problems in eliciting reflexes associated with generalized CNS dysfunction:

   a. All of the abnormal reflexes are rarely present in the same patient; the reliability of each reflex as an indication of CNS dysfunction largely depends on the skill and experience of the examiner.

   b. The significance of the abnormal reflex must be viewed in the context of the patient's history and examination; e.g., some normal patients who are very nervous may have an easily elicitable jaw reflex.

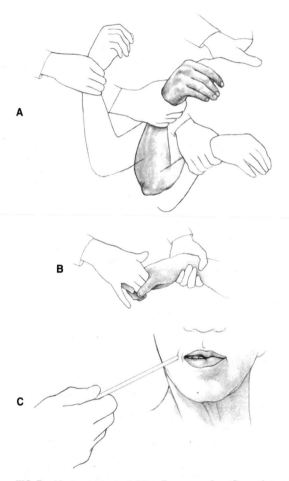

FIG B–41. A, paratonic rigidity; **B,** grasp reflex; **C,** rooting reflex; **D,** snout reflex; **E,** jaw reflex. *(Continued.)*

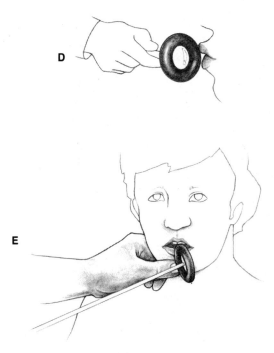

FIG B–41 (cont'd.).

E. **Important disorders of higher cortical function due to focal lesions.**
1. *Aphasia:* disturbance of comprehension or expression of language.
2. *Apraxia:* difficulty in performing a motor task in the absence of any significant weakness or sensory loss.
3. *Agnosia:* failure to interpret sensory information despite primary sensory modalities being intact.

4. Short examination of higher cortical functions for aphasia, apraxia, and agnosia:

 a. Listen for abnormalities of spontaneous speech: word output, rhythm, effort, syntax, paraphasias.

 b. Evaluate speech flow by having the patient name the days of the week and months of the year.

 c. Evaluate repetition by having the patient repeat a sentence (e.g., "The weather is nice outside today").

 d. Assess reading ability and comprehension of written material by having the patient read several sentences or a paragraph aloud (a page from a magazine is useful) and discuss what was read.

 e. Evaluate naming ability by asking the patient to name several objects pointed out by the examiner (e.g., coins, pen, comb, button).

 f. Determine whether singing is performed better than ordinary speech by having the patient sing a familiar melody such as "Happy Birthday" either without or with prompting.

 g. Evaluate the ability of the patient to understand and follow one-, two-, and three-step oral instructions (e.g., "Stand up," "Go to the door," "Take the glass, fill it with water, and put the glass on the table in the corner of the room").

 h. Assess the ability of the patient to follow written instructions ("Stand up," "Sit down," "Take the glass and fill it with water").

 i. Evaluate writing ability by having the patient write several sentences spontaneously (e.g., ask the patient to write a description of the weather); then have the patient copy several short sentences written by the examiner.

 j. Evaluate spatial abilities by having the patient draw a house, a clock, and a cube.

 k. Evaluate the patient for evidence of agnosia and right-left disorientation by giving the patient complex body instructions (e.g., "Put your right thumb on your nose and your left thumb on your right ear").

 l. Evaluate the patient for evidence of apraxia by instructing the patient to perform a variety of motor tasks spontaneously and following the examiner's demonstration (e.g., "Stick out your tongue," "Stand up," "Pretend to use a hammer," "Show me how you comb your hair;" "Show me how to pound a nail into a board").

5. Common problems:
   a. Many patients have elements of several aphasic syndromes due to involvement of several focal brain areas involved in language function.
   b. The aphasic patient is mistakenly considered to be demented; the aphasic patient has difficulty only in communication, but other cognitive functions are intact.
   c. The speech abnormality of Wernicke's aphasia is confused with the "word salad" characteristic of schizophrenia.
   d. Mutism is mistaken for aphasia.

6. Common abnormalities:
   a. Broca's aphasia (anterior, motor, or expressive aphasia).
      1) Quantity of speech is reduced ("nonfluent" aphasia).
      2) Conversational speech requires extra effort.
      3) Prepositions, articles, and conjunctions are often omitted (telegraphic speech).
      4) The patient is aware of the deficit and often is embarrassed and frustrated.
      5) Comprehension is intact, but repetition is poor.
      6) Emotional speech, including profanity, is often preserved.
      7) Naming of objects may be intact or impaired.
   b. Wernicke's aphasia (posterior, sensory, or receptive aphasia).
      1) Total quantity of speech is normal or increased ("fluent" aphasia).
      2) Meaningless, nonsense, or inappropriate words are substituted for correct words (paraphasias, such as desk for table or phone for stone). Often referred to as jargon speech.
      3) The patient has difficulty understanding the

   examiner's words and has difficulty repeating
   them.
   4) Speech intonation and rhythm are intact (normal
      speech melody).
   5) The patient is often unaware of the deficit.
   6) Writing: letters are well formed but content is ab-
      normal with normal words mixed with unintelli-
      gible words.
   c. Conduction or anomic aphasia.
      1) Comprehension is normal (in contrast to
         Wernicke's aphasia).
      2) Excessive use of paraphasias, but with excellent
         articulation (in contrast to Broca's aphasia).
      3) Difficulty in naming objects and difficulty with
         repetition.
      4) The patient can often sing better than speak.
   d. Apraxia.
      1) Ideomotor apraxia: patient has difficulty with
         simple motor tasks, but improves on repetition,
         particularly after the examiner demonstrates the
         task.
      2) Ideational apraxia: patient can perform simple
         motor tasks and individual steps of complex mo-
         tor task, but has difficulty performing correct se-
         quence of steps of complex motor task.
      3) Constructional apraxia: patient has difficulty
         drawing or copying two-dimensional or three-
         dimensional objects or arranging or building
         puzzles.
   e. Alexia without agraphia:
      1) The patient can write, but cannot read what has
         just been written.
      2) Usually associated with a right homonymous
         hemianopia.

XII. EXAMINATION OF THE PATIENT SUSPECTED OF HAVING A NONORGANIC PROCESS.

A. **Suspect that a patient may have a nonorganic ("func-tional") lesion under the following circumstances:**
   1. The motor or sensory deficit is not accompanied by *ob-jective* abnormalities, e.g., reflex changes.

2. The pattern of motor or sensory deficit violates known anatomic principles.
3. The patient shows no concern over the deficit, and may even seem pleased about being disabled.
4. The deficit potentially could result in considerable financial or psychological gain for the patient.
5. The patient has a history of multiple hospitalizations or complaints without *objective* pathologic findings.
6. The patient dresses inappropriately for the occasion (e.g., a female excessively groomed in a provocative negligee, presenting with a hemiparesis).

B. **Procedures which may help in identifying a nonorganic complaint.**
   1. If one leg is paralyzed (Fig B–42):
      a. With the patient supine, the examiner places both palms beneath the heels of the patient (Fig. B–42,A). The patient is asked to lift the paralyzed leg. Then when asked to lift the nonparalyzed leg, the patient will unconsciously increase the pressure on the examiner's palm beneath the supposedly paralyzed leg (Fig B–42,B).
      b. The patient is then asked to press down with both heels (Fig B–42,A). If pressure to the examiner's palm is not equal to that applied when the patient lifted the nonparalyzed leg, a conversion reaction can be suspected.
   2. If the patient complains of sensory disturbance in one hand: Have the patient clasp together inverted hands (Fig B–43,A) and bring the arms upward; this places the right hand on the left side of the body (and vice versa) and distorts a person's sense of which hand is which; thus, quickly reexamining the patient's sensibility to pinprick or a cotton wisp will give different results if the sensory disturbance is due to a conversion reaction (Fig B–43,B).
   3. When the hand of a comatose patient is lifted above the face and then dropped, it will strike the face (Fig B–44,A); the hand of the patient with a nonorganic abnormality will veer to the side to avoid striking the face (Fig B–44,B).

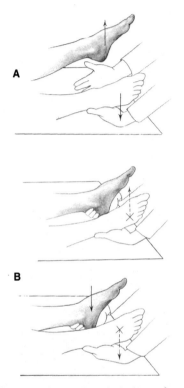

FIG B–42. Testing for pseudoparalysis due to conversion reaction.

4. The patient with hemiparesis will have weakness in turning the head *away* from the paralyzed side due to paresis of the sternocleidomastoid muscle (Fig. B–45). The patient with a nonorganic hemiparesis will often have normal strength turning to the opposite side but weakness turning to the same side.

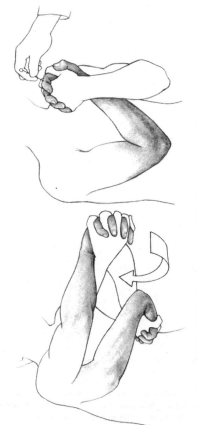

FIG B–43. Testing for sensory disturbance in conversion reaction.

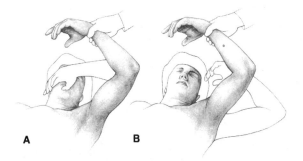

FIG B–44. Demonstrating pseudocoma due to conversion reaction.

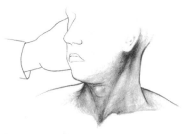

FIG B–45. Testing for hemiparesis by evaluating weakness in head turning.

5. A patient with a nonorganic positive straight leg raising test will complain of pain in the supine position (Fig. B–46,A), but not when the leg is straightened by the examiner to the same angle in the sitting position, even though the geometry is the same in both positions (Fig B–46,B).

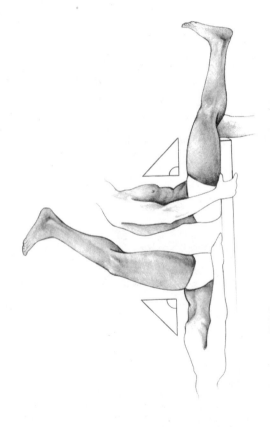

FIG B–46. Nonorganic positive straight leg raising test.

6. If a patient complains of weakness on one side of the body, test strength on both sides simultaneously. It is difficult to "give way" with one muscle group while maintaining normal strength on the opposite side (Fig B–47).

7. If the patient complains of an area of anesthesia: instruct the patient to close the eyes and answer "yes" if feeling the pinprick, or "no" if not (obviously the only appropriate answer is silence when the supposedly anesthetic area is touched).

8. A patient with an organic hemisensory deficit in the face can still feel the vibrations of a tuning fork placed on either side of the face owing to the conductive properties of bone; a patient with a nonorganic lesion will often report no vibratory feeling at all on the affected side (Fig B–48). This test also works on the sternum.

9. If the patient complains of total blindness in one eye, the lesion must be anterior to the optic chiasm and a Marcus-Gunn pupil or other pupillary abnormality must be present.

10. If the patient complains of a visual field defect, plot the defect on a tangent screen at two different distances; with an organic lesion, the field defect should increase as the distance from the patient to the chart increases.

11. A patient with bilateral blindness will not blink when the examiner's hand is suddenly thrust at the patient's face in a threatening manner; the patient with nonorganic blindness often will blink.

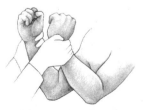

FIG B–47. Simultaneous bilateral testing of muscle strength to demonstrate weakness due to conversion reaction.

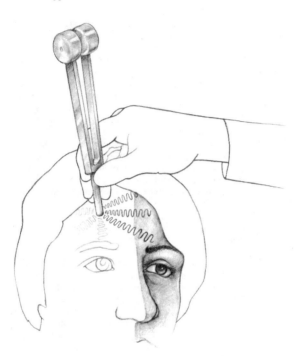

FIG B−48. Testing for nonorganic hemisensory deficit on the face.

    12. The patient with nonorganic total blindness will not be able to suppress the nystagmus induced by an opticokinetic tape.

C. Common problems.

    1. The examiner does not appreciate that many patients with *organic* lesions elaborate on symptoms and appear to have a psychiatric disturbance.

2. The examiner hastily makes a diagnosis on subjective findings and submits the patient to dangerous and expensive tests.
3. The examiner becomes angry with the patient with nonorganic complaints and fails to appreciate that the patient is in distress and needs sympathy and understanding, along with referral to a psychiatrist or psychologist.
4. The examiner feels insecure in his or her knowledge of psychiatry and neurology and considers a psychiatric diagnosis only after organic causes are ruled out.

   Caveat: Psychiatric diagnoses, like neurologic diagnoses, should be made only on the basis of objective evidence and should never be made simply by exclusion.

XIII. EXAMINING THE COMATOSE PATIENT.

A. **Before examining the comatose patient,** make certain that respirations and circulation are adequate. In the emergency room, an intravenous infusion should have been started and glucose and thiamine given. If there is a history of trauma, a fracture of the cervical spine must be excluded by radiographic studies. The general physical examination may give clues as to the causes of coma: jaundice of hepatic failure, bleeding ear or Battle's sign of trauma, petechiae of infections, or neoplastic and bleeding disorders. Check for characteristic breath odor (alcohol or diabetic ketoacidosis).

B. **Obtain blood pressure and pulse.**
   1. An elevated blood pressure is commonly found in patients with intracranial hemorrhage or cerebral edema.
   2. Increasing blood pressure and slowing of the pulse can be associated with medullary compression from cerebral herniation caused by increased intracranial pressure.
   3. Low blood pressure is often associated with toxic-metabolic coma.
   4. A rapid pulse may indicate severely depleted blood volume.

C. Observe the character of the breathing pattern (Fig B-49).

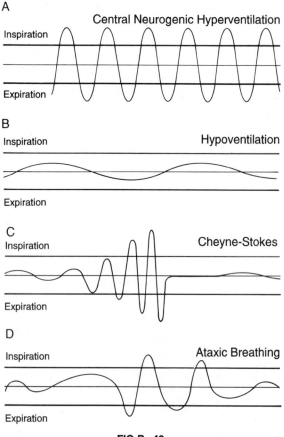

A

Central Neurogenic Hyperventilation

Inspiration

Expiration

B

Inspiration

Hypoventilation

Expiration

C

Inspiration

Cheyne-Stokes

Expiration

D

Inspiration

Ataxic Breathing

Expiration

FIG B-49.

D. **Record rectal temperature.**
   1. Temperature is usually normal or decreased in metabolic coma.
   2. Temperature is often increased in structural CNS coma, meningitis, and heat stroke.

   Caveat: Infants and the elderly may not have elevated temperatures with infection.

E. **If the patient is spontaneously moving,** note whether the movements are symmetric or asymmetric. Asymmetric movements are suggestive of a structural CNS lesion.

F. **Determine the level of consciousness according to the Glasgow Coma Scale** (Table B–6).

G. **The type of movement in response to painful stimulation can suggest the site of the lesion.** To produce the painful stimulation, stand behind the patient and apply pressure to the styloid process.
   1. Symmetric decerebrate posturing (Fig B–50,A) or decorticate posturing (Fig B–50,B) is suggestive of metabolic coma or of central rostral-caudal brain herniation.
   2. Asymmetric posturing (Fig B–50,C) is suggestive of coma from a structural CNS lesion.

H. **Check for neck suppleness** by placing one hand under the occiput and attempting to flex the patient's neck.

   Caveat: Do not manipulate the neck if cervical fracture is a possibility.

FIG B–49. Common abnormal breathing patterns include: **A,** central neurogenic hyperventilation (deep, rapid, regular); **B,** hypoventilation (shallow, slow, regular); **C,** Cheyne-Stokes (apneic spells followed by respiration that gradually increases in rate and depth and then gradually decreases in rate and depth until apnea again occurs); **D,** ataxic breathing (respirations totally unpredictable as to depth, rate, or rhythm; this is the only respiratory pattern diagnostic of a CNS lesion).

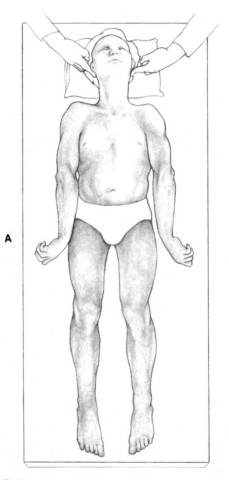

FIG B–50. A, symmetric decerebrate posturing in response to painful stimulation.

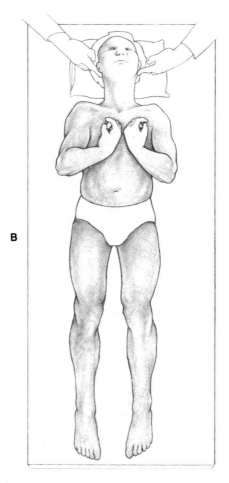

FIG B–50. B, symmetric decorticate posturing in response to painful stimulation.

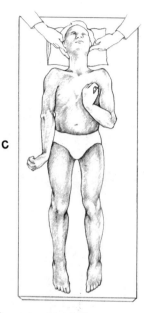

FIG B–50. C, asymmetric posturing in response to painful stimulation.

  1. Common Observations:
     a. Normal responses: chin should easily touch the chest.
     b. Stiff neck: with subarachnoid hemorrhage or meningitis examiner often can raise the upper part of the body without inducing neck flexion.

I.   Check for muscle tone.
  1. Lift both arms together above the chest and let them fall simultaneously. The hypotonic arm will fall faster.

TABLE B–6.
Glasgow Coma Scale (Circle the appropriate number and compute the total)

	Eyes Open
Never	1
To pain	2
To verbal stimuli	3
Spontaneously	4
	Best Verbal Response
No response	1
Incomprehensible sounds	2
Inappropriate words	3
Disoriented and converses	4
Oriented and converses	5
	Best Motor Response
No response	1
Extension (decerebrate rigidity)	2
Flexion abnormal (decorticate rigidity)	3
Flexion withdrawal	4
Localizes pain	5
Obeys	6
Total Score (range)	3–15

*Sum of highest value in each category is coma score: full mental capacity = 15; highest level of coma = 8; brain death = 3.

2. Lift both lower extremities at the knees so that both knees and hips are flexed. When released the hypotonic leg will externally rotate and extend faster.
3. The resistance to passive movement should be tested separately in each limb.

J. **Evaluation of cranial nerves and brainstem integrity.**
   1. Examine the optic fundus (see section IV. A). Papill-edema is usually associated with structural CNS lesions but can also occur with metabolic abnormalities that cause cerebral edema.
   2. Observe pupils for size, symmetry, and reaction to light (see section IV. B).

Note: Use a bright, pinpoint source of light; when there is doubt about whether the pupils are reactive, observing the pupil through the magnification lens of the otoscope may be helpful.

3. Common abnormalities:
   a. Pinpoint pupils: suggestive of pontine hemorrhage, narcotic overdose, or cholinergic drugs.
   b. Unilaterally dilated and fixed or poorly reactive pupils: suggestive of intracerebral hemorrhage or tumor resulting in transtentorial herniation causing damage to cranial nerve III.
   c. Bilaterally large and poorly reactive pupils: suggestive of anoxia or anticholinergic or adrenergic drugs.
   d. Asymmetric pupils: suggestive of coma from a structural CNS lesion (symmetric pupils suggest metabolic coma).
4. Oculocephalic (doll's-eyes) reflex: Holding the eyelids open, passively rotate the patient's head rapidly to each side (Fig B–51,A). In the comatose patient with an intact brainstem, the eyes deviate away from the direction of rotation, then return to the neutral "straight ahead" position. Awake patients have no oculocephalic reflex.

Caveat: This should *never* be done in comatose patients with head trauma until a neck fracture has been ruled out.

   a. Common observations:
      1) No response (eyes turn with head) occurs in both severe metabolic and CNS structural coma.
      2) Dysconjugate movement of the eyes is seen in coma from CNS structural lesion damaging the brainstem.
      3) Response present: this indicates that the brainstem is intact from cranial nerves III to VIII and that the coma is probably due to a metabolic abnormality.
5. Oculovestibular (caloric) reflex (Fig B–51,B) (performed if there is suspicion of a neck fracture or if the

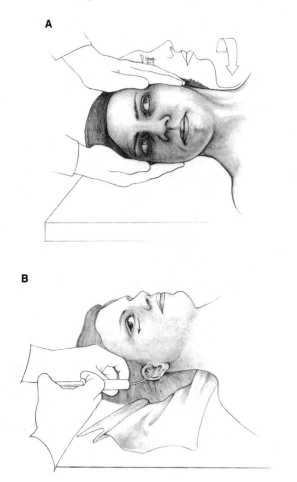

FIG B−51. A, oculocephalic reflex; **B,** oculovestibular reflexes.

oculocephalic reflex is equivocal): Check to see that the tympanic membrane is intact and that the external auditory canal is not blocked by wax or blood; inject at least 10 mL of ice water through a small polyethylene catheter into the external auditory canal and then immediately elevate the head to approximately 30 degrees from the horizontal.

Caveat: If a neck fracture is suspected, do not move the head or neck. Instead, tilt the table to elevate the head.

    a. Common observations:
        1) In a comatose patient with an intact brainstem from cranial nerves III to VIII, there is conjugate deviation of the eyes toward the cooled ear and no nystagmus occurs.
        2) No response suggests either severe metabolic or a structural CNS lesion, while dysconjugate eye movement indicates a structural lesion damaging the brainstem.
6. Corneal reflex (see section IV. C).
    a. Common observations:
        1) No response is seen in patients with deep coma from any cause.
        2) Symmetric response indicates the brainstem between cranial nerves V and VII is intact.
        3) Asymmetric response is seen in structural CNS coma.
7. Evaluation of facial symmetry (cranial nerve VII): With facial asymmetry, as the patient breathes a paralyzed cheek will exhibit more movement than the nonparalyzed cheek. This is seen in coma from structural CNS lesions.
8. Evaluation of the pharyngeal reflex (refer back above to testing of cranial nerve X).
    a. Common observations:
        1) No response is seen in patients in deep coma from any cause.
        2) Asymmetric response indicates structural CNS coma.

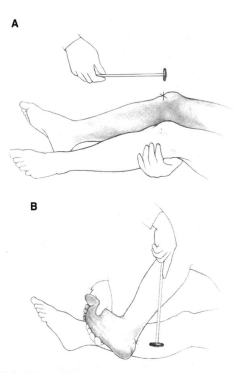

FIG B–52. A, eliciting patellar reflexes in a comatose patient. Place an arm under both knees so that the knees are slightly flexed and then strike the patellar tendon with a reflex hammer. Pay close attention to reflex asymmetries and crossed adductor responses. **B,** in the comatose patient, the Achilles reflex is elicited by crossing the legs as illustrated and slightly dorsiflexing the foot before tapping the Achilles tendon.

K. Evaluation of muscle stretch reflexes and plantar response (Fig B–52).
   1. Common problems:
      a. An acutely paralyzed limb may exhibit either absent or hypoactive reflexes even if the paralysis is due to an upper motor neuron lesion.
      b. Occasionally patients may have asymmetric posturing, movement, or reflexes when the cause of the coma is metabolic; this is especially true if there is an old injury to the CNS system.
   2. Common observations:
      a. Symmetric reflexes (hyperactive, hypoactive, or absent) are seen primarily in metabolic coma.
      b. Asymmetric reflexes are seen most often in structural CNS coma.

XIV. THE NEUROVASCULAR EXAMINATION.
A. Determine blood pressure.
   1. Blood pressure cuff should be of suitable size (a normal-size blood pressure cuff on an obese patient may give a falsely high reading).
   2. Brachial blood pressure is measured in both arms, usually both in supine and erect positions.
      a. Asymmetric blood pressures of more than 10 mm Hg (torr) suggest occlusive disease in the proximal artery, usually the subclavian artery.
      b. Blood pressure change of 30 mm Hg (torr) or more in systolic pressure in assuming the erect from the supine position suggests peripheral autonomic dysfunction; lack of compensatory tachycardia substantiates autonomic dysfunction.
   3. Common problems:
      a. Blood pressure changes must be correlated with the patient's symptoms.
      b. Especially in the elderly, blood pressure changes may vary; orthostatic hypotension is usually more prominent in the morning because of dehydration.
      c. The patient must be protected from falling.
      d. The examiner should perform the measurements

(rather than relying on nurses or technicians) in order to correlate the symptoms with the measurements.

    e. An accurate handheld manometer is more convenient to use than a mercury manometer.

B. **Examine blood vessels:** Palpate the superficial temporal, radial, femoral, and dorsalis pedis arteries to evaluate collateral circulation and find evidence of atherosclerosis or emboli.

    1. Common abnormalities:

        a. Reduced or absent pulse in superficial temporal artery is seen in occlusion of the common carotid artery.

        b. Tenderness and beading of the superficial temporal artery suggest temporal arteritis.

        c. An irregular pulse suggests the possibility of emboli originating in the heart.

        Caveat: Palpation of the carotid artery may cause bradycardia and has the potential of dislodging a clot. An occluded artery may appear to have a relatively normal pulsation, and therefore palpation is of limited value.

C. **Auscultation.**

    1. Carotid artery bruits are best heard at the bifurcation.

    2. Subclavian artery bruits are best detected in the supraclavicular fossa.

    3. Intracranial bruits are best heard over the orbits.

    Note: Bruits are best heard by using the bell of the stethoscope.

    4. Common problems:

        a. Transmitted heart murmurs may be mistaken for bruits.

        b. Too firm pressure from the stethoscope bell may create an artificial bruit.

        c. Fluttering of the eyelids can be mistaken for a bruit.

        d. The loudness of the bruit does not correlate with the degree of stenosis or pathologic condition.

5. Common abnormalities:
   a. Carotid or subclavian bruits suggest arterial stenosis.
   b. Orbital bruits suggest intracranial arteriovenous malformation or carotid-cavernous fistula.
D. **Retinal examination.** Funduscopic vascular findings are presented in Table B–7.

TABLE B–7.
Funduscopic Vascular Findings

Lesion	Findings
Subarachnoid hemorrhage	Subhyaloid hemorrhage (between retina and vitreous)
Hollenhorst plaques	Yellow refractile cholesterol emboli in retinal arterioles
Fibrin-platelet emboli	White emboli in retinal arterioles
Septic emboli	Small retinal hemorrhages with a central white spot (Roth's spots)
Central retinal artery occlusion	Pale retina, attenuated arterioles, and red macula
Diabetic retinopathy	Microaneurysms, hard exudates, neovascularization, vitreous hemorrhage, retinal detachment
Hypertensive retinopathy	Copper- or silver-wiring appearance of narrowed arterioles, flame hemorrhages, cotton-wool exudates, and (in later stages) papilledema

INDEX